AF327400

Monokines and Other Non-Lymphocytic Cytokines

PROGRESS IN LEUKOCYTE BIOLOGY

Series Editor

Sherwood M. Reichard, Medical College of Georgia, Augusta, Georgia

Advisory Board

Hillel S. Koren, Environmental Protection Agency, Chapel Hill, North Carolina
Ronald B. Herberman, National Cancer Institute, Frederick, Maryland
Frank Collins, Trudeau Institute, Saranac Lake, New York
Emil Unanue, Harvard Medical School, Boston, Massachusetts
Philip D. Stahl, Washington University School of Medicine, St. Louis, Missouri
Carleton Stewart, Los Alamos National Laboratory, Los Alamos, New Mexico
Emil Skamene, Montreal General Hospital, Montreal, Quebec, Canada
Dolph O. Adams, Duke University Medical Center, Durham, North Carolina
Joost J. Oppenheim, National Cancer Institute, Frederick, Maryland
Siamon Gordon, Oxford University, Oxford, England
Ralph van Furth, University Hospital, Leiden, The Netherlands
Klaus Resch, Hannover Medical School, Hannover, FRG
Michael Feldman, Weizmann Institute of Science, Rehovot, Israel
David S. Nelson, Royal North Shore Hospital, Sydney, Australia

TITLES IN THE SERIES

Volume 1

Viral Mechanisms of Immunosuppression
Norbert Gilmore and Mark A. Wainberg, *Editors*

Volume 2

The Physiologic, Metabolic, and Immunologic Actions of Interleukin-1
Matthew J. Kluger, Joost J. Oppenheim, and
Michael C. Powanda, *Editors*

Volume 3

Genetic Control of Host Resistance to Infection and Malignancy
Emil Skamene, *Editor*

Volume 4

Macrophage Biology
Sherwood Reichard and Mizu Kojima, *Editors*

Volume 5

Leukocytes and Host Defense
Joost J. Oppenheim and Diane M. Jacobs, *Editors*

Volume 6

Immunopharmacology of Infectious Diseases:
Vaccine Adjuvants and Modulators of Non-Specific Resistance
Jeannine A. Majde, *Editor*

Volume 7

Antigen Presenting Cells: Diversity, Differentiation, and Regulation
Lawrence B. Schook and John G. Tew, *Editors*

Volume 8

Monokines and Other Non-Lymphocytic Cytokines
Michael C. Powanda, Joost J. Oppenheim, Matthew J. Kluger, and
Charles A. Dinarello, *Editors*

Monokines and Other Non-Lymphocytic Cytokines

Proceedings of an International Workshop sponsored by the Society for Leukocyte Biology (a Reticuloendothelial Society) and the Biological Response Modifier Program, National Cancer Institute, held at Hilton Head Island, South Carolina, December 6–10, 1987

Editors

Michael C. Powanda
Division of Cutaneous Hazards
Letterman Army Institute of Research
Presidio of San Francisco, California

Joost J. Oppenheim
Laboratory of Immunoregulation
Biological Response Modifier Program
National Cancer Institute
Frederick Cancer Research Facility
Frederick, Maryland

Matthew J. Kluger
Department of Physiology
University of Michigan Medical School
Ann Arbor, Michigan

Charles A. Dinarello
Department of Medicine
New England Medical Center
Boston, Massachusetts

Alan R. Liss, Inc., New York

Address all Inquiries to the Publisher
Alan R. Liss, Inc., 41 East 11th Street, New York, NY 10003

Library of Congress Cataloging-in-Publication Data

Monokines and other non-lymphocytic cytokines

   (Progress in leukocyte biology ; v. 8)
   Bibliography: p.
   Includes index.
   1. Cytokines—Congresses. 2. Monokines—Congresses.
I. Powanda, M. C. (Michael C.) II. Reticuloendothelial
Society. II. Biological Response Modifier Program
(U.S.) IV. Series.
QR185.8.C95M66 1988   616.07′9   88-12637
ISBN 0-8451-4107-4

Contents

Contributors . . . . *xiii*

Foreword
Sherwood M. Reichard . . . . *xxv*

Preface
Michael C. Powanda, Joost J. Oppenheim, Matthew J. Kluger, and
Charles A. Dinarello . . . . *xxvii*

Acknowledgments . . . . *xxix*

Section I.   Interferon-β_2 /HSF/IL-6

Interleukin-6: Structure, Production, and Actions
A. Billiau *3*

Interferon $\beta2$ Is Identical to Monocytic HSF and Regulates the Full
Acute Phase Protein Response in Liver Cells
Jack Gauldie, Carl Richards, Del Harnish, and Heinz Baumann *15*

Human IFN-Beta-2: A Cytokine With Multiple Functions in
Infections and Inflammation
Michel Revel, Asher Zilberstein, Rosa-Maria Ruggieri, Louisa Chen,
Yves Mory, Menachem Rubinstein, and Rita Michalevicz *21*

Structure, Genetics, and Function of Human "β_2-Interferon/
B-Cell Stimulatory Factor-2/Hepatocyte Stimulating Factor"
(Interleukin-6)
Uma Santhanam, Stephen B. Tatter, David C. Helfgott, Anuradha Ray,
John Ghrayeb, Lester T. May, and Pravinkumar B. Sehgal *29*

Induction of the Acute-Phase Response in Rat Hepatocyte/
Hepatoma Cells: Effects of Different Mediators
H. Northoff, T. Andus, T. Geiger, J. Bauer, D. Männel, T. Hirano,
T. Kishimoto, and P.C. Heinrich *35*

vi   **Contents**

Section II.   Gene Expression

Restriction Fragment Length Polymorphisms and Linkage of
Murine IL-1α and β Genes on Chromosome 2
*David D. Chaplin, Robert C. Fuhlbrigge, Shirin Jadidi,
Kathleen C. Sheehan, Robert D. Schreiber, Patrick W. Gray,
Emil R. Unanue, and Peter D'Eustachio* *41*

Characterization of *Cis* and *Trans* Acting Elements Involved in
Human proIL-1 Beta Gene Expression
*Burton D. Clark, Matthew J. Fenton, Homero L. Rey, Andrew C. Webb,
and Philip E. Auron* *47*

Control of LPS Induced Interleukin-1 and Tumor Necrosis Factor
mRNAs Expression by Inhibitors of Second Messenger Pathways in
Murine Macrophages
*Elizabeth J. Kovacs, Danuta Radzioch, Howard A. Young, and
Luigi Varesio* *55*

Dynamics and Regulation of Macrophage Tumor Necrosis Factor-α
(TNF), Interleukin-1α (IL-1α), and Interleukin-1β (IL-1β) Gene
Expression by Arachidonate Metabolites
*Steven L. Kunkel, Wendy E. Scales, Robert Spengler, Mary Spengler, and
Jim Larrick* *61*

Regulation of TNF Gene Expression by Lipopolysaccharide, Cyclic
AMP, and Interferon
Steven M. Taffet *67*

Cloning of the cDNAs for Rat Interleukin-1α and β
*Tsutomu Nishida, Tohru Hirato, Naoki Nishino, Keiko Mizuno,
Yasuyo Sekiguchi, Masaaki Takano, Kazuyoshi Kawai, Satoru Nakai,
and Yoshikatsu Hirai* *73*

Quantitative Analysis of IL-1α and β mRNA in Human Monocytes
and Macrophages
*Michael F. Smith, Jr., Friedrich R. Kueppers, Peter R. Young, and
John C. Lee* *79*

Transcription and Translation of IL-1α and IL-1β Genes in the
Presence of the Glucocorticoid Hormone Dexamethasone
*Peter R. Young, Daria J. Hazuda, Janice R. Connor, and
Barbara J. Dalton* *83*

Detection of IL-1 Gene Expression by In-Situ Hybridization
Histochemistry: Tissue Localization of IL-1 mRNA in the Normal
C57BL/6 Mouse
*Laszlo Takacs, Elizabeth J. Kovacs, Mark R. Smith, Howard A. Young,
and Scott K. Durum* *89*

Section III.   Regulation of Synthesis/Release of Cytokines

The Kinetics of IL-1 Secretion From Activated Monocytes—
Differences Between IL-1α and IL-1β
Daria Hazuda, John Lee, and Peter Young *97*

A Plasma Membrane Anchoring Mechanism for IL-1
Dan T. Brody and Scott K. Durum *101*

Autoregulation of IL-1 Protein Production
*Jean C. Manson, Julian A. Symons, Francesco S. di Giovine, Stephen Poole,
and Gordon W. Duff* *109*

Mechanisms of Interferon-γ and Cyclohexamide Enhancement of
Interleukin-1 Production in Cultured Human Monocytes
*William P. Arend, Fenneke G. Joslin, Shahid Jameel, and
Donald B. Carter* *113*

Differential Effects of Human Monokine Transcription and
Translation Following Stimulation With LPS Plus γ-Interferon
Mary W. Vermeulen and Heinz G. Remold *119*

β-Endorphin Inhibits Interleukin-1β Release by Human Peripheral
Blood Mononuclear Cells
*Charles F. Brummitt, Burt Sharp, Genya Gekker, William F. Keane, and
Phillip K. Peterson* *125*

Generation of Interleukin-1 in a Macrophage Cell Line and
Enhancement of Interleukin-1 Fibroblast Proliferative Activity by
Substance P
*Edward S. Kimball, Jeffry L. Vaught, Francis J. Persico, and
M. Carolyn Fisher* *131*

Interleukin-1 Secretion by Human Peripheral Blood Mononuclear
Cells in Response to Interleukin-2
Robert P. Numerof, Charles A. Dinarello, and James W. Mier *137*

Liposomal Muramyl Dipeptide Is More Potent Than Free Muramyl
Dipeptide in Inducing IL-1 Secretion From Macrophages
Nigel C. Phillips *141*

Cachectin/TNF and IL-1 Synthesis and Secretion Are Induced by
Glucose-Modified Protein Binding to High-Affinity Macrophage
Receptor
*Helen Vlassara, Michael Brownlee, Kirk Manogue, Araxi Pasagian,
Charles Dinarello, and Anthony Cerami* *145*

Humans Taking Dietary Omega-3 Fatty Acids Have Decreased
In Vitro Production of Interleukin-1
*Stefan Endres, Reza Ghorbani, Joseph G. Cannon, Gerhard Lonnemann,
Jos W.M. van der Meer, Sheldon M. Wolff, and Charles A. Dinarello* *153*

viii   **Contents**

Regulation of Gamma Interferon Production by EGF: Evidence for
a Novel Inducible EGF Receptor on Lymphocytes
N.A. Abdullah, B.A. Torres, and H.M. Johnson 159

Section IV.   Receptors and Post-Receptor Events

Immunoprecipitation of Interleukin-1 Receptors From Murine
Cell Lines
Janet M.D. Plate and Vivek M. Rangnekar 167

Structure and Properties of the Receptor for Interleukin-1
Michael Martin, Roswitha Kroggel, Marta Szamel, and Klaus Resch 175

Evidence for Differences in the Molecular Properties of
Interleukin-1 Receptors
*Richard Horuk, James J. Huang, Maryanne Covington, and
Robert C. Newton* 179

Evidence for an Essential Disulfide Bond Required for Binding
Activity of the Interleukin-1 Receptor
Kathryn Paganelli Parker and Patricia L. Kilian 185

Mapping the Receptor Binding Site of Human Interleukin-1β
James J. Huang, Robert C. Newton, Richard Horuk, and Yuan Lin 191

Monoclonal Antibodies to Human Interleukin-1β for Analysis of the
Structure-Function Relationship
*Diana Boraschi, Gianfranco Volpini, Stefano Censini, Paolo Bossù,
Paolo Ghiara, Giuseppe Scapigliati, Annalisa Massone, Cosima Baldari,
John L. Telford, and Aldo Tagliabue* 197

Effect of Trans-Retinoic Acid on Interleukin-1 Receptor Activity
Patricia L. Kilian 203

Covalent Disulfide Binding of IL-1 to α_2-Macroglobulin
*Marius Teodorescu, John L. Skosey, Carol Schlesinger, and
Jeanette Wallman* 209

Kinetics of Growth Inhibition and Receptor Binding by Interleukin-1
Edwin Gaffney, Shiow Tsai, George Koch, and Richard Malovarca 213

Signal Requirement for Interleukin-1-Dependent IL-2 Production
and IL-2 Receptor Induction by Human Leukemia-Derived HSB.2
Subclones
*Tadashi Kasahara, Naofumi Mukaida, Hitoshi Yagisawa, Tadashi Kawai,
and Kohei Shioiri-Nakano* 217

Interleukin-1-Stimulated EL-4 Cells Release Linoleic Acid, Which
Augments Translocation of Protein Kinase C and Production of
Interleukin-2
Philip L. Simon, Mike A. Clark, Linda S. Henderson, and Shouki Kassis . 223

Detection of Protein Phosphorylation in Human Peripheral Blood
Mononuclear Cells in Response to Interleukin-1 (IL-1)
*Kouji Matsushima, Masahiro Shiroo, Wook Lew, Yoshiro Kobayashi,
Tohru Akahoshi, and Joost J. Oppenheim* 229

Recombinant Human Granulocyte-Macrophage Colony-
Stimulating Factor (rh GM-CSF) Induces Different Intracellular
Signals in Mature and Immature Myeloid Cells
*A.F. Lopez, S.J. Hardy, J. Eglinton, J. Gamble, L.B. To, P. Dyson,
G. Wong, S. Clark, A.W. Murray, and M.A. Vadas* 235

Studies on the NIH 3T3 Cells Sensitized to Tumor Necrosis Factor
by the Expression of Adenovirus E1A Oncogene
*M.-J. Chen, C.Q. Earl, B. Holskin, M. Anzano, D. Shalloway, and
J.L. Cook* 243

Section V.   Cytokine Activities and Interactions In Vitro
Biological Activities and Production of TNF-α
Grace H.W. Wong and David V. Goeddel 251

Actions of IL-1 and TNF on Human Osteoblast-Like Cells:
Similarities and Synergism
Maxine Gowan 261

Inhibited Steroid Induction of PEPCK in Hepatoma Cells Treated
With HurIL-1 and HurTNF
R.E. McCallum, M.R. Hill, and R.D. Stith 267

Induction of IL-2 Receptor Expression by Interleukin-1 and Tumor
Necrosis Factor on YT Cells
J.C. Lee, A. Truneh, M.F. Smith, M.-J. Chen, and K.Y. Tsang 273

Interleukin-1 Effects on Monocyte Receptor Expression
William P. Arend, J. Timothy Ammons, and Brian L. Kotzin 281

In TNF Mediated Cytolysis Apoptosis Can Occur in the Absence of
Nuclear Disintegration
Scott M. Laster, Mary Scanlon, John G. Wood, and Linda R. Gooding . . . 285

Potentiating Effects of Tumor Necrosis Factor on Interleukin-1
Mediated Pancreatic Beta-Cell Toxicity
*Thomas Mandrup-Poulsen, Klaus Bendtzen, Charles A. Dinarello, and
Jorn Nerup* 291

Influence of Interleukin-1 on Human Bone Marrow Blast
Progenitor Cells In Vitro
Jan Moreb, James Zucali, Mary Ann Gross, and Charles A. Dinarello 297

Recombinant Human Monocyte Specific Colony-Stimulating Factor
Stimulates Both Immature and Mature Cells of Human Monocyte
Lineage
*K. Motoyoshi, K. Yoshida, K. Hatake, N. Yanai, T. Kawashima,
M. Saito, Y. Miura, G.G. Wong, M. Fujisawa, A. Yuo, T. Okabe, and
F. Takaku* 301

Transforming Growth Factor β: A Selective Growth Inhibitor for
Hematopoietic Progenitor Cells
*Francis Ruscetti, Garwin Sing, Larry Ellingsworth, Sandra Ruscetti, and
Jonathan Keller* 307

Transforming Growth Factor-β Induces Persistent and Coordinate
Increase in Collagens Type I and III and Fibronectin Gene
Expression
John Varga, Joel Rosenbloom, and Sergio A. Jimenez 313

Section VI.   Cytokine Activities and Interactions In Vivo
Interleukin-1's Role in the Increased Vascular Permeability of
Inflammation
Gail S. Habicht and Gregory Beck 319

Isolation and Characterization of a Vascular Permeability Factor
From Stimulated U937 Cells
Gregory Beck and Gail S. Habicht 325

Interleukin-1 Induces Chronic Granulomatous Inflammation
*Colin J. Dunn, Marilyn M. Hardee, Anna J. Gibbons, Nigel D. Staite, and
Karen A. Richard* 329

Interleukin-1 and Tumor Necrosis Factor Depress Cytochrome
P-450 Dependent Liver Drug Metabolism in Mice
*Pietro Ghezzi, Riccardo Bertini, Marina Bianchi, Annalaura Erroi,
Pia Villa, and Alberto Mantovani* 337

Amplification of Antibody Mediated Glomerulonephritis by Tumor
Necrosis Factor and Interleukin-1
Andrew J. Rees, Steve Cashman, and Nao Tomosugi 343

TNF-α and IFN-γ Have Alternate Effects on the Immune System
In Vivo
Chaim O. Jacob, May Koo, and Hugh O. McDevitt 349

Effects of Recombinant Murine Interleukin-1α on the Pathogenesis
of Murine Listeriosis
*Charles J. Czuprynski, James F. Brown, Karen M. Young, A. James Cooley,
and Robin S. Kurtz* 355

Synergistic Activity of IL-1 With TNF and IL-1 With CSF in
Radioprotection
Ruth Neta and J.J. Oppenheim *359*

Effect of a Synthetic Nonapeptide of Human IL-1β on the Cellular
Immunoreactivity and In Vivo Growth of a Fibrosarcoma of
BALB/c Mice
Tiziana Musso, Mirella Giovarelli, Cristina Jemma, Guido Forni,
G. Antoni, D. Boraschi, P. Bossú, S. Censini, P. Ghiara, L. Nencioni,
G. Scapigliati, A. Tagliabue, and G.F. Volpini *365*

**Section VII.   Assays for and Detection of Cytokines in Cells,
Tissues, and Body Fluids**

Interleukin-1 in Human Blood: Chloroform Extraction and
Radioimmunoassay
Joseph G. Cannon, Jos W.M. van der Meer, Stefan Endres,
Gerhard Lonnemann, and Charles A. Dinarello *373*

A RIA for Tumor Necrosis Factor (TNFα) and Interleukin-1β
(IL-1β) and Their Direct Determination in Serum
Aimée Reuter, Jacques Bernier, Philippe Gysen, Yvonne Gevaert, Renée Gathy,
Miguel Lopez, Ginette Dupont, Pierre Damas, and Paul Franchimont *377*

Generation of Neutralizing Monoclonal Antibodies Specific for
Human Interleukin-1 Beta
David A. Wunderlich, Thomas J. Lobl, Jefferson W. Paslay,
and Ann E. Berger *383*

Immunoassay, Bioassay, and In Situ Hybridization of Monokines in
Human Arthritis
G.W. Duff, E. Dickens, N. Wood, J. Manson, J. Symons, S. Poole, and
F. di Giovine *387*

An Enzyme Immunoassay for Platelet-Derived Growth Factor
(PDGF): Application to the Measurement of Macrophage-Derived
PDGF
R.K. Kumar, R.A. Bennett, and A.R. Brody *393*

A Fluorometric Enzyme-Linked Immunosorbent Assay (F ELISA)
for TGF-Beta
Benjamin S. Leung and Li Zhou *397*

Epilogue
Michael C. Powanda *401*

Index *405*

Contributors

N.A. Abdullah, Department of Comparative and Experimental Pathology, University of Florida, Gainesville, FL 32610 **[159]**

Tohru Akahoshi, Laboratory of Molecular Immunoregulation, Biological Response Modifiers Program, Division of Cancer Treatment, National Cancer Institute, Frederick, MD 21701 **[229]**

J. Timothy Ammons, Division of Rheumatology, Department of Medicine, University of Colorado Health Sciences Center, Denver, CO 80262 **[281]**

T. Andus, Department of Biochemistry, University of Freiburg, D-7800 Freiberg, Federal Republic of Germany **[35]**

G. Antoni, Sclavo Research Center, 53100 Siena, Italy **[365]**

M. Anzano, Smith Kline and French Laboratories, King of Prussia, PA 19406 **[243]**

William P. Arend, Division of Rheumatology, Department of Medicine, University of Colorado Health Sciences Center, Denver, CO 80262 **[113, 281]**

Philip E. Auron, Division of Health Sciences and Technology, Massachusetts Institute of Technology, Cambridge, MA 02139 **[47]**

Cosima Baldari, Sclavo Research Center, 53100 Siena, Italy **[197]**

J. Bauer, Department of Biochemistry, University of Freiberg, D-7800 Freiberg, Federal Republic of Germany **[35]**

Heinz Baumann, Department of Molecular and Cellular Biology, Roswell Park Memorial Institution, Buffalo, NY 14263 **[15]**

Gregory Beck, Department of Pathology, State University of New York at Stony Brook, Stony Brook, NY 11794 **[319,325]**

Klaus Bendtzen, University Hospital of Copenhagen, DK-2200 Copenhagen, Denmark **[291]**

R.A. Bennett, Laboratory of Pulmonary Pathobiology, National Institute of Environmental Health Sciences, Research Triangle Park, NC 27709 **[393]**

Ann E. Berger, Department of Cell Biology, The Upjohn Company, Kalamazoo, MI 49001 **[383]**

The numbers in brackets are the opening page numbers of the contributors' articles.

Jacques Bernier, Radioimmunoassay Laboratory, University of Liege, B-4000 Liege, Belgium **[377]**

Riccardo Bertini, Istituto di Ricerche Farmacologiche "Mario Negri," 20157 Milano, Italy **[337]**

Marina Bianchi, Istituto di Ricerche Farmacologiche "Mario Negri," 20157 Milano, Italy **[337]**

A. Billiau, Rega Institute, University of Leuven, B-3000 Leuven, Belgium **[3]**

Diana Boraschi, Sclavo Research Center, 53100 Siena, Italy **[197,365]**

Paola Bossù, Sclavo Research Center, 53100 Siena, Italy **[197,365]**

A.R. Brody, Laboratory of Pulmonary Pathobiology, National Institute of Environmental Heath Sciences, Research Triangle Park, NC 27709 **[393]**

Dan T. Brody, Biological Carcinogenesis Development Program, Program Resources, Inc., NCI-Frederick Cancer Research Facility, Frederick, MD 21701 **[101]**

James F. Brown, Department of Pathobiological Sciences, School of Veterinary Medicine, University of Wisconsin, Madison, WI 53706 **[355]**

Michael Brownlee, Laboratory of Medical Biochemistry, The Rockefeller University, New York, NY 10021 **[145]**

Charles F. Brummitt, Department of Medicine, Hennepin County Medical Center, and the University of Minnesota Medical School, Minneapolis, MN 55415 **[125]**

Joseph G. Cannon, Department of Medicine, New England Medical Center Hospitals and Tufts University School of Medicine, Boston, MA 02111 **[153,373]**

Donald B. Carter, Department of Molecular Biological Research, The Upjohn Company, Kalamazoo, MI 49001 **[113]**

Steve Cashman, Renal Unit, Department of Medicine, The Royal Postgraduate Medical School, Hammersmith Hospital, London W12 ONN, United Kingdom **[343]**

Stefano Censini, Sclavo Research Center, 53100 Siena, Italy **[197,365]**

Anthony Cerami, Laboratory of Medical Biochemistry, The Rockefeller University, New York, NY 10021 **[145]**

David D. Chaplin, Department of Medicine, Washington University School of Medicine, St. Louis, MO 63110 **[41]**

Louisa Chen, Department of Virology, Weizmann Institute of Science, Rehovot, 76100 Israel **[21]**

M.-J. Chen, Department of Molecular Genetics, Smith Kline and French Laboratories, King of Prussia, PA 19406 **[243,273]**

Burton D. Clark, Division of Health Sciences and Technology, Massachusetts Institute of Technology, Cambridge, MA 02139 **[47]**

Mike A. Clark, Department of Molecular Pharmacology, Smith Kline and French Laboratories, King of Prussia, PA 19406 **[223]**

S. Clark, Genetics Institute, Cambridge, MA **[235]**

Janice R. Connor, Smith Kline and French Laboratories, King of Prussia, PA 19406 **[83]**

J.L. Cook, Department of Medicine, National Jewish Center for Immunology and Respiratory Medicine, Denver, CO 80206 **[243]**

A. James Cooley, Department of Pathobiological Sciences, School of Veterinary Medicine, University of Wisconsin, Madison, WI 53706 **[355]**

Maryanne Covington, Medical Products Division, E.I. du Pont de Nemours & Company, Glenolden Laboratory, Glenolden, PA 19036 **[179]**

Charles J. Czuprynski, Department of Pathobiological Sciences, School of Veterinary Medicine, University of Wisconsin, Madison, WI 53706 **[355]**

Barbara J. Dalton, Department of Immunology, Smith Kline and French Laboratories, King of Prussia, PA 19406 **[83]**

Pierre Damas, Radioimmunoassay Laboratory, University of Liege and IRE-MEDGENIX, Fleurus, Belgium **[377]**

Peter D'Eustachio, Department of Biochemistry, New York University Medical Center, New York, NY 10016 **[41]**

E. Dickens, Department of Medicine, University of Edinburgh, Rheumatic Diseases Unit, Northern General Hospital, Edinburgh EH5 2DQ, United Kingdom **[387]**

Francesco S. di Giovine, Department of Medicine, University of Edinburgh, Rheumatic Diseases Unit, Northern General Hospital, Edinburgh EH5 2DQ, United Kingdom **[109,387]**

Charles A. Dinarello, Department of Medicine, New England Medical Center, Boston, MA 02111 **[137,145,153,291,297,373]**

Gordon W. Duff, Department of Medicine, University of Edinburgh, Rheumatic Diseases Unit, Northern General Hospital, Edinburgh EH5 2DQ, United Kingdom **[109,387]**

Colin J. Dunn, Department of Hypersensitivity Diseases Research, The Upjohn Company, Kalamazoo, MI 49001 **[329]**

Ginette Dupont, Radioimmunoassay Laboratory, University of Liege and IRE-MEDGENIX, Fleurus, Belgium **[377]**

Scott K. Durum, Laboratory of Molecular Immunoregulation, National Cancer Institute, Frederick Cancer Research Facility, Frederick, MD 21701 **[89,101]**

P. Dyson, Department of Hematology, Institute of Medical and Veterinary Science, Adelaide, Australia **[235]**

C.Q. Earl, Smith Kline and French Laboratories, King of Prussia, PA 19406 **[243]**

J. Eglinton, Department of Human Immunology, Institute of Medical and Veterinary Science, Adelaide, Australia **[235]**

Larry Ellingsworth, Department of Immunology, Collagen Corp., Palo Alto, CA **[307]**

Stefan Endres, Department of Medicine, New England Medical Center, Boston, MA 02111 **[153,373]**

Annalaura Erroi, Istituto di Ricerche Farmacologiche "Mario Negri," 20157 Milano, Italy **[337]**

Matthew J. Fenton, Division of Health Sciences and Technology, Massachusetts Institute of Technology, Cambridge, MA 02139 **[47]**

M. Carolyn Fisher, Department of Biological Research, Janssen Research Foundation, Spring House, PA 19477 **[131]**

Guido Forni, Institute of Microbiology, University of Torino, 10126 Torino, Italy **[365]**

Paul Franchimont, Radioimmunoassay Laboratory, University of Liege, B-4000 Liege, Belgium **[377]**

Robert C. Fuhlbrigge, Department of Medicine, Washington University School of Medicine, St. Louis, MO 63110 **[41]**

M. Fujisawa, University of Tokyo, Tokyo 113, Japan **[301]**

Edwin Gaffney, Department of Molecular and Cell Biology, The Pennsylvania State University, University Park, PA 16802 **[213]**

J. Gamble, Department of Human Immunology, Institute of Medical and Veterinary Science, Adelaide, Australia **[235]**

Renée Gathy, Radioimmunoassay Laboratory, University of Liege and IRE-MEDGENIX, Fleurus, Belgium **[377]**

Jack Gauldie, Department of Pathology, McMaster University, Hamilton, Ontario, Canada L8N 3Z5 **[15]**

T. Geiger, Department of Biochemistry, University of Freiberg, D-7800 Freiberg, Federal Republic of Germany **[35]**

Genya Gekker, Department of Medicine, Hennepin County Medical Center, Minneapolis, MN 55415 **[125]**

Yvonne Gevaert, Radioimmunoassay Laboratory, University of Liege and IRE-MEDGENIX, Fleurus, Belgium **[377]**

Pietro Ghezzi, Istituto di Ricerche Farmacologiche "Mario Negri," 20157 Milano, Italy **[337]**

Paolo Ghiara, Sclavo Research Center, 53100 Siena, Italy **[197,365]**

Reza Ghorbani, Department of Medicine, New England Medical Center Hospitals and Tufts University School of Medicine, Boston, MA 02111 **[153]**

John Ghrayeb, Centocor, Malvern, PA 19355 **[29]**

Anna J. Gibbons, Department of Hypersensitivity Diseases Research, The Upjohn Company, Kalamazoo, MI 49001 **[329]**

Mirella Giovarelli, Institute of Microbiology, University of Torino, 10126 Torino, Italy **[365]**

David V. Goeddel, Department of Molecular Biology, Genetech, Inc., South San Francisco, CA 94080 **[251]**

Linda R. Gooding, Department of Microbiology and Immunology, Emory University School of Medicine, Atlanta, GA 30322 **[285]**

Maxine Gowen, Department of Human Metabolism and Clinical Biochemistry, University of Sheffield Medical School, Sheffield S10 2RX, United Kingdom **[261]**

Patrick W. Gray, Department of Developmental Biology, Genentech Inc., South San Francisco, CA 94080 **[41]**

Mary Ann Gross, Department of Medicine, University of Florida, Gainesville, FL 32610 **[297]**

Philippe Gysen, Radioimmunoassay Laboratory, University of Liege and IRE-MEDGENIX, Fleurus, Belgium **[377]**

Gail S. Habicht, Department of Pathology, State University of New York at Stony Brook, Stony Brook, NY 11794 **[319,325]**

Marilyn M. Hardee, Department of Hypersensitivity Diseases Research, The Upjohn Company, Kalamazoo, MI 49001 [329]

S.J. Hardy, The School of Biological Sciences, Flinders University, Bedford Park, South Australia [235]

Del Harnish, Department of Pathology, McMaster University, Hamilton, Ontario, Canada L8N 3Z5 [15]

K. Hatake, Jichi Medical School, Tochigi-ken 329-04, Japan [301]

Daria J. Hazuda, Department of Molecular Genetics, Smith Kline and French Laboratories, King of Prussia, PA 19406 [83,97]

P.C. Heinrich, Department of Biochemistry, University of Freiberg, D-7800 Freiberg, Federal Republic of Germany [35]

David C. Helfgott, The Rockefeller University, New York, NY 10021 [29]

Linda S. Henderson, Department of Pharmacology, Smith Kline and French Laboratories, King of Prussia, PA 19406 [223]

M.R. Hill, Department of Microbiology and Immunology, University of Oklahoma Health Sciences Center, Oklahoma City, OK 73190 [267]

Yoshikatsu Hirai, Laboratories of Cellular Technology, Otsuka Pharmaceutical Co., Ltd., Tokushima 771-01, Japan [73]

T. Hirano, Institute of Molecular and Cellular Biology, Osaka University, Osaka 565, Japan [35]

Tohru Hirato, Laboratories of Cellular Technology, Otsuka Pharmaceutical Co., Ltd., Tokushima 771-01, Japan [73]

B. Holskin, Smith Kline and French Laboratories, King of Prussia, PA 19406 [243]

Richard Horuk, Medical Products Division, E.I. du Pont de Nemours & Company, Glenolden Laboratory, Glenolden, PA 19036 [179,191]

James J. Huang, Medical Products Division, E.I. du Pont de Nemours & Company, Glenolden Laboratory, Glenolden, PA 19036 [179,191]

Chaim O. Jacob, Department of Medical Microbiology, Stanford University School of Medicine, Stanford, CA 94305 [349]

Shirin Jadidi, Department of Medicine, Washington University School of Medicine, St. Louis, MO 63110 [41]

Shahid Jameel, Division of Rheumatology, Department of Medicine, University of Colorado Health Sciences Center, Denver, CO 80262 [113]

Cristina Jemma, Institute of Microbiology, University of Torino, 10126 Torino, Italy [365]

Sergio A. Jimenez, Department of Medicine, Thomas Jefferson University, Philadelphia, PA 19107 [313]

H.M. Johnson, Department of Comparative and Experimental Pathology, University of Florida, Gainesville, FL 32610 [159]

Fenneke G. Joslin, Division of Rheumatology, Department of Medicine, University of Colorado Health Sciences Center, Denver, CO 80262 [113]

Tadashi Kasahara, Department of Medical Biology and Parasitology, Jichi Medical School, Tochigi-ken 329-04, Japan [217]

Shouki Kassis, Department of Immunology, Smith Kline and French Laboratories, King of Prussia, PA 19406 **[223]**

Kazuyoshi Kawai, Laboratories of Cellular Technology, Otsuka Pharmaceutical Co., Ltd., Tokushima 771-01, Japan **[73]**

Tadashi Kawai, Department of Clinical Pathology, Jichi Medical School, Tochigi-ken 329-04, Japan **[217]**

T. Kawashima, Morinaga Milk Industry, Tokyo 153, Japan **[301]**

William F. Keane, Department of Medicine, Hennepin County Medical Center, and the University of Minnesota Medical School, Minneapolis, MN 55415 **[125]**

Jonathan Keller, Program Resources, Inc., NCI-Frederick Cancer Research Facility, Frederick, MD 21701 **[307]**

Patricia L. Kilian, Department of Immunopharmacology, Hoffmann-La Roche Inc., Nutley, NJ 07110 **[185,203]**

Edward S. Kimball, Department of Biological Research, Janssen Research Foundation, Spring House, PA 19477 **[131]**

T. Kishimoto, Institute of Molecular and Cellular Biology, Osaka University, Osaka 565, Japan **[35]**

Yoshiro Kobayashi, Laboratory of Molecular Immunoregulation, Biological Response Modifiers Program, Division of Cancer Treatment, National Cancer Institute, Frederick, MD 21701 **[229]**

George Koch, Cistron Biotechnology, Pine Brook, NJ 07058 **[213]**

May Koo, Department of Medical Microbiology, Stanford University School of Medicine, Stanford, CA 94305 **[349]**

Brian L. Kotzin, Division of Rheumatology, Department of Medicine, University of Colorado Health Sciences Center, Denver, CO 80262 **[281]**

Elizabeth J. Kovacs, Department of Anatomy, Loyola University, Stritch School of Medicine, Maywood, IL 60153 **[55,89]**

Roswitha Kroggel, Institute of Molecular Pharmacology, Medical School Hannover, D-3000 Hannover 61, Federal Republic of Germany **[175]**

Friedrich R. Kueppers, Department of Microbiology and Immunology, Temple University School of Medicine, Philadelphia, PA 19140 **[79]**

R.K. Kumar, Laboratory of Pulmonary Pathobiology, National Institute of Environmental Health Sciences, Research Triangle Park, NC 27709 **[393]**

Steven L. Kunkel, Department of Pathology, University of Michigan Medical School, Ann Arbor, MI 48109 **[61]**

Robin S. Kurtz, Department of Pathobiological Sciences, School of Veterinary Medicine, University of Wisconsin, Madison, WI 53706 **[355]**

Jim Larrick, Department of Immunology, Cetus Corporation, Palo Alto, CA 94303 **[61]**

Scott M. Laster, Department of Microbiology and Immunology, Emory University School of Medicine, Atlanta, GA 30322 **[285]**

John C. Lee, Department of Immunology, Smith Kline and French Laboratories, King of Prussia, PA 19406 [79,97,273]

Benjamin S. Leung, Department of Obstetrics and Gynecology, University of Minnesota Medical School, Minneapolis, MN 55455 [397]

Wook Lew, Laboratory of Molecular Immunoregulation, Biological Response Modifiers Program, Division of Cancer Treatment, National Cancer Institute, Frederick, MD 21701 [229]

Yuan Lin, Medical Products Division, E.I. du Pont de Nemours & Company, Glenolden Laboratory, Glenolden, PA 19036 [191]

Thomas J. Lobl, Department of Biopolymer Chemistry, The Upjohn Company, Kalamazoo, MI 49001 [383]

Gerhard Lonnemann, Department of Medicine, New England Medical Center Hospitals and Tufts University School of Medicine, Boston, MA 02111 [153,373]

A.F. Lopez, Department of Human Immunology, Institute of Medical and Veterinary Science, Adelaide, Australia [235]

Miguel Lopez, Radioimmunoassay Laboratory, University of Liege and IRE-MEDGENIX, Fleurus, Belgium [377]

Richard Malovarca, Cistron Biotechnology, Pine Brook, NJ 07058 [213]

Thomas Mandrup-Poulsen, Steno Memorial Hospital, DK-2820 Gentofte, Denmark [291]

D. Männel, German Cancer Research Center, D-6900 Heidelberg, Federal Republic of Germany [35]

Kirk Manogue, Laboratory of Medical Biochemistry, The Rockefeller University, New York, NY 10021 [145]

Jean C. Manson, Department of Medicine, University of Edinburgh, Rheumatic Diseases Unit, Northern General Hospital, Edinburgh EH5 2DQ, United Kingdom [109,387]

Alberto Mantovani, Istituto di Ricerche Farmacologiche "Mario Negri," 20157 Milano, Italy [337]

Michael Martin, Institute of Molecular Pharmacology, Medical School Hannover, D-3000 Hannover 61, Federal Republic of Germany [175]

Annalisa Massone, Sclavo Research Center, 53100 Siena, Italy [197]

Kouji Matsushima, Laboratory of Molecular Immunoregulation, Biological Response Modifiers Program, Division of Cancer Treatment, National Cancer Institute, Frederick, MD 21701 [229]

Lester T. May, Department of Virology, The Rockefeller University, New York, NY 10021 [29]

R.E. McCallum, Department of Microbiology and Immunology, University of Oklahoma Health Sciences Center, Oklahoma City, OK 73190 [267]

Hugh O. McDevitt, Department of Medical Microbiology, Stanford University School of Medicine, Stanford, CA 94305 [349]

Rita Michalevicz, Department of Hematology, Ichilov Hospital, Tel Aviv, Israel [21]

James W. Mier, Department of Medicine, New England Medical Center, Boston, MA 02111 [137]

Y. Miura, Jichi Medical School, Tochigi-ken 329-04, Japan [301]

Keiko Mizuno, Laboratories of Cellular Technology, Otsuka Pharmaceutical Co., Ltd., Tokushima 771-01, Japan **[73]**

Jan Moreb, Department of Medicine, University of Florida, Gainesville, FL 32610 **[297]**

Yves Mory, Department of Virology, Weizmann Institute of Science, Rehovot, 76100 Israel **[21]**

K. Motoyoshi, Division of Hemopoiesis, Institute of Hematology, Jichi Medical School, Tochigi-ken 329-04, Japan **[301]**

Naofumi Mukaida, Department of Clinical Pathology, Jichi Medical School, Tochigi-ken 329-04, Japan **[217]**

A.W. Murray, The School of Biological Sciences, Flinders University, Bedford Park, South Australia **[235]**

Tiziana Musso, Institute of Microbiology, University of Torino, 10126 Torino, Italy **[365]**

Satoru Nakai, Laboratories of Cellular Technology, Otsuka Pharmaceutical Co., Ltd., Tokushima 771-01, Japan **[73]**

L. Nencioni, Sclavo Research Center, 53100 Siena, Italy **[365]**

Jørn Nerup, Steno Memorial Hospital, DK-2820 Gentofte, Denmark **[291]**

Ruth Neta, Armed Forces Radiobiology Research Institute, Bethesda, MD 20814 **[359]**

Robert C. Newton, Medical Products Division, E.I. du Pont de Nemours & Company, Glenolden Laboratory, Glenolden, PA 19036 **[179,191]**

Tsutomu Nishida, Laboratories of Cellular Technology, Otsuka Pharmaceutical Co., Ltd., Tokushima 771-01, Japan **[73]**

Naoki Nishino, Laboratories of Cellular Technology, Otsuka Pharmaceutical Co., Ltd., Tokushima 771-01, Japan **[73]**

H. Northoff, DRK Blood Center, D-7900 Ulm, Federal Republic of Germany **[35]**

Robert P. Numerof, Department of Medicine, New England Medical Center, Boston, MA 02111 **[137]**

T. Okabe, University of Tokyo, Tokyo 113, Japan **[301]**

Joost J. Oppenheim, Laboratory of Molecular Immunoregulation, Biological Response Modifier Program, National Cancer Institute, Frederick Cancer Research Facility, Frederick, MD 21701 **[229,359]**

Kathryn Paganelli Parker, Department of Immunopharmacology, Hoffmann-La Roche Inc., Nutley, NJ 07110 **[185]**

Araxi Pasagian, Laboratory of Medical Biochemistry, The Rockefeller University, New York, NY 10021 **[145]**

Jefferson W. Paslay, Department of Hypersensitivity Diseases, The Upjohn Company, Kalamazoo, MI 49001 **[383]**

Francis J. Persico, Department of Biological Research, Janssen Research Foundation, Spring House, PA 19477 **[131]**

Phillip K. Peterson, Department of Medicine, Hennepin County Medical Center, and the University of Minnesota Medical School, Minneapolis, MN 55415 **[125]**

Nigel C. Phillips, Department of Medicine, Montreal General Hospital Research Institute/McGill University, Montreal, Quebec H3G 1A4, Canada **[141]**

Janet M.D. Plate, Section of Medical Oncology, Department of Internal Medicine, Rush-Presbyterian-St. Luke's Medical Center, Chicago, IL 60612 **[167]**

Stephen Poole, National Institute for Biological Standards and Controls, Potters Bar EN6 3QG, United Kingdom **[109,387]**

Michael C. Powanda, Division of Cutaneous Hazards, Letterman Army Institute of Research, Presidio of San Francisco, CA 94129 **[401]**

Danuta Radzioch, Program Resources, Inc., National Cancer Institute, Frederick Cancer Research Facility, Frederick, MD 21701 **[55]**

Vivek M. Rangnekar, Section of Medical Oncology, Department of Internal Medicine, Rush-Presbyterian-St. Luke's Medical Center, Chicago, IL 60612 **[167]**

Anuradha Ray, The Rockefeller University, New York, NY 10021 **[29]**

Andrew J. Rees, Renal Unit, Department of Medicine, The Royal Postgraduate Medical School, Hammersmith Hospital, London W12 0NN, United Kingdom **[343]**

Heinz G. Remold, Department of Rheumatology and Immunology, Brigham and Women's Hospital, and Harvard Medical School, Boston, MA 02115 **[119]**

Klaus Resch, Institute of Molecular Pharmacology, Medical School Hannover, D-3000 Hannover 61, Federal Republic of Germany **[175]**

Aimée Reuter, Radioimmunoassay Laboratory, University of Liege, B-4000 Liege, Belgium **[377]**

Michel Revel, Department of Virology, Weizmann Institute of Science, Rehovot, 76100 Israel **[21]**

Homero L. Rey, Division of Health Sciences and Technology, Massachusetts Institute of Technology, Cambridge, MA 02139 **[47]**

Karen A. Richard, Department of Hypersensitivity Diseases Research, The Upjohn Company, Kalamazoo, MI 49001 **[329]**

Carl Richards, Department of Pathology, McMaster University, Hamilton, Ontario, Canada L8N 3Z5 **[15]**

Joel Rosenbloom, School of Dental Medicine, University of Pennsylvania, Philadelphia, PA 19104 **[313]**

Menachem Rubinstein, Department of Virology, Weizmann Institute of Science, Rehovot, 76100 Israel **[21]**

Rosa-Maria Ruggieri, Department of Virology, Weizmann Institute of Science, Rehovot, 76100 Israel **[21]**

Francis Ruscetti, Laboratory of Molecular Immunoregulation, Frederick Cancer Research Facility, Frederick, MD 21701 **[307]**

Sandra Ruscetti, National Cancer Institute, Bethesda, MD **[307]**

M. Saito, Jichi Medical School, Tochigi-ken 329-04, Japan **[301]**

Uma Santhanam, Department of Virology, The Rockefeller University, New York, NY 10021 **[29]**

Wendy E. Scales, Department of Pathology, University of Michigan Medical School, Ann Arbor, MI 48109 **[61]**

Mary Scanlon, Department of Anatomy and Cell Biology, Emory University School of Medicine, Atlanta, GA 30322 **[285]**

Giuseppe Scapigliati, Sclavo Research Center, 53100 Siena, Italy **[197, 365]**

Carol Schlesinger, Department of Microbiology/Immunology, University of Illinois College of Medicine, Chicago, IL 60612 **[209]**

Robert D. Schreiber, Department of Pathology, Washington University School of Medicine, St. Louis, MO 63110 **[41]**

Pravinkumar B. Sehgal, Department of Virology, The Rockefeller University, New York, NY 10021 **[29]**

Yasuyo Sekiguchi, Laboratories of Cellular Technology, Otsuka Pharmaceutical Co., Ltd., Tokushima 771-01, Japan **[73]**

D. Shalloway, Molecular and Cell Biology Program, The Pennsylvania State University, University Park, PA 16802 **[243]**

Burt Sharp, Department of Medicine, Hennepin County Medical Center, and the University of Minnesota Medical School, Minneapolis, MN 55415 **[125]**

Kathleen C. Sheehan, Department of Pathology, Washington University School of Medicine, St. Louis, MO 63110 **[41]**

Kohei Shioiri-Nakano, Department of Medical Biology and Parasitology, Jichi Medical School, Tochigi-ken 329-04, Japan **[217]**

Masahiro Shiroo, Laboratory of Molecular Immunoregulation, Biological Response Modifiers Program, Division of Cancer Treatment, National Cancer Institute, Frederick, MD 21701 **[229]**

Philip L. Simon, Department of Immunology, Smith Kline and French Laboratories, King of Prussia, PA 19406 **[223]**

Garwin Sing, Laboratory of Molecular Immunoregulation, Frederick Cancer Research Facility, Frederick, MD 21701 **[307]**

John L. Skosey, Department of Medicine, University of Illinois College of Medicine, Chicago, IL 60612 **[209]**

Mark R. Smith, Laboratory of Molecular Biochemistry, Program Resources Inc., NCI-Frederick Cancer Research Facility, Frederick, MD 21701 **[89]**

Michael F. Smith, Jr., Department of Microbiology and Immunology, Temple University School of Medicine, Philadelphia, PA 19140 **[79,273]**

Mary Spengler, Department of Pathology, University of Michigan Medical School, Ann Arbor, MI 48109 **[61]**

Robert Spengler, Department of Pathology, University of Michigan Medical School, Ann Arbor, MI 48109 **[61]**

Nigel D. Staite, Department of Hypersensitivity Diseases Research, The Upjohn Company, Kalamazoo, MI 49001 **[329]**

R.D. Stith, Department of Physiology and Biophysics, University of Oklahoma Health Sciences Center, Oklahoma City, OK 73190 **[267]**

Julian A. Symons, Department of Medicine, University of Edinburgh, Rheumatic Diseases Unit, Northern General Hospital, Edinburgh EH5 2DQ, United Kingdom **[109,387]**

Marta Szamel, Institute of Molecular Pharmacology, Medical School Hannover, D-3000 Hannover 61, Federal Republic of Germany **[175]**

Steven M. Taffet, Departments of Microbiology/Immunology and Biochemistry/Molecular Biology, SUNY Health Science Center at Syracuse, Syracuse, NY 13210 **[67]**

Aldo Tagliabue, Sclavo Research Center, 53100 Siena, Italy **[197, 365]**

László Takács, Laboratory of Molecular Immunoregulation, National Cancer Institute, Frederick Cancer Research Center, Frederick, MD 21701 **[89]**

F. Takaku, Third Department of Internal Medicine, Faculty of Medicine, University of Tokyo, Tokyo 113, Japan **[301]**

Masaaki Takano, Laboratories of Cellular Technology, Otsuka Pharmaceutical Co., Ltd., Tokushima 771-01, Japan **[73]**

Stephen B. Tatter, Department of Virology, The Rockefeller University, New York, NY 10021 **[29]**

John L. Telford, Sclavo Research Center, 53100 Siena, Italy **[197]**

Marius Teodorescu, Department of Microbiology/Immunology, University of Illinois College of Medicine, Chicago, IL 60612 **[209]**

L.B. To, Department of Hematology, Institute of Medical and Veterinary Science, Adelaide, Australia **[235]**

Nao Tomosugi, Renal Unit, Department of Medicine, The Royal Postgraduate Medical School, Hammersmith Hospital, London W12 0NN, United Kingdom **[343]**

B.A. Torres, Department of Comparative and Experimental Pathology, University of Florida, Gainesville, FL 32610 **[159]**

A. Truneh, Department of Immunology, Smith Kline and French Laboratories, King of Prussia, PA 19406 **[273]**

Shiow Tsai, Department of Molecular and Cell Biology, The Pennsylvania State University, University Park, PA 16802 **[213]**

K.Y. Tsang, Medical University of South Carolina, Charleston, SC 29425 **[273]**

Emil R. Unanue, Department of Pathology, Washington University School of Medicine, St. Louis, MO 63110 **[41]**

M.A. Vadas, Department of Human Immunology, Institute of Medical and Veterinary Science, Adelaide, Australia **[235]**

Jos W.M. van der Meer, Department of Medicine, New England Medical Center Hospitals and Tufts University School of Medicine, Boston, MA 02111 **[153,373]**

Luigi Varesio, Laboratory of Molecular Immunoregulation, BRMP, National Cancer Institute, Frederick Cancer Research Facility, Frederick, MD 21701 **[55]**

John Varga, Department of Medicine, Thomas Jefferson University, Philadelphia, PA 19107 **[313]**

Jeffry L. Vaught, Department of Biological Research, Janssen Research Foundation, Spring House, PA 19477 **[131]**

Mary W. Vermeulen, Department of Rheumatology and Immunology, Brigham and Women's Hospital, and Harvard Medical School, Boston, MA 02115 **[119]**

Pia Villa, Istituto di Ricerche Farmacologiche "Mario Negri," 20157 Milano, Italy **[337]**

Helen Vlassara, Laboratory of Medical Biochemistry, The Rockefeller University, New York, NY 10021 **[145]**

Gianfranco Volpini, Sclavo Research Center, 53100 Siena, Italy **[197, 365]**

Jeanette Wallman, Department of Microbiology/Immunology, University of Illinois College of Medicine, Chicago, IL 60612 **[209]**

Andrew C. Webb, Department of Biological Sciences, Wellesley College, Wellesley, MA 02181 **[47]**

Sheldon M. Wolff, Department of Medicine, New England Medical Center Hospitals and Tufts University School of Medicine, Boston, MA 02111 **[153]**

G. Wong, Genetics Institute, Cambridge, MA **[235,301]**

Grace H.W. Wong, Department of Molecular Biology, Genetech, Inc., South San Francisco, CA 94080 **[251]**

John G. Wood, Department of Anatomy and Cell Biology, Emory University School of Medicine, Atlanta, GA 30322 **[285]**

N. Wood, Department of Medicine, University of Edinburgh, Rheumatic Diseases Unit, Northern General Hospital, Edinburgh EH5 2DQ, United Kingdom **[387]**

David A. Wunderlich, Department of Cell Biology, The Upjohn Company, Kalamazoo, MI 49001 **[383]**

Hitoshi Yagisawa, Department of Medical Biology and Parasitology, Jichi Medical School, Tochigi-ken 329-04, Japan **[217]**

N. Yanai, Biomedical Research Laboratory, Morinaga Milk Industry, Tokyo 153, Japan **[301]**

K. Yoshida, Morinaga Milk Industry, Tokyo 153, Japan **[301]**

Howard A. Young, Laboratory of Molecular Immunoregulation, National Cancer Institute, Frederick Cancer Research Facility, Frederick, MD 21701 **[55,89]**

Karen M. Young, Department of Pathobiological Sciences, School of Veterinary Medicine, University of Wisconsin, Madison, WI 53706 **[355]**

Peter R. Young, Department of Molecular Genetics, Smith Kline and French Laboratories, King of Prussia, PA 19406 **[79,83,97]**

A. Yuo, University of Tokyo, Tokyo 113, Japan **[301]**

Li Zhou, Department of Obstetrics and Gynecology, University of Minnesota Medical School, Minneapolis, MN 55455 **[397]**

Asher Zilberstein, Department of Virology, Weizmann Institute of Science, Rehovot, 76100 Israel **[21]**

James Zucali, Department of Medicine, University of Florida, Gainesville, FL 32610 **[297]**

Foreword

This series of books, PROGRESS IN LEUKOCYTE BIOLOGY, and the *Journal of Leukocyte Biology* are published by Alan R. Liss, Inc., for the Society for Leukocyte Biology (a Reticuloendothelial Society).

The series focuses on the biology of granulocytes, lymphocytes, and mononuclear phagocytes. This includes topics relating to the origins and developmental biology of these cells, their mechanism(s) of interpopulation communication, and the means by which they destroy infectious organisms, foreign tissue, or neoplastic cells.

In order to maintain the highest quality possible, there is an advisory board that recommends and approves publications in this series. The Publication Committee of the Society for Leukocyte Biology serves as the core of the board. In addition, a small number of key people throughout the world have been invited who are recognized for their expertise in granulocyte, lymphocyte, and macrophage biology.

This is an exciting area and it is growing in importance. We hope to capture the essence of this dialogue and continue to provide state-of-the-art coverage of this unfolding story.

Sherwood M. Reichard

Preface

By way of introduction to the International Workshop on Monokines and Other Non-Lymphocytic Cytokines, let us propose that at present we are confronted with a cornucopia, one might venture to say, a confusion, of cytokines. Taken together these cytokines are apparently capable of affecting the function of virtually every cell, tissue, and organ system.

Why are there so many cytokines? Many have similar, or at least overlapping, activities such as the colony stimulating factors. But even molecules that have a multiplicity of activities in common may have different consequences to the host. For example, interleukin-1 appears to participate in protecting the organism from an array of insults, whereas tumor necrosis factor, not only may be lethal to tumor cells, but, in some instances, to the host itself.

What roles do these cytokines, in concert or confrontation, play in the regulation of the organism in health, following injury, during infection, in the presence of neoplasia? Is there a prime mover monokine, or are cytokines existentialists, adapting their actions to circumstance such as concentration of self, the presence of antagonists, the target cell? Or rather is homeostasis a variant of democracy, with two houses, mind and body, and an evolutionally as well as situationally defined separation of powers among diverse constituents?

Whether one fancies the philosophical or political analogy, or neither, their function is to remind us that in molecular biology, as in atomic physics, when one intensely focuses on a single component of a complex, interactive system, one may alter the reality and lose sight of the system as a whole. In arranging this meeting, we tried not to focus on one cytokine, but rather to achieve a broad perspective. We therefore were immensely gratified by the variety of topics, as well as the quantity and quality of the abstracts received.

The papers published here by no means include all of the 240 presentations, oral and poster, but rather convey the direction and sense of the workshop. We hope that this selection of papers will provide a better sense of how cytokines cooperate to maintain multicellular organisms, in particular ourselves, in health, and enable them to confront disease, illness and injury.

Michael C. Powanda
San Francisco, CA
Joost J. Oppenheim
Frederick, MD
Matthew J. Kluger
Ann Arbor, MI
Charles A. Dinarello
Boston, MA

Acknowledgments

The organizers are most grateful for the generous financial support provided by the following companies:

Ayerst Laboratories
Boehringer Ingelheim
Bristol-Myers Company
Cetus Corporation
Ciba-Geigy Corporation
Cistron Biotechnology, Inc.
E.I. duPont de Nemours & Company
Eli Lilly and Company
Genentech, Inc.
Hoffman-La Roche Inc.
Immunex Corporation
Interferon Sciences, Inc.
Johnson & Johnson International
McNeil Pharmaceutical
Merck Sharpe & Dohme Research Laboratories
Monsanto Company
Pfizer Central Research
G.D. Searle & Company
Smith Kline & French Laboratories
Syntex Research
The Upjohn Company

The Biological Response Modifier Program, NCI, and the U.S. Army Medical Research and Development Command provided support through grants and a contribution was made in memory of his father (1906–1987) by Michael C. Powanda.

Section I. Interferon-β_2/HSF/IL-6

Monokines and Other Non-Lymphocytic Cytokines, pages 3–13
© 1988 Alan R. Liss, Inc.

INTERLEUKIN-6 : STRUCTURE, PRODUCTION AND ACTIONS

A. Billiau

Rega Institute, University of Leuven, Belgium

INTRODUCTION

The newest candidate for taking rank as an interleukin is a molecule that, in the human system, has sofar been known as 26kDa-protein, IFN-β_2 (for interferon-β_2), HGF or HPGF (for hybridoma/plasmacytoma growth factor)[2] or BSF-2 (for B-cell stimulatory factor-2). Investigators of this cytokine have already suggested to resolve the prevailing confusion in nomenclature by calling this molecule IL-6. For convenience, this designation will be used here whenever reference is made to the molecule in general rather than to one of its specific properties.

As suggested by the multiplicity in names, the cytokine was independently discovered by several research teams, each interested in related, but different biological activities. Identity of the factors responsible for these activities did not appear until, after several years of research, their molecular structure became known.

26kDa PROTEIN/IFN-β_2

The molecule was first associated with <u>interferon-like antiviral activity</u>, when two groups of investigators (Weissenbach <u>et al.</u>, 1980; Content <u>et al.</u>, 1982) isolated and cloned a mRNA, which was found to occur in association with the mRNA of human IFN-β. The anti-IFN-β antisera of that day were found to precipitate the translation products of one as well as the other mRNA, so that initially these products seemed to be serologically related. In addition, the observations of one of the two research teams (Weissenbach et al., 1980) indicated that the translation products of both mRNAs possessed antiviral activity, that could be neutralized by antibodies against IFN-β. These observations were at the origin of the designation "IFN-β$_2$". The second research team (Content et al., 1982), found antiviral activity associated with the translation products of only one of the two mRNAs (that of IFN-β) and introduced the designation "26kDa protein" for the translation product(s) of the other mRNA.

It is not an exaggeration to say that, in connection with these translation products, two issues (serological relationship to classical IFN-β and presence of antiviral activity) have kept the interferon community in suspense for more than 5 years. The first issue was partially resolved when it appeared that the apparent cross-reactivity in immunoprecipitation reactions was simply due to nonspecificity of the early antisera. It remained a problem why the antiviral activity was neutralized by even the most specific antisera available. However, this question is now loosing importance, as it is becoming clear that the antiviral effect found in the preparations coming from a single laboratory is increasingly outbalanced by the lack of antiviral activity of preparations from other laboratories. An additional mortgage weighing on the interferon-status of IL-6 is that any resemblance between its primary structure and that of known human interferons (α, β or γ) is at best inferential (Haegeman et al., 1986).

In summary then, studies on IFN-β were at the basis of the first discovery of IL-6. This association between the two cytokines is merely historical and has its origin in the fact that they are sometimes co-induced in cells. Although there may be a molecular-biological basis for this frequent co-induction, there are sofar no other biological properties shared by the two molecules. Hence there is no reason to let them share a name that hints at a specific biological activity.

An important point revealed by these early studies is the fact that the IL-6 gene can be expressed into its mRNA in "ordinary" fibroblasts after stimulation with the double-stranded RNA, poly-rI.rC (Weissenbach et al., 1980; Content et al., 1982), or cycloheximide (Poupart et al., 1984). Later studies revealed that similar stimulation of expression can be obtained by exposing the fibroblasts to IL-1 (Content et al., 1985), or (less so) to TNF (Kohase et al., 1986).

HYBRIDOMA GROWTH FACTOR

IL-6 was discovered a second time by investigators who where interested in a hybridoma growth factor (HGF). This episode started in 1980, when Astaldi et al. (1980) described that supernatant from human endothelial cell cultures could replace feeder cells as promotors for the outgrowth of mouse hybridomas. A similar activity was subsequently found in crude preparations of human IL-2, produced by a heterogenous population of mononuclear cells (Aarden, 1985). This HGF was found to be different from IL-2 but difficult to distinguish from IL-1, since (among other things) it proved to be produced by the monocytes. A possible relationship or identity between this HGF and 26kDa protein was surmised when it appeared that human fibroblasts, exposed to any of the agents which stimulate 26kDa protein mRNA expression, produce HGF activity (Van Damme et al., 1987a,d).

Several lines of evidence supported identity between the two proteins. The availability of murine hybridoma cell lines which are strictly dependent on HGF (Aarden, 1985; Van Snick, 1986) greatly facilitated analytical and preparative work, which ultimately led to sequencing of the N-terminus of both fibroblast and monocyte-derived HGF (Van Damme et al., 1987b,d,e). Both molecules were identical to each other and their amino acid sequence matched that of the 26kDa protein. A potentially important point, noted early on by investigators of HGF (Aarden, 1985), is the fact that most murine hybridomas are independent of and insensitive to the growth promoting effect of HGF. In addition, cell lines which are factor-dependent, easily become independent. Another important point is the fact that mouse plasmacytomas which can normally only be maintained by in vivo passage, will grow in vitro if the culture medium is supplemented with human HGF (Van Damme et al., 1987d).

B CELL STIMULATING FACTOR-2 (BSF-2)

Human IL-6 was discovered a third time, independently, by investigators studying the regulation of B-cells by T-cells. T-cells produce BCDF's (B-cell differentiation factors), i.e. factors detectable by their ability to induce high rate secretion of Ig by Staphylococcus aureus Cowan I (SAC)-stimulated normal B blasts or CESS cells (an EBV-transformed human B-cell line). Analysis of these factors led to the isolation of one particular human BCDF, called BSF-2 (Hirano et al., 1985) which was originally found in supernatants of mitogen-stimulated T lymphocytes (Muraguchi et al., 1981), but also as a constitutive product of an IL-2-dependent T-cell clone, d4 (Kaieda et al., 1982), and of several HTLV-transformed T-cell lines (Kishimoto, 1985). Intriguingly, a factor apparently identical with BSF-2 was found to be constitutively produced by various non-T-cell lines, such as cardiac myxoma, cervical carcinoma and bladder carcinoma cell lines (Hirano et al., 1986, 1987). Another potentially important point revealed by investigations on BSF-2 is the fact that the factor seems to have no growth promoting effect on "normal" human B cells (Okada et al., 1983; Hirano et al., 1985). While BSF-2 was originally discovered in 1982, its primary structure became known in 1986 as a result of successful cDNA cloning work (Hirano et al., 1986). Although there may be minor differences in truncation at the N-terminus, the amino acid sequence of BSF-2 is otherwise strictly identical with that of 26kDa protein/HGF, as derived from the DNA sequence (Haegeman et al., 1986; Zilberstein et al., 1986).

IL-6 OF THE MOUSE

A murine HGF has already been isolated (Van Snick et al., 1986). The factor is identical (Van Snick et al., 1987) to a factor which had earlier been described (Nordan et al., 1987a,b) as a growth promotor for mouse plasmacytoma cells. Intriguingly, the N-terminal amino acid sequence of this murine hybridoma/plasmacytoma growth factor is quite different from that of human IL-6.

DISCUSSION

The identity between the three factors allows us to combine all the information (see Tables 1 and 2) gathered by several research groups, and to speculate on the specific biological function(s) of the protein.

The physicochemical properties of the molecule are summarized in Table 1. The protein is synthesized as a pre-polypeptide of 212 amino acids, of which the 21 to 23 first ones constitute the signal peptide. The natural products have molecular weights (Van Damme _et al._, 1987b,d,e) that show some heterogeneity and that are slightly higher than the molecular weight predicted from the amino-acid sequence. This, as well as the heterogeneity in charge and the presence in the amino acid sequence of two potential glycosylation sites indicates that the molecule is secreted as a glycoprotein.

The known biological properties of IL-6 are summarized in Table 2. A salient point is that IL-6 is produced by many different cell types including normal fibroblasts, endo-

Table 1. Physicochemical properties of human IL-6

Molecular weight

     polypeptide : native 212 residues
              mature 189-199 residues

natural product (HGF) :	from fibroblasts	from leukocytes
gel filtration	27 kDa	32 kDa
SDS-PAGE	23 kDa	24 & 28 kDa

Glycosylation
     2 potential N-sites
     heterogeneous cation exchange profile

N-terminus of natural product (HGF)
     ALA-PRO-VAL-PRO-PRO-GLY-...
           VAL-PRO-PRO-GLY-...
        PRO-VAL-PRO-PRO-GLY-...

Table 2. Biological properties of human IL-6

Inducible in :
-   normal skin fibroblasts
-   osteosarcoma cell line (MG-63)
-   blood monocytes
-   endothelial cells

Spontaneous production by cell lines :
-   T-cell hybridoma (d4)
-   HTLV-transformed T-cells
-   cardiac myxoma
-   cervical carcinoma

Inducing agents :
-   IL-1α
-   IL-1β
-   TNF
-   viruses
-   dsRNA
-   cycloheximide

Activities :   stimulation of
-   Ig-secretion by human B-cells
    (normal SAC-stimulated; EBV-transformed CESS-cells)
-   growth of murine B-cell hybridomas and plasmacytomas
-   proliferation of mouse thymocytes (LAF assay)
-   secretion of acute phase reactant by hepatocytes

---

thelial cells and monocytes, as well as cell lines of T, B, sarcomatous or carcinomatous origin. In addition, a multiplicity of agents can induce IL-6: endogenous factors such as IL-1 and TNF, and exogenous agents such as viruses, foreign RNA and metabolic inhibitors. These observations suggest that IL-6 may appear at any time or any place in any tissue. Thus, the induction of the factor seems to be less specific than that of IL-1, suggesting that IL-6 fulfills a need for amplification of a function that is triggered in a more specific way.

About the actions of IL-6 in homologous cell systems, we know little more than that it acts as a terminal differentiation factor for B-cells, converting the latter to

high-rate Ig producers. Could it be that connective or pa-
renchymatous tissues use IL-6 as a means to influence local
antibody production ? Such influence might be merely quantitative (simple enhancement) or qualitative. For instance,
IL-6 might direct Ig class and isotype specificity in much
the same way as this is done by IL-4 and IFN-γ (for review
see Kishimoto, 1985; Snapper and Paul, 1987). It is not un-
logical to postulate that non-lymphoid components of the
tissues have the means to select Ig class and isotype, so
that they suit the proper local needs. Along this line it
has also been suggested (Hirano et al., 1987) that the
auto-antibodies found in certain patients with cardiac myxoma or cervical carcinoma are due to in vivo secretion by
these tumors of IL-6.

Taking into account the fact that, among endogenous
stimulators of IL-6 production, IL-1 is sofar the most potent one, one might find physiological functions for the
molecule by asking the question which IL-1 effects are mediated by IL-6.

For instance, it has become known recently that human
IL-6 is active in the mouse thymocyte proliferation assay
(LAF assay) (Van Damme et al., 1987e), thereby mimicking
the action of IL-1 and raising the question, unanswered sofar, whether perhaps the LAF activity of IL-1 is mediated
by IL-6. Clarity in this question may come as soon as the
mouse equivalent of human IL-6 will be identified unequivocally (see above).

A well-known function of IL-1 is its ability to induce
production of acute phase proteins in vivo and by hepatocytes. It has recently been reported (Gauldie et al., 1987)
that human IL-6 possesses similar hepatocyte stimulating
activity. Another well-known function of IL-1 is its antiviral effect in certain cells (Van Damme et al., 1985).
However, this effect is mediated by IFN-γ, not by IL-6 (Van
Damme et al., 1987c). IL-1 is believed to play an important
role in the pathogenesis of inflammation, e.g. by inducing
production of proteases and prostaglandins. Experiments in
our laboratory, testing the ability of IL-6 to stimulate
proteases and prostaglandins, failed to support the idea
that local inflammation may be mediated by IL-6. IL-1 also
induces granulocyte-macrophage (GM) colony formation in
bone-marrow cultures, an effect which depends on the presence of monocytic adherent cells (Fibbe et al., 1986); it

is not known sofar wether this requirement reflects production of IL-6 by these monocytes.

REFERENCES

Aarden L, Lansdorp P, De Groot E (1985). A growth factor
    for B cell hybridomas produced by human monocytes. In
    Pick E, Landy M (eds): "The Lymphokines", Vol. 10, New
    York: Academic Press, pp 175-185.
Astaldi GCB, Janssen MC, Lansdorp P, Willems C, Zeijlemaker
    WP, Oosterhof F (1980) Human endothelial culture superna-
    tant (HECS): a growth factor for hybridomas. J Immunol
    125: 1411-1414.
Content J, De Wit L, Pierard D, Derynck R, De Clercq E,
    Fiers W (1982) Secretory proteins induced in human fibro-
    blasts under conditions used for the production of inter-
    feron β. Proc Natl Acad Sci USA 79:2768-2772.
Content J, Dewit L, Poupart P, Opdenakker G, Van Damme J,
    Billiau A (1985) Induction of a 26-kDa-protein mRNA in
    human cells treated with an interleukin-1-related, leuko-
    cyte-derived factor. Eur J Biochem 152:253-257.
Fibbe WE, Van Damme J, Billiau A, Voogt PJ, Duinkerken N,
    Kluck PMC, Falkenburg JHF (1986) Interleukin-1 (22-K fac-
    tor) induces release of granulocyte-macrophage colony-
    stimulating activity from human mononuclear phagocytes.
    Blood 68:1316-1321.
Gauldie J, Richards C, Harnish D, Lansdorp P, Baumann H
    (1987) Interferon-β$_2$/BSF-2 shares identity with monocyte-
    derived hepatocyte stimulating factor (HSF) and regulates
    the major acute phase response in liver cells. Proc Natl
    Acad Sci USA: in press.
Haegeman G, Content J, Volckaert G, Derynck R, Tavernier
    J, Fiers W (1986) Structural analysis of the sequence co-
    ding for an inducible 26-kDa protein in human fibro-
    blasts. Eur J Biochem 159:625-632.
Hirano T, Teranishi T, Lin B, Onoue K (1984) Human helper T
    cell factor(s). IV. Demonstration of a human late-acting
    B cell differentiation factor acting on Staphylococcus
    aureus Cowan I-stimulated B cells. J Immunol 133:798-802.
Hirano T, Taga T, Nakano N, Yasukawa K, Kashiwamura S, Shi-
    mizu K, Nakajima K, Pyun KH, Kishimoto T (1985) Purifica-
    tion to homogeneity and characterization of human B-cell
    differentiation factor (BCDF or BSFp-2). Proc Natl Acad
    Sci USA 82:5490-5494.

Hirano T, Yasukawa K, Harada H, Taga T, Watanabe Y, Matsuda T, Kashiwamura S-I, Nakajima K, Koyama K, Iwamatsu A, Tsunasawa S, Sakiyama F, Matsui H, Takahara Y, Taniguchi T, Kishimoto T (1986) Complementary DNA for a novel human interleukin (BSF-2) that induces B lymphocytes to produce immunoglobulin. Nature 324:73-76.

Hirano T, Taga T, Yasukawa K, Nakajima K, Nakano N, Takatsuki F, Shimizu M, Murashima A, Tsunasawa S, Sakiyama F, Kishimoto T (1987) Human B-cell differentiation factor defined by an anti-peptide antibody and its possible role in autoantibody production. Proc Natl Acad Sci USA 84: 228-231.

Kaieda T, Okada M, Yoshimura N, Kishimoto S, Yamamura Y, Kishimoto T (1982) A human helper T cell clone secreting both killer helper factor(s) and T cell-replacing factor(s). J Immunol 129:46-51.

Kishimoto T (1985) Factors affecting B-cell growth and differentiation. Ann Rev Immunol 3:133-157

Kohase M, Henriksen-De Stefano D, May LT, Vilcek J, Sehgal P (1986) Induction of beta-2 interferon by tumor necrosis factor: a homeostatic mechanism in the control of cell proliferation. Cell 45:659-669.

Muraguchi A, Kishimoto T, Miki Y, Kuritani T, Kaieda T, Yoshizaki K, Yamamura Y (1981) T cell-replacing factor-(TRF) induced IgG secretion in a human B blastoid cell line and demonstration of acceptors for TRF. J Immunol 127:412-416.

Nordan RP, Potter M (1986) A macrophage-derived factor required by plasmacytomas for survival and proliferation in vitro. Science 233:566-569.

Nordan RP, Pumphrey JG, Rudikoff S (1987) Purification and NH_2-terminal sequence of a plasmacytoma growth factor derived from the murine macrophage cell line P388D1. J Immunol 139:813-817.

Okada M, Sakaguchi N, Yoshimura N, Hara H, Shimizu K, Yoshida N, Yoshizaki K, Kishimoto S, Yamamura Y, Kishimoto T (1983) B cell growth factors and B cell differentiation factor from human T hybridomas. Two distinct kinds of B cell growth factor and their synergism in B cell proliferation. J Exp Med 157:583-590.

Poupart P, De Wit L, Content J (1984) Induction and regulation of the 26-kDa protein in the absence of synthesis of beta-interferon mRNA in human cells. Eur J Biochem 143: 15-21.

Snapper CM, Paul WE (1987) Interferon-γ and B-cell stimulatory factor-1 reciprocally regulate Ig isotype production. Science 236:944-947.

Van Damme J, De Ley M, Opdenakker G, Billiau A, De Somer P, Van Beeumen J (1984) Homogeneous interferon-inducing 22K factor is related to endogenous pyrogen and interleukin-1. Nature 314:266-268.

Van Damme J, Cayphas S, Opdenakker G, Billiau A, Van Snick J (1987a) Interleukin 1 and poly(rI).(rC) induce production of a hybridoma growth factor by human fibroblasts. Eur J Immunol 17:1-7.

Van Damme J, Cayphas S, Van Snick J, Conings R, Put W, Lenaerts J-P, Simpson RJ, Billiau A (1987b) Purification and characterization of human fibroblast-derived hybridoma growth factor identical to T-cell-derived B-cell stimulatory factor-2 (interleukin-6). Eur J Biochem 168: 543-550.

Van Damme J, De Ley M, Van Snick J, Dinarello CA, Billiau A (1987c) The role of interferon-β_1 and the 26-kDa protein (interferon-β_2) as mediators of the antiviral effect of interleukin-1 and tumor necrosis factor. J Immunol 139: 1867-1872.

Van Damme J, Opdenakker G, Simpson RJ, Rubira MR, Cayphas S, Vink A, Billiau A, Van Snick J (1987d) Identification of the human 26-kD protein, interferon β_2 (IFN-β_2), as a B cell hybridoma/plasmacytoma growth factor induced by interleukin 1 and tumor necrosis factor. J Exp Med 165:914-919.

Van Damme J, Van Beeumen J, Decock B, Van Snick J, De Ley M, Billiau A (1987e) Separation and comparison of two monokines with LAF activity (interleukin-1β and hybridoma growth factor): identification of leukocyte-derived HGF as interleukin-6. J Immunol: in press.

Van Snick J, Cayphas S, Vink A, Uyttenhove C, Coulie P, Simpson RJ (1986) Purification and NH_2-terminal amino acid sequence of a new T cell-derived lymphokine with growth factor activity for B cell hybridomas. Proc Natl Acad Sci USA 83:9679-9683.

Van Snick J, Vink A, Cayphas S, Uyttenhove C (1987) Interleukin-HP1, a T cell-derived hybridoma growth factor that supports the in vitro growth of murine plasmacytomas. J Exp Med 165:641-649.

Weissenbach J, Chernajovsky Y, Zeevi M, Shulman L, Soreq H,
  Nir U, Wallach D, Perricaudet M, Tiollais P, Revel M
  (1980) Two interferon mRNAs in human fibroblasts: in vitro translation and Escherichia coli cloning studies.
  Proc Natl Acad Sci USA 77:7152–7156.
Zilberstein A, Ruggieri R, Korn JH, Revel M (1986) Structure and expression of cDNA and genes for human interfe-
  ron-β-2, a distinct species inducible by growth-stimula-
  tory cytokines. EMBO J 5:2529–2537.

Monokines and Other Non-Lymphocytic Cytokines, pages 15–20

INTERFERON $\beta2$ IS IDENTICAL TO MONOCYTIC HSF AND REGULATES THE FULL ACUTE PHASE PROTEIN RESPONSE IN LIVER CELLS

Jack Gauldie, Carl Richards, Del Harnish and Heinz Baumann
Dept. of Pathology, McMaster University, Hamilton, Ontario, Canada L8N 3Z5 (J.G., C.R.,D.H.), Dept. of Molecular and Cellular Biology, Roswell Park Memorial Inst., Buffalo, New York USA (H.B.)

INTRODUCTION

One of the oldest and most preserved of the homeostatic responses of the body to injury and infection is the acute phase response. This includes leukocytosis, fever, and a characteristic increase in a group of liver-derived plasma proteins called acute phase (AP) reactants (Koj 1985).These include $\alpha1$ acid glycoprotein ($\alpha1$AGP), haptoglobin (HPT), fibrinogen (FBG), hemopexin (HPX), ceruloplasmin (CER), $\alpha1$ antichymotrypsin ($\alpha1$ACY), C3 and $\alpha1$ proteinase inhibitor ($\alpha1$PI) in most species, along with C reactive protein (CRP), Factor B complement component and serum amyloid A and P proteins (SAA & SAP) in man and cysteine proteinase inhibitor (CPI) and $\alpha2$ macroglobulin ($\alpha2$M) in the rat. The changes seen in the acute phase can be attributed to the action of a group of protein hormones (cytokines) released from activated monocytes, which includes Hepatocyte stimulating factor (HSF), IL-1 and TNF. Among these monocytic cytokines, HSF plays the most prominent role in the stimulation of hepatic cells. The human factor was characterized as a 30 kD, pI5 peptide (Ritchie and Fuller 1983; Koj et al 1984; Baumann et al 1984), and was active in primary cultures of rat hepatocytes and human (HepG2) and rat (H35) hepatoma cells (Koj et al 1985; Woloski and Fuller 1985; Baumann et al 1987a). Here we show that the monocytic cytokine HSF shares identity with a previously characterized and cloned molecule known variously as Interferon $\beta2$ (IFN$\beta2$), B cell stimulatory factor (BSF2), Hybridoma growth factor, 26-kd protein and Il-6 (summarized in Billiau 1987; Sehgal et al 1987).

Materials and Methods

The activity of HSF, stimulation of AP protein synthesis, in primary rat hepatocytes and human and rat hepatoma cells, was determined as described. Human peripheral blood monocyte (LPS stimulated) conditioned medium (PBM-CM) and human lung fibroblast conditioned medium (FBL-CM) were prepared as described (Baumann et al 1987a,b; Gauldie et al 1987). Recombinant human IL-1β (2×10^8 U/mg) was provided by Dr. Urdal,Immunex corp.; recombinant human BSF2 (E. coli-2×10^5 U/ml) was supplied by Drs Hirano and Kishimoto; and recombinant human IL-6 (COS cell-10^6 U/mg) was supplied by Dr. Wong, Genetics Inst. Antisera to Interferon β was from NIH and anti-rhIFNβ2 was provided by Drs May and Sehgal.

Results and Discussion

When PBM-CM was size fractionated by HPLC (TSK3000) the main HSF activity emerged at 30kD, clearly separable from IL-1. For instance, α2 Macroglobulin and CPI were induced by HSF only, while α1AGP and albumin were affected by both cytokines. Analysis of PBM-CM on PAGE under non-denaturing conditions showed the main HSF activity migrating as a protein with Mr of 25-28 kD and pI of 5. These properties were similar to those of Hybridoma growth factor (Aarden et al 1987) and thus to IFNβ2. To examine this relationship we carried out antibody absorptions of PBM-CM. Antibodies recognizing fibroblast-derived IFNβ2 and rhIFNβ2, but not IFNβ1 or other interferons, neutralized the HSF-specific activity in PBM-CM. The combination of anti-IL-1β and anti-IFNβ2 neutralized all hepatocyte stimulating activity in PBM-CM. Unstimulated fibroblasts (FBL-CM) were a potent source of HSF (no IL-1) which was neutralized by anti-IFNβ2. Thus monocyte HSF was serologically related to fibroblast HSF and to IFNβ2.

Anti-IFNβ2 immunoprecipitates 23- and 26-kD proteins from PBM-CM and the precipitation is inhibited by rhIFNβ2. A cDNA probe for IFNβ2 (pβ2.15, Sehgal et al 1987) identified a 1.3 kb mRNA in stimulated PBM. By a combination of column chromatography, gel electrophoresis and western blot analysis with anti-rhIFNβ2, we showed that HSF migrating at 30 kD under non-denaturing conditions is identical to the IFNβ2 25-26 kD protein and that the 23 kD protein is also active as HSF.   We have further shown that rhBSF2/IFNβ2/IL-6 from both sources stimulates the increased expression of the same spectrum of acute phase proteins as monocyte HSF at both the mRNA and protein level (Gauldie et al 1987; Prowse & Baumann 1988).   Figure 1 shows that rhIFNβ2/BSF2 combined with glucocorticoid (dexamethasone 1μM) can regulate most if not all of the AP proteins in HepG2 cells. Maximum response was achieved with 25–50 U/ml (picomolar).

Having identified IFNβ2 as a major regulator of AP protein genes in hepatocytes, and knowing that IL-1, TNF and glucocorticoid are also able to induce a limited set of AP proteins (Baumann et al 1987a; Gauldie et al 1987; Darlington et al 1986), we then defined the hormone combinations necessary to accomplish an optimal hepatic acute phase response <u>in vitro</u>. The effect of glucocorticoid, rhIL-1β, rhIFNβ2/IL-6 in the various hepatocyte assays are summarized in Table 1. Several concepts emerge: rhIFNβ2 can regulate all acute phase protein genes, some more strongly than others, while rhIL-1β regulates only a subset of the genes and the two cytokines in the presence of glucocorticoid are needed to elicit the full hepatic acute phase protein response. The most striking example of <u>in vitro</u> protein regulation by IFNβ2/HSF is hemopexin in rat H35 cells. There are examples of synergy between IFNβ2 and IL-1β (α1AGP – rat and human) and between glucocorticoid and IFNβ2 (α2M – rat) and examples of inhibitory activity of IL-1β

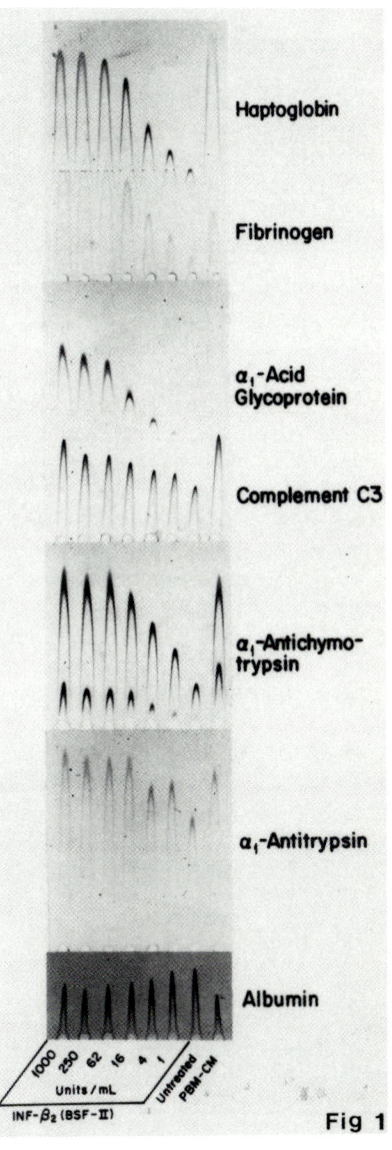

Fig 1

on the action of IFNβ2 (FBG -human) as demonstrated in Fig.2. The additive effect between the inhibitory action of IL-1β and stimulating action of IFNβ2 on FBG expression accounts for the relatively lower stimulation induced by PBM-CM than by IFNβ2 alone. IFNβ2/IL-6 is active in different species, the response however is species specific. Examination of other interferons (α,β1 or τ) or other growth factors (CSF-1) showed no HSF activity. Thus it appears that the three hormones can account for all liver stimulating activity derived from monocytes or fibroblasts. In addition, by examining multiple proteins in several hepatocyte systems, we have been able to classify the proteins into those stimulated by IFNβ2 only (type II) and those stimulated by both IFNβ2 and IL-1β (type I) as well as those showing synergy and additive actions (Table 2)

TABLE 1.   REGULATION OF ACUTE PHASE PROTEIN SYNTHESIS (µg/24h/10^6 cells)

TREATMENT	RAT HEPATOCYTES			H35 RAT HEPATOMA				
	α2M	CPI	ALB	α1AGP	α2M	CPI	C3	HPX
Media	-	-	-	ND	ND	0.01	0.01	0.5
Media & dex	7	25	40	ND	ND	0.02	0.01	0.7
IL-1β & dex	8	23	33	0.03	ND	ND	0.12	-
IFNβ2	-	-	-	ND	ND	0.2	0.05	-
IFNβ2 & dex	46	38	14	0.02	0.25	0.60	0.07	8.6
IL-1β+IFNβ2 & dex	-	-	-	0.3	0.17	0.58	0.19	-
PBM-CM & dex	50	30	13	0.36	0.06	0.38	0.20	-
FBL-CM & dex	42	33	29	-	-	-	-	-

Dexamethasone (dex) - 1µM; IL-1β - 250 U/ml; IFNβ2 - 50 U/ml
(Gauldie et al 1987: Baumann et al 1987a,b; Baumann and Müller-Eberhard 1978)

TABLE 2   SUBSETS OF ACUTE PHASE PROTEINS

TYPE I - INDUCED BY IL-1,TNF & HSF/IFNβ2		TYPE II - INDUCED ONLY BY HSF/IFNβ2		DEPENDENT ON BOTH IL1β & HSF/IFNβ2	
				SYNERGY	INHIBITION
α1AGP	HPT	FBG	HPX	α1AGP	FBG
C3	FACTOR B	α2M	CPI	HPT	CPI
SAA	SAP?	α1PI	α1ACHY	C3	
		CER	CRP?		

(ND, not detected; -, not done)

Human squamous carcinoma (COLO-16) cells produce 2 structurally distinct HSF forms which induce similar sets of AP proteins as IL-1 and IFNβ2/HSF, but do not share immunologic identity and must be considered an additional set of HSF's.   The relationship of keratinocyte-HSF's to monocyte/fibroblast cytokines awaits sequence comparisons.

In summary, IFNβ2/HSF acts as an anabolic hormone having regulatory elements on the genes it modulates (Prowse & Baumann, 1988).   Its function is to regulate the expression of the major group of acute phase proteins and acting in conjunction with IL-1 and glucocorticoid, in both a synergistic and additive manner, can account for all liver stimulating activity derived from activated monocytes similar to the acute phase protein response seen <u>in vivo</u>.

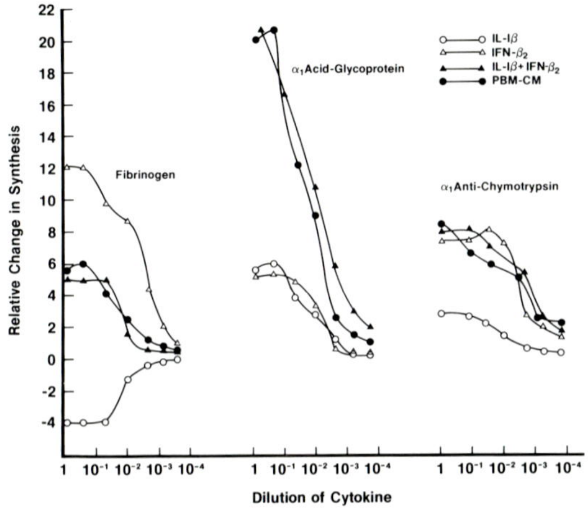

Figure 2 Human Hep G2 cells stimulated with various combinations of cytokines (Baumann et al 1987b).

REFERENCES

Aarden LA, DeGroot E, Schaap OL, Lansdorp PM (1987). Production of hybridoma growth factor by human monocytes. Eur J Immunol 17:1411-1416.

Baumann H, Jahreis GP, Sauder DN, Koj A (1984). Human keratinocytes and monocytes release factors which regulate the synthesis of major acute phase plasma proteins in hepatic cells from man, rat and mouse. J Biol Chem 259:7331-7342.

Baumann H, Muller-Eberhard U (1987).   Synthesis of hemopexin and cysteine protease inhibitor is coordinately regulated by HSF-II and interferon-β2 in rat hepatoma cells.   Biochem Biophys Res Comm 146:1218-1226.

Baumann H, Onorato V, Gauldie J, Jahreis GP (1987a). Distinct sets of acute phase plasma proteins are stimulated by separate human hepatocyte-stimulating factors and monokines in rat hepatoma cells. J Biol Chem 262:9756-9768.

Baumann H, Richards C, Gauldie J (1987b). Interaction between hepatocyte-stimulating factors, IL-1 and glucocorticoids for regulation of acute phase plasma proteins in human HepG2 cells. J Immunol (in press).

Billiau A (1987). Interferon β2 as a promoter of growth and differentiation of B cells. Immunol Today 8:84-87.

Darlington GJ, Wilson DR, Lachman LB (1986). Monocyte-conditioned medium, interleukin-1 and tumor necrosis factor stimulate the acute phase response in human hepatoma cells in vitro. J Cell Biol 103:787-799.

Gauldie J, Richards C, Harnish D, Lansdorp P, Baumann H (1987). Interferon β2/B-cell stimulatory factor type 2 shares identity with monocyte-derived hepatocyte-stimulating factor and regulates the major acute phase protein response in liver cells. Proc Natl Acad Sci USA 84:7251-7255.

Koj A (1985). In Gordon AH, Koj A (eds): "The Acute Phase Response to Injury and Infection" New York: Elsevier, pp 139-144.

Koj A, Gauldie J, Regoeczi E, Sauder DN, Sweeney GD (1984). The acute-phase response of cultured rat hepatocytes. Biochem J 224:505-514.

Prowse KR, Baumann H (1988) Hepatocyte-stimulating factor, β2 IFN, and IL-1 enhance expression of the rat α1-acid glycoprotein gene via a distal upstream regulatory region. Mol Cell Biol (in press).

Ritchie DG, Fuller GM (1983) Hepatocyte-stimulating factor: a monocyte-derived acute-phase regulatory protein. Ann NY Acad Sci 408:490-496.

Sehgal PB, May LT, Tamm I, Vilcek J (1987) Human β2 interferon and B-cell differentiation factor BSF-2 are identical. Science 235:731-732.

Woloski BMRNJ, Fuller GM (1985) Identification and partial characterization of hepatocyte-stimulating factor from leukemia cell lines: comparison with interleukin 1. Proc Natl Acad Sci USA 82:1443-1447.

Monokines and Other Non-Lymphocytic Cytokines, pages 21–27
© 1988 Alan R. Liss, Inc.

HUMAN IFN-Beta-2: A CYTOKINE WITH MULTIPLE FUNCTIONS
IN INFECTIONS AND INFLAMMATION.

Michel Revel, Asher Zilberstein, Rosa-
Maria Ruggieri, Louisa Chen, Yves Mory,
Menachem Rubinstein, Rita Michalevicz (*)

Department of Virology, Weizmann Institute
of Science, Rehovot and Department of
Hematology (*) Ichilov Hospital, Tel Aviv,
Israel

INTRODUCTION.

IFN-β2 is a cytokine originally described as
the product of a 1.3 kb RNA encoding IFN-β type
activity, induced in human fibroblasts by poly
(rI)(rC) or by a superinduction regimen (Weissenbach et al, 1980; Sehgal and Sagar, 1980).
Fibroblasts were shown to secrete several forms of
the protein, mainly of 21-26 Kd, which appear to be
processed from a 212 aminocids-long precursor. The
cDNA sequence shows 15-20% homology with other type
I IFNs, with the conservation of several clusters
of aminoacids (Zilberstein et al, 1985, 1986). Two
forms of the IFN-β2 gene, both with introns, were
cloned and mapped to chromosome 7 (Sehgal et al,
1987). In addition to viral inducers, the cytokine
is also produced by fibroblasts in response to
bacterial LPS (Sehgal and May, 1987), and to other
cytokines as IL-1, TNF and PDGF (Kohase et al,
1986; Zilberstein et al, 1986;). Several other
activities have been associated with this cytokine,
including 1) BSF-2: B-plasma cells differentiation
(Hirano et al, 1986), 2) HGF: growth stimulation
of plasmacytomas, hybridomas, EBV-transformed
B-lymphocytes and thymocytes (Van Damme et al,1987;
Tosato et al, 1987), 3) hepatocyte stimulation
factor (HSF) activity (Gauldie et al, 1987)
and 4) a hemopoietic progenitor cell stimulating
activity (Revel et al, 1987a). The different

activities observed probably result from
interaction with different receptors, since some
(antiviral and antigrowth effects) are species
specific, while others (HGF and HSF) are seen in
rodent cells as well. Preparations of this
cytokine (also refered to as IL-6) from different
laboratories appear to differ in these multiple
activities, generating controversy about its
genuine functions. We describe here our results
using both recombinant IFN-β2 produced in mammalian
cells (CHO) and in E.coli.

RESULTS

     Constitutive production of glycosylated and
processed recombinant HuIFN-β2 was obtained by
cotransfecting Hamster CHO DHFR$^-$ cells with a
full-length cDNA fused to the SV40 early promoter
together with pSV-DHFR DNA, and amplifying the
transgenes through selection in Metho- trexate.
From two separate series of transformants, clones
producing IFN-β2 activity were isolated
(Zilberstein et al, 1986). Purification of the
antiviral activity (AV) produced by CHO subclone
B-131-5-017 is shown in Table 1. Two ion-exchange

TABLE 1.   Purification of recombinant CHO HuIFN-β2

Fraction	Total IFN AV units	IFN[a] AV U/ml	Specific Activity AV units/mg
input[b]	172,500	15,000	$3x10^2$
DEAE-Seph.	140,000	8,000	$2x10^3$
CM-Seph.	54,000	8,000	$1x10^5$
DEAE-Seph.	50,000	4,000	$6x10^3$
CM-Seph.	64,000	8,000	$1x10^4$
Superose-12	20,000	10,000	$8x10^5$
Mono-P	900	100	$1x10^6$

a/ Antiviral activity on VSV in FS11 cells. Titer
in peak fractions.
b/ 3 trays of $12x10^6$ CHO-B131-5-017 cells. Medium
harvested daily for 3 days. Concentrated 10 fold.
Fractions: DEAE, 100 mM NaCl; CM, 250 mM NaCl.

and two HPLC were used. Specific activities of 10^6
AV units/mg protein were obtained in the most
purified fractions. The AV activity in crude CHO
culture medium was often variable and was unmasked
by the DEAE-Sephadex step which appears to remove
inhibitors. Purified CHO rIFN-B2 also induced
typical IFN-activated genes (such as the (2'-5')
oligo A synthetase and MHC class I) and had anti-
proliferative activity (AP) on human fibroblasts
and Breast carcinoma cells (Zilberstein et al,
1985; Revel et al, 1987b). When tested for the
other IFN-B2/IL-6 activities, the DEAE-fractionated
CHO rIFN-Beta-2 showed BSF-2 titers (stimulation if
IgG secretion by human lymphoblastoid CESS cells)
and HGF titers (^{3}H-Thymidine incorporation by
murine T1165 plasmacytoma cells) which were 10-100
times lower than the AV titers (Fig. 1). While
HGF activity coeluted with the AV activity, about
half of the HGF activity was the protein fraction
unbound to DEAE-Sephadex and without AV activity
suggesting the existence of different subforms of

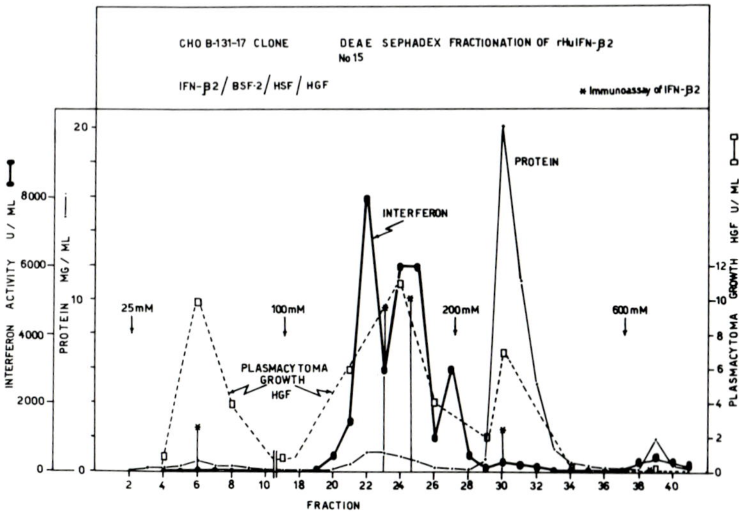

Fig. 1. Distribution of IFN (antiviral activity)
and HGF activity on DEAE-Sephadex. Immunoassay of
IFN-Beta-2 protein is shown.

the cytokine. Immunoassays detected the IFN-Beta-2
protein in both fractions (Fig.1). Immunoblots
reveal several bands of 21-26 Kd as well as larger
(multimeric) forms. Baumann et al (1987) also
observed that HSF activity separates in two similar
fractions on DEAE-Sephadex.

Another form of rIFN-β2 was produced in E.
coli by fusing the coding region (starting at
Pro-Val-Pro, the N-terminus defined for BSF-2
[Hirano et, 1986]) to a bacterial tryplac promoter
inducible by IPTG. This E.coli rIFN-β2 of 20 Kd,
was found to have high BSF-2 and HGF titers of
10-20,000 U/ml)(Table 2), the amplitude of the IgG
increase in CESS cultures being also larger than
what was observed with CHO material. AV activities
of 2-6,000 U/ml were found (versus 500 induced by
parallel extracts not IPTG-induced or of control
bacterias), but on DEAE-Sephadex the bulk of the
BSF-2/HGF was in the DEAE-unbound fraction without
significant AV activity; about 10% of the BSF-2
activity coeluted from DEAE with some AV activity,
again suggesting two subforms of the protein.
Other groups have obtained BSF-2 activity (10[7]
U/mg) without AV activity (Hirano et al, 1986;
Poupart et al,1987). Both in our work and that of
Sehgal and May (1987), the AV activity of E.coli
rIFN-β2 differed from that of the CHO rIFN-β2 by a
requirement for 7-days aged fibroblasts. While
aged cells are known to have a better AV response
to IFNs (but also to LPS), the reason for the
difference is not known. At the 1987 ISIR meeting,
J. Wintzerbin et al reported that an antiviral
effect of E.coli rBSF-2/IFN-β2 is observed in Wish
cells treated by low amounts of TNF. The antigrowth
activity on Breast carcinoma T47 cells (AP activity
of IFN-β2) was clearly seen in the DEAE-unbound
fraction of E.coli rIFN-β2 (Table 2). This effect
was blocked by antibodies to a N-terminal 20-mer
peptide from the IFN-β2 sequence, and also by
antibodies to purified IFN-Beta-1 (Table 2), as
previously found for the AV activity (Zilberstein
et al, 1986).

The cytokine is clearly not a lymphocyte-
specific factor but regulates gene activity in many
cells. In collaboration with Dr G. Darlington, a

Table 2. Activities of E.coli produced Hu rIFN-β2.

rIFN-β-2 dilution	CESS cells BSF-2 IgG ng/ml	Plasmacytoma T1165 (HGF) 3H-Td cpm	Breast carcinoma T47 cells (AP) 3H-Td cpm	Colonies Number
No factor	235	800	18,800	110
1/31,250	450	16,650	9,250	–
1/12,000	525	24,600	–	–
1/ 6,250	–	32,600	3,700	50
1/ 1,250	775	36,250	1,700	18
1/ 400	825	–	–	5
1/ 10			1,800	
1/ 10 with antipeptide IFN-β-2:			10,400	
1/ 10 with anti-IFN-B1 :			16,200	

E.coli rIFN-β2, DEAE-Sephadex unbound, 275 ug/ml.
BSF-2 and HGF assays as described (Revel et al,
1987b). The 50% effect (1U) indicates 20,000 U/ml.
For AP, serum-refed T47 cells were treated 24 hrs,
and pulsed 1 hr by Td, or seeded at 200 cells/plate
and cultured 15 days. Mock rIFN-β2 did not inhibit.

Table 3. Liquid Culture Assay for Hemopoietic
Progenitors

Additions	Number of colonies LGEMM	LGM	BFU-E
None	2	3	2
rIFN-β2, 0.3 U/ml	23	16	16
rIL-1, 20 U/ml	19	19	11
rIL-3 + GM-CSF	3	5	1
PHA-LCM, 7.5%	35	15	42

PBMC from hairy cell leukemia donor were cultured 1
week in Iscove-Medium with 10% fetal calf serum and
indicated additions. Cells were then plated in
0.9% methylcellulose complete medium with PHA-
conditioned LCM. After 14 days, LGEMM (mixed), LGM
(myelogranulocytic) and BFU-E (erythroid) colonies
were counted (Michalevicz and Revel, 1987).

5Ø fold increase in fibrinogen,15 fold increase in
Complement C3 and 2-fold decrease in albumin
production were demonstrated in Hep3B2 cells
treated with 4Ø BSF-2 U/ml of E.coli rIFN-β2, confirming the HSF activity. Furthermore, rIFN-β2
stimulates also the hematopoietic system. In
particular, we found that CHO rIFN-β2 stimulates
the early progenitors in blood of hairy cell
leukemia patients, a system we have shown to be
rich in early lymphomyeloid stem cells (Michalevicz
and Revel, 1987). The increase in clonogenic cells
was studied in two-stage assays: blood mononuclear
cells were first cultured for 1 week in suspension
and then plated in methylcellulose with PHA-
conditioned medium as source of CSF. Addition of
Ø.3 AV U/ml CHO rIFN-β2 in the first stage produces
a marked stimulation of myeloid, erythroid and
mixed colonies progenitors (Table 3). The effect
is comparable to that of IL-1 (hemopoietin), but
IL-3 and GM-CSF have no such effect alone (Table
3). Similar effects were seen with normal bone
marrow but the cell target remains to be precisely
determined.

In conclusion, IFN-β2/IL-6 is a cytokine with
multiple functions which can be viewed as providing
an integrated defense against infections and
inflammations. Being induced in fibroblasts,
epithelial cells and in monocytes (but not
lymphocytes) (Sanceau et al, 1987) by viral dsRNA,
bacterial LPS and PHA, the cytokine may locally 1)
act against viruses and bacteria (AV effect and
complement formation), 2) regulate cell growth and
prevent sclerosis (AP effect), and at distance 3)
expand plasma cells and stimulate antibody
production, 4) stimulate hematopoiesis, 5) induce
complement, clot proteins and other acute phase
reactants favoring tissue repair and healing.

REFERENCES.

Baumann, H., Onorato, V., Gauldie, J. and
  Jahreis, G.P. (1987) J. Biol. Chem. 262:
  9756-9768.

Gauldie, J., Richards, C., Harnish, D., Landsdorp, P. and Baumann, H. (1987) Proc. Natl. Acad. Sci. USA, in press.

Hirano, T., Yasukawa, K., Harada, H. et al. (1986) Nature 234:73-76.

Kohase, M., Henrikson-Destefano, D., May, L.T., Vilcek, J. and Sehgal, P.B. (1986) Cell 45: 659-666.

Michalevicz, R. and Revel, M. (1987) Proc. Natl. Acad. Sci. USA 84: 2307-2311.

Poupart, P., Vandenabeele, P. Cayphas, S., Van Snick, J et al. (1987) EMBO J. 6:1219-1224.

Revel, M., Zilberstein, A., Ruggieri, R., et al. (1987a) in Kirchner, Tumor Necrosis Factor, in press (Karger, Basel).

Revel, M., Zilberstein, A., Ruggieri, R., Rubinstein, M., Chen, L. (1987b) J. Interferon Res 7:529-536.

Sanceau, J., Falcoff, R., Zilberstein, A. et al. (1987) J. Interferon Res. in press.

Sehgal, P.B. and May L.T. (1987) J. Interferon Res. 7:521-527.

Sehgal, P.B. and Sagar, A.D. (1980) Nature 287:95-97.

Sehgal, P.B., Zilberstein, A., Ruggieri, R., et al. (1986) Proc. Natl. Acad. Sci. USA 83:5219-5222.

Tosato, G., Seamon, K.B., Goldman, N.D., Sehgal, P.B. et al (1987) Science, in press.

VanDamme, J., Opdenakker, G., Simpson, R.J., et al. (1987) J. Exptl. Med. 165:914-919.

Weissenbach, J., Chernajovsky, Y., Zeevi, M. et al. (1980) Proc. Natl. Acad. Sci USA 77:7152-7156.

Zilberstein, A., Ruggieri R., and Revel, M. (1985) in Rossi and Dianzani, The IFN system, Serono Symposia 24, pp 73-83 (Raven Press, New York).

Zilberstein, A., Ruggieri, R., Korn, J.H. and Revel, M. (1986) EMBO J. 5:2529-2537.

Zilberstein, A., Ruggieri, R., Korn, J.H., Chen, L., Mory, Y., Shulman, L. and Revel, M., (1987) in Cantell and Schellekens, The Biology of the Interferon System, pp 165-171 (Martinus Nijhoff, Boston).

Monokines and Other Non-Lymphocytic Cytokines, pages 29–34
© 1988 Alan R. Liss, Inc.

STRUCTURE, GENETICS AND FUNCTION OF HUMAN "β_2-INTERFERON/B-CELL STIMULATORY FACTOR-2/ HEPATOCYTE STIMULATING FACTOR" (INTERLEUKIN-6)

Uma Santhanam, Stephen B. Tatter, David C. Helfgott, Anuradha Ray, John Ghrayeb[*], Lester T. May, and Pravinkumar B. Sehgal
The Rockefeller University, New York, NY 10021, and
[*]Centocor, Malvern, PA 19355.

Introduction

During the last year there has occured a remarkable confluence of research in three separate disciplines. It has become clear that for the last 5-7 years investigators in the interferon field, in the B-cell growth factor field and in the hepatic acute phase response field have been studying the biological properties of the same set of proteins derived from the same gene. It is now established that "interferon-β_2", "B-cell differentiation factor BSF-2" and "hepatocyte stimulating factor" are terms that refer to products from the same human gene on chromosome 7p15-21 (reviewed in Sehgal *et al.*, 1987a; Gauldie *et al.*, 1987; May *et al.*, 1988 a,b). These recent insights have led to the realization that IFN-β_2/BSF-2/HSF is the mediator of a phenomenon that was at the heart of the Hippocratic system of medicine (the alterations in the separation properties of blood during acute illness) (reviewed in May *et al.*, 1988 a,b). IFN-β_2/BSF-2/HSF are proteins that mediate the alterations in the chemistry of the blood in response to tissue injury or damage. The elemental property of polypeptides derived from the IFN-β_2/BSF-2/HSF gene appears to be hormone-like communication between peripheral damaged tissues and the hepatocyte.

Multiple forms of IFN-β_2

We isolated full-length cDNA clones corresponding to the 1.3 kb IFN-β_2 mRNA from a cDNA library prepared from polyadenylated RNA obtained from tumor necrosis factor (TNF) and cycloheximide induced human diploid fibroblasts (FS-4 strain; May *et al.*, 1986). The IFN-β_2 cDNA was inserted into an expression plasmid which when introduced into *E. coli* yields large amounts of an IFN-β_2 fusion protein (May *et al.*, 1988b). We have prepared a rabbit polyclonal antibody to the human rIFN-β_2 protein and have used this antiserum in immunoprecipitation and Western blot experiments to characterize at least six distinct forms of IFN-β_2 in the size range 23 kDa to 30 kDa secreted by human fibroblasts and monocytes induced with TNF or interleukin-1 (IL-1) or bacterial lipopolysaccharide (LPS). The synthesis of the upper triplet is inhibited by tunicamycin (gp 28, gp29 and gp30) whereas the synthesis of the lower triplet is resistant to tunicamycin (p23, p25 and p25.5). Figure 1 illustrates Western blot analyses of IFN-β_2 species present in protein fractions eluted off a DEAE-

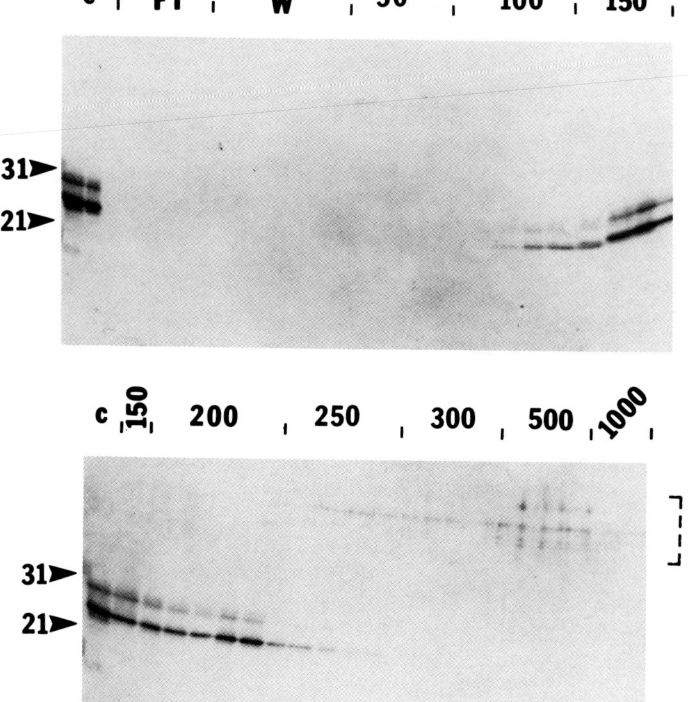

Figure 1. DEAE-Sephacel fractionation of medium from IL-1 induced fibroblasts (FS-4 cells). Medium was concentrated by 75% $(NH_4)_2SO_4$ precipitation and dialyzed against 5mM Tris buffer (pH 7.5) and applied to a 10 cm DEAE-Sephacel column. Aliquots of all fractions eluting off the column were run on 17.5% SDS-PAGE and Western blotted. The primary antibody has been characterized elsewhere (May *et al.*, 1988b). C represents control illustrating major immunoreactive bands. FT is the flow-through fractions, W is the 5mM Tris (pH 7.5) wash fractions and all of NaCl elutions re marked above their respective fractions (50mM-1000mM).

Sephacel column using a NaCl gradient.   In addition to the monomer set at 23-30 kDa, immunoreactive material in the 70-80 kDa range (presumably multimers) is clearly eluted at high salt. We are in the process of purifying each of the monomer species separately as well as the "multimer" material in order to determine their chemical and biological characteristics.

Genetics of human IFN-β_2

The human IFN-β_2 gene was assigned by us almost two years ago to chromosome 7 (Sehgal *et al.*, 1986).   Drs. Y. Chen, Anne Ferguson-Smith and Frank Ruddle, in collaboration with us, have obtained a regional localization of this gene to 7p15-21 using procedures that included *in situ* hybridization of chromosome spreads (manuscript in preparation).   Drs. Anne Bowcock, Luigi L. Cavalli-Sforza, Judith Kidd and Kenneth Kidd, in collaboration with us, have obtained evidence for a high frequency of restriction fragment length polymorphisms at the IFN-β_2 locus in the human population detected using numerous restriction enzymes (MspI, BanII, BstNI, HaeIII, HinfI, BglI, etc.) (manuscript in preparation).   The biological and clinical consequences of these polymorphisms remain to be evaluated.

Regulation of expression of the IFN-β_2 gene

The regulation of expression of the IFN-β_2 gene is superbly tailored to its primary function of serving as a means of communication between damaged tissues and the hepatocyte. If one were to intentionally design the principles governing the regulation of expression of such an "alarm" gene, one would make sure that the gene be turned on by inflammatory cytokines (TNF, IL-1, PDGF, other interferons) but not by "physiological" cytokines such as EGF and TGF-β, that it be turned on by bacterial products such as LPS, and that it be turned on by a variety of different viruses as well as abnormal nucleic acids such as dsRNA (Table 1; Content *et al.*, 1985; Kohase *et al.*, 1986, 1987a,b; Helfgott *et al.*, 1987; Walther *et al.*, 1988; Y. Zhang *et al.* personal communication; and our unpublished data). One would ensure that a variety of different second messenger systems enhanced transcription of such an "alarm" gene (Sehgal *et al.*, 1987b; and unpublished data). It would also be necessary to ensure that the IFN-β_2 gene were turned on in a wide variety of different tissues (Table 2; reviewed in Sehgal *et al.*, 1987a; May *et al.*, 1988b). The ubiquitous stromal fibroblast, the keratinocyte (the skin is the largest organ in the body)(our observations in collaboration with Dr. Thomas Kupper) and cells of the monocyte/ macrophage lineage (Gauldie *et al.*, 1987; Tosato *et al.*, 1988).

This would ensure that tissue damage anywhere in the body rapidly delivers the alarm signal to the hepatocyte. In the overall response to tissue damage it is a clear advantage that the same hormone which stimulates the liver to alter plasma protein composition also stimulates human B cells to proliferate and secrete immunoglobulins (Tosato *et al.*, 1988) and stimulates T cell function (our observations in collaboration with Dr. Thomas Kupper).

Table 1. Reagents that enhance IFN-β_2/BSF-2/HSF transcription

IL-1	TPA
TNF	DiC$_8$
PDGF	OAG
IFN-β_1	A23187
Bacterial LPS	dbcAMP
Viruses (Sendai, EMC, VSV)	Poly(I)·Poly(C)

Perhaps the most remarkable adaptation of the IFN-β_2 gene to the "alarm" function is the phenomenon of cycloheximide super-induction (Weissenbach *et al.*, 1980; Content *et al.*, 1985; Kohase *et al.*, 1986, 1987a). As macromolecular synthesis is compromised, as in fibroblasts or keratinocytes (due to tissue damage), there is an increase in the stability of IFN-β_2 mRNA resulting in the net sustained and high level of secretion of IFN-β_2 proteins (May *et al.*, 1988b).

Table 2. Cells that express IFN-β_2/BSF-2/HSF

Fibroblasts
Epithelial Cells
Keratinocytes
Endothelial Cells
Monocytes/Macrophages
T-Cell Lines

Table 3. Cells affected by IFN-β_2/BSF-2/HSF

Hepatocytes
Fibroblasts
B-Cells
T-Cells

Dexamethasone inhibits the enhancement of IFN-β_2 mRNA levels in fibroblasts induced with IL-1, TNF or LPS (Kohase *et al.*, 1987b, Helfgott *et al.*, 1987). However, other anti-inflammatory drugs such as indomethacin or acetylsalicylic acid do not affect IFN-β_2 expression in LPS-treated human fibroblasts (our unpublished data).

We have prepared plasmid constructs containing the 1200-bp DNA immediately 5' to the RNA start site in the IFN-β_2 gene fused upstream to the chloramphenical acetyltransferase (CAT) gene coding region. HeLa cells transiently transfected with this plasmid contain high levels of CAT when induced with IL-1 or TNF. These experiments will make possible a detailed dissection of the promoter elements involved in the regulation of transcription of the IFN-β_2 gene (see also Walther *et al.*, 1988).

The recent observation that elevated levels of serum IFN--β_2 precede the increase in serum levels of C-reactive protein and α_1-antitrypsin in patients with sereve burns (Nijsten *et al.*, 1987) attests to the central role of IFN-β_2 in the acute phase response.

Acknowledgements

We thank Dr. Igor Tamm for his enthusiastic support and for numerous helpful discussions. We also thank Robert Clarick for his excellent technical assistance. Supported by research grants AI-16262 and CA-44365 from the National Institutes of Health, a contract from the National Foundation for Cancer Research and an Established Investigatorship from the American Heart Association (P. B. S.).

REFERENCES

Content J, De Wit L, Poupart P, Opdenakker G, Van Damme J, and Billiau A (1985). Induction of a 26-kDa-protein mRNA in human cells treated with interleukin-1-related, leukocyte-derived factor. *Eur J Biochem* **152:** 253-257.

Gauldie J, Richards C, Harnish D, Lansdorp P, and Baumann H (1987). Interferon β_2/B-cell stimulatory factor type 2 shares identity with monocyte-derived hepatocyte-stimulating factor and regulates the major acute phase protein response in liver cells. *Proc Natl Acad Sci USA* **84:** 7251-7255.

Helfgott DC, May LT, Sthoeger Z, Tamm I, and Sehgal PB (1987). Bacterial lipopolysaccharide (endotoxin) enhances expression and secretion of β_2 interferon by human fibroblasts. *J Exp Med* **166:** 1300-1309.

Kohase M, Henriksen-DeStefano D, May LT, Vilcek J, and Sehgal PB (1986). Induction of β_2-interferon by tumor necrosis factor: a homeostatic mechanism in the control of cell proliferation. *Cell* **45:** 659-666.

Kohase M, May LT, Tamm I, Vilcek J, and Sehgal PB (1987a). A cytokine network in human diploid fibroblasts: interactions of βinterferons, tumor necrosis factor, platelet-derived growth factor, and interleukin-1. *Mol Cell Biol* **7:** 273-280.

Kohase M, Henriksen-DeStefano D., Sehgal PB, and Vilcek J

(1987b). Dexamethasone inhibits feedback regulation of the mitogenic activity of tumor necrosis factor, interleukin-1, and epidermal growth factor in human fibroblasts. *J Cell Physiol* **132:** 271-278.

May LT, Helfgott DC, and Sehgal PB (1986). Anti-β-interferon antibodies inhibit the increased expression of HLA-B7 mRNA in tumor necrosis factor-treated human fibroblasts: structural studies of the β_2-interferon involved. *Proc Natl Acad Sci USA* **83:** 8957-8961.

May LT, Santhanam U, Tatter SB, Ghrayeb J, and Sehgal PB (1988a). Interferon-β_2/B-cell differentiation factor BSF-2/hepatocyte stimulating factor: A major mediator of the "acute phase response." In Bonavida B, Kirchner H (eds): *Tumor Necrosis Factor/Cachectin, Lymphotoxins and Related Cytokines.* Basel: S. Karger, in press.

May LT, Ghrayeb J, Santhanam U, Tatter SB, Sthoeger Z, Helfgott DC, Chiorazzi N, Grieninger G, and Sehgal PB (1988b). Synthesis and secretion of multiple forms of "β_2-interferon/B-cell differentiation factor BSF-2/ hepatocyte stimulating factor" by human fibroblasts and monocytes. *J Biol Chem,* submitted.

Nijsten, MWN, De Groot ER, Ten Duis HJ, Klasen HJ, Hack CE, and Aarden LA (1987). Serum levels of interleukin-6 and acute phase responses. *The Lancet* **ii:** 921.

Sehgal PB, Zilberstein A, Ruggieri M-R, May LT, Ferguson-Smith A, Slate DL, Revel M, and Ruddle FH (1986). Human chromosome 7 carries the β_2 interferon gene. *Proc Natl Acad Sci* **83:** 5219-5222.

Sehgal PB, May LT, Tamm I, and Vilcek J (1987a). Human β_2 interferon and B-cell differentiation factor BSF-2 are identical. *Science* **235:** 731-732.

Sehgal PB, Walther Z and, Tamm I (1987b). Rapid enhancement of β_2-interferon/B-cell differentiation factor BSF-2 gene expression in human fibroblasts by diacylglycerols and the calcium ionophore A23187. *Proc Natl Acad Sci USA* **84:** 3663-3667.

Tosato G, Seamon KB, Goldman ND, Sehgal PB, May LT, Washington GC, Jones KD, and Pike SE (1988) Identification of a monocyte derived human B-cell growth factor as in interferon-β_2 (BSF-2, IL-6) *Science,* in press.

Walther Z, May LT, and Sehgal PB (1988) Transcriptional regulation of the "β_2-interferon/B-cell differentiation factor BSF-2-/hepatocyte stimulating factor HSF" gene in human fibroblasts by other cytokines. *J Immunol,* in press.

Weissenbach J, Chernajovsky Y, Zeevi M, Shulman L, Soreq H, Nir U, Wallach D, Perricaudet M, Tiollais P, and Revel M (1980). Two interferon mRNAs in human fibroblasts: *in vitro* translation and *Escherichia coli* cloning studies. *Proc Natl Acad Sci USA* **77:** 7152-7156.

Monokines and Other Non-Lymphocytic Cytokines, pages 35–38
© 1988 Alan R. Liss, Inc.

INDUCTION OF THE ACUTE-PHASE RESPONSE IN RAT HEPATOCYTE/ HEPATOMA CELLS: EFFECTS OF DIFFERENT MEDIATORS

H. Northoff, T. Andus, T. Geiger, J. Bauer, D. Männel, T. Hirano, T. Kishimoto and P.C. Heinrich

DRK Blood Center (H.N.), D-7900 Ulm, FRG, Dept. Biochem. Univ. Freiburg, D-7800 Freiburg (T.A., T.G.,J.B.,P.C.H), Germ. Canc. Res. Center (D.M.) D-6900 Heidelberg, FRG, and Inst. Mol. Cell. Biol., Osaka Univ., Osaka 565, Japan

INTRODUCTION

The acute-phase response of rat liver cells is characterized by an increase in the production of several proteins, like a2-macroglobulin (a2M), ß-fibrinogen, a1-acid glycoprotein (AGP), cysteine protease inhibitor (CPI) and by a concommitant decrease in albumin synthesis. Synthesis of virtually all known acute-phase proteins can be elicited in primary rat hepatocyte cultures by supernatants of stimulated human monocytes. We have shown earlier that hepatocyte-stimulating factor (HSF), which seems to be a rather universal stimulator of the acute-phase response, is a LPS-inducible monokine different from interleukin-1 (IL-1) and tumor necrosis factor a (TNFa) (Northoff et al., 1987; Andus et al., 1987). Recently, it has been proposed that HSF is functionally and antigenically identical with interferon-ß2 (Gauldie et al., 1987). Here we confirm these findings using recombinant B-cell-stimulating factor 2 (BSF-2), which in turn is identical with IFN-ß2 (IFN-ß2/ interleukin-6 (IL-6)). We further demonstrate (i) that other cytokines of monocyte origin like TNFa and IL-1 each do stimulate an individual spectrum of acute-phase proteins, (ii) that IL-1a and IL-1ß show differing activity, and (iii) that interferons a, ß1, and γ are unable to stimulate fibrinogen or a2M mRNA synthesis.

RESULTS

The action of different interferons on Fao rat hepatoma cells was studied by measuring mRNA levels of fibrinogen and albumin (Fig. 1A,B). Only natural IFNß, which is

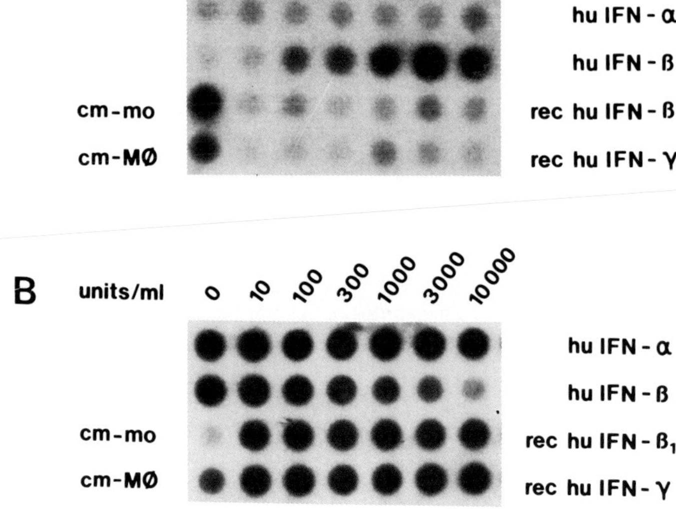

Fig. 1. Induction of rat ß-fibrinogen mRNA by human inter-
feron-ß. Fao cells (5×10^5 cells/well) were incubated
with purified human IFNα, purified hIFN-ß, rhIFN-ß1 and
rhIFN at the indicated concentrations or with conditioned
media from human monocytes (cm-mo) or macrophages (cm-Mø)
in the presence of 10^{-6} M dexamethasone for 12 h. Cells
were lysed, the cytoplasmic RNA extracts blotted to a gene
screen membrane and hybridized with ^{32}P-labeled ß-fibrinogen cDNA (A) or albumin cDNA (B).

known to contain contaminating IFNß2 (IL-6) led to an
increase in fibrinogen mRNA and to a decrease in albumin
mRNA. Recombinant human IL-6 (rhIL-6) however exhibited
the same effect in very low concentrations (Fig. 2).
Activity of natural IL-6 in supernatants from monocytes
could be blocked by a specific antibody to IL-6. When the
effect of interferons and IL-6 on α2M synthesis was stu-

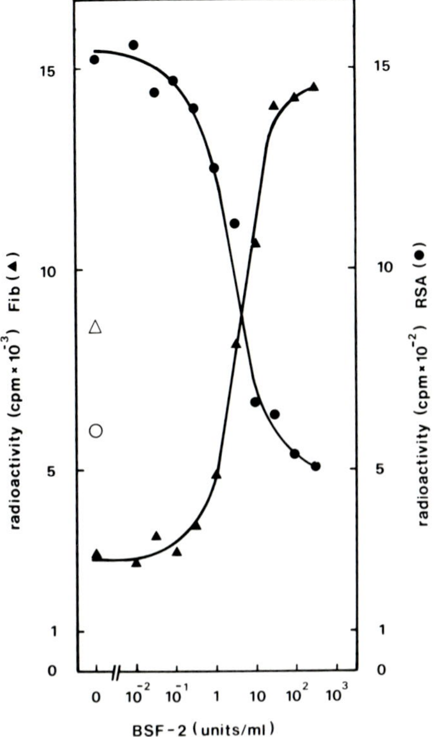

Fig. 2. Regulation of ß-fibrinogen (▲) and albumin mRNA (●) levels by recombinant human BSF-2/IL-6

died in primary rat hepatocytes, the same pattern of reaction evolved. In the Fao system rhIL-1α or ß were unable to induce fibrinogen mRNA and induced only marginal levels of a2M mRNA. This corresponds well to the only marginal induction of a2M synthesis by primary rat hepatocytes in response to murine IL-1, which we have described earlier, and to the rather weak induction of some other acute-phase proteins described in the literature.

Murine IL-1 and human IL-1, however, could effectively stimulate the synthesis of AGP (Fig. 3). RhIL-1α was two orders of magnitude less effective than rhIL-1ß. This finding is unique, since in most systems IL-1α and ß seem to be functionally indistinguishable. Finally, the effect of TNFα which has been reported to induce the synthesis of several acute-phase proteins in HepG2 hepatoma cells was tested in primary rat hepatocytes using a2M, albumin, CPI, and AGP synthesis as read-out. Only AGP was weakly en-

hanced by TNFa, whereas the other proteins were unaffected.
   In summary, we have shown that HSF is functionally
identical with BSF-2/IL-6. While BSF-2/IL-6 may be the
major inducer of the acute-phase response, IL-1 and TNFa
each can stimulate an individual spectrum of acute-phase
proteins. IL-1a and ß show differing activity in this
system and IFNs are negative as measured by a2M and fibrinogen mRNA induction.

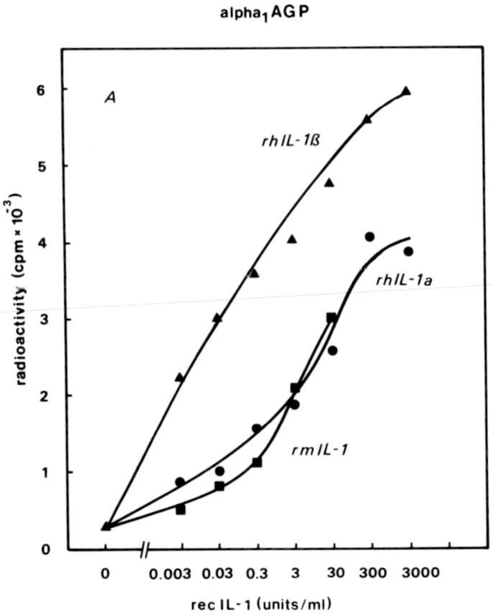

Fig. 3.   Induction   of al-acid glycoprotein mRNA   by
recombinant   human   interleukin-la,   recombinant   human
interleukin-1ß and murine interleukin-1

REFERENCES

Andus T, Heinrich PC, Bauer J, Tran-Thi TA, Decker K,
   Männel D, Northoff H (1987a) Discrimination of hepatocyte-stimulating activity from human recombinant tumor
   necrosis factor a. Eur. J. Immunol. 17: 1193-1197.
Gauldie J, Richards C, Harnish D, Lansdorp P, Baumann H
   (1987) Interferon ß2/BSF-2 shares identity with monocyte
   derived hepatocyte-stimulating factor (HSF) and regulates the major acute phase protein response in liver
   cells. Proc. Natl. Acad. Sci. USA, in press.
Northoff H, Andus T, Tran-Thi TA, Bauer J, Decker K,
   Kubanek B, Heinrich PC (1987) The inflammation mediators
   interleukin1 and hepatocyte-stimulating factor are differently regulated in human monocytes. Eur. J. Immunol.
   17: 707-711.

Section II. Gene Expression

Monokines and Other Non-Lymphocytic Cytokines, pages 41–46
© 1988 Alan R. Liss, Inc.

RESTRICTION FRAGMENT LENGTH POLYMORPHISMS AND LINKAGE OF
MURINE IL-1 α AND β GENES ON CHROMOSOME 2

David D. Chaplin, Robert C. Fuhlbrigge, Shirin
Jadidi, Kathleen C. Sheehan, Robert D. Schreiber,
Patrick W. Gray, Emil R. Unanue, and
Peter D'Eustachio

Depts. of Medicine (D.D.C, R.C.F., S.J.) and
Pathology (K.C.S., R.D.S., E.R.U.), Washington
Univ. Sch. of Med., St. Louis, MO 63110; Dept.
of Developmental Biol. (P.W.G.), Genentech Inc.,
South San Francisco, CA 94080; and Dept. of
Biochemistry (P.D.), New York Univ. Medical
Center, New York, NY 10016

INTRODUCTION

Interleukin 1 (IL-1) designates a family of cytokines
that are produced primarily by monocytes and macrophages
and that possess potent activity in a broad range of in
vitro and in vivo assay systems. IL-1 functions as a costimulator of T cell activation and appears to be required
for the normal cooperation between antigen presenting cells
and lymphocytes at the initiation of an immune response.
IL-1 also serves as an important mediator in inflammatory
reactions and wound repair where it demonstrates diverse
effects on brain, liver, endothelia, myeloid cells, and
fibroblasts promoting acute phase responses and
proliferation (Durum et al., 1985).

Molecular cloning analysis of human IL-1 has
indicated that IL-1 bioactivity is encoded by two discrete
genes termed IL-1α and IL-1β (Auron et al., 1984; March et
al., 1985). Both genes encode an approximately 32 kd pro-
molecule which is found intracellularly. Extracellularly,
both gene products are detected as 17 kd molecules derived
from the carboxyl half of the respective precursors. The
extracellular form of human IL-1α has pI ~5.0 and IL-1β has
pI ~7. Both 17 kd molecules bind to the same receptor,
with apparently equivalent affinity. Two IL-1 genes have
also been defined in mice (Lomedico et al., 1984;

Gray et al., 1986); however, biochemical analysis has been limited to the IL-1α homologue (Mizel, 1979). Both IL-1α and IL-1β mRNA are found in murine peritoneal macrophages, with their levels of expression regulated in parallel (Fuhlbrigge et al., 1987). Comparison of the predicted amino acid sequences of the mouse IL-1α and IL-1β molecules shows only scattered conservation with 23% identical residues. A similar comparison of the human IL-1α and IL-1β amino acid sequences shows only 20% identical residues. Sequence analysis shows that the IL-1α polypeptides of mice and humans are, in contrast, 62% identical, with the IL-1β molecules being 68% conserved, indicating that the creation of two IL-1 genes antedates mouse/human speciation. In order to define more completely the evolutionary relationship of the IL-1α and IL-1β genes, we have determined their chromosomal location (D'Eustachio et al., 1987).

RESULTS AND DISCUSSION

To determine the chromosomal locations of the IL-1α and IL-1β genes, we analyzed by Southern blotting somatic hybrid cell lines carrying various combinations of mouse chromosomes on a constant Chinese hamster background. cDNA clones (Gray et al., 1986) of each gene were used as probes (Table 1). Only the four hybrid cell lines that had retained mouse chromosome 2 yielded mouse-specific IL-1α and IL-1β fragments, indicating that both IL-1 genes are situated on chromosome 2 in the mouse.

TABLE 1. Chromosomal Mapping of the IL-1α and IL-1β Genes in Somatic Cell Hybrids

Hybrid	Mouse Chromosomes Retained																				Reaction with Probe α	β
BEMI-4	1	2	3		5	6		8				12	13	14	15	16	17	18	19	X	+	+
MACH4B31Az3		2					7	8				12			15	16	17		19		+	+
MACH2A2B1	1	2	3	4		6	7	8	9	10		12		14	15	16	17			X	+	+
MACH2A2C2	1	2	3				7	8	9	10		12	13		15	16	17		19	X	+	+
MACH2A2H3	1		3			6	7	8	9	10		12	13	14	15	16	17	18	19	X	-	-
MAE28												12								X	-	-
R44-1																	17				-	-
ECm4e														14	15						-	-

(adapted from D'Eustachio et al., 1987)

More complete linkage analysis was possible because of the existence of restriction fragment length polymorphisms (RFLP) of the IL-1α and IL-1β genes. When the IL-1α probe was used to analyze Msp I- or Taq I-digested genomic DNA from eight different inbred mouse strains, six RFLP alleles were observed (Fig. 1 and Table 2). Using the IL-1β probe, only two RFLP were identified (Fig. 1 and Table 2). The locations of the polymorphic restriction sites relative to the coding portions of the genes has not yet been determined. Additionally, the detailed nature of the sequence changes which produce the RFLP are not known. It is of interest that the RFLP observed in both the SJL and BALB/c strains might represent gene duplications. Further studies to clarify these issues are underway. The biologic consequences of the observed RFLP are unclear. There is to date no evidence for structural or functional alleles of the IL-1 polypeptides in either mouse or man.

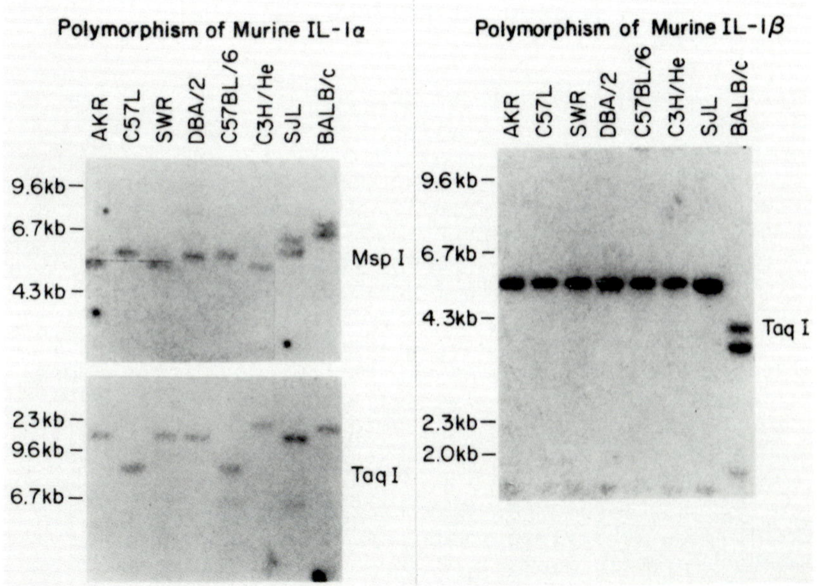

Figure 1. Southern blot analysis of mouse IL-1α (left panel) and IL-1β (right panel) gene restriction fragment length polymorphisms using IL-1α and IL-1β cDNAs as probes (adapted from D'Eustachio et al., 1987).

TABLE 2. DNA Restriction Fragment Length Polymorphisms
Associated with the IL-1α and IL-1β Genes

| | | Restriction Fragments | |
Allele	Strains	Msp I	Taq I
IL-1α			
a	BALB/cJ	7.1, 6.6	~23
b	C57BL/6J, C57L/J	6.2	8.4
c	AKR/J, SWR/J	6.0	~18
d	DBA/2J	6.2	~18
e	C3H/HeJ	6.0	~23
f	SJL/J	6.6, 6.3	~18
IL-1β			
a	BALB/cJ	–	4.2, 3.8, 1.9
b	C57BL/6J, AKR/J, C57L/J, SWR/J, DBA/2J, C3H/HeJ, SJL/J	–	5.6, 1.7

(adapted from D'Eustachio et al., 1987)

To localize the IL-1α and IL-1β genes on chromosome
2, recombinant inbred strains of mice were scored for
inheritance of the IL-1 RFLPs. Of fifteen strains
informative for both IL-1 genes, none was recombinant,
indicating that the two IL-1 genes are less than 8 cM
apart. Because of the greater polymorphism detected for
IL-1α, 76 strains were informative in localizing IL-1
relative to other known loci on chromosome 2. These data
yielded the map:

   B2m – 3.2 cM – **Hdc** – 1.5 cM – **Il-1a** – 11.0 cM – **Psp**

where B2m represents the β_2-microglobulin locus, Hdc the
histidine decarboxylase locus, and Psp the parotid
secretory protein locus.

The close chromosomal linkage of IL-1α and IL-1β
strongly supports their evolution by sequence divergence
following duplication of an ancestral gene. Also
supporting such an evolutionary relationship is the finding
by several groups, including our own, that the exon
structures of the IL-1α and IL-1β genes are strongly

conserved. Analysis of the evolutionary lineage of the
IL-1 genes has, therefore, demonstrated the following:
1) duplication of an ancestral gene occurred to produce two
IL-1 genes (α and β); 2) sequence analysis shows that the
two IL-1 genes have diverged at 75-80% of their amino acid
residues; 3) in spite of this sequence divergence, both
IL-1 molecules appear to bind with essentially identical
activity to the same IL-1 receptor and to demonstrate
identical bioactivities. We feel that the conservation of
IL-1 bioactivity by two molecules which have diverged so
substantially in their primary structure indicates that
there is strong selective pressure for the presence of two
functional genes. We also feel that an understanding of
the nature of this genetic selection will be required for a
complete understanding of the role of IL-1 in the
regulation of immune and inflammatory responses.

In order to be able to discriminate mouse IL-1α from
IL-1β in vitro as well as in vivo, we are generating
specific monoclonal anti-IL-1 antibodies. The immunogens
are being prepared using the pJG200 E. coli expression
vector (Germino and Bastia, 1984). A fragment of the
murine IL-1α cDNA encoding amino acid residues 99-270 was
cloned into this vector, resulting in the expression of a
tri-partite fusion protein comprised of the 172 amino acid
IL-1α polypeptide followed by a chicken α-procollagen
linking peptide and the E. coli β-galactosidase. The
fusion protein was purified from bacterial cell lysates
using an anti-β-galactosidase affinity column. The
isolated fusion protein was digested with collagenase and
the recombinant IL-1α (rIL-1α) polypeptide was purified by
gel filtration HPLC. This material was homogeneous by SDS-
PAGE and showed a specific activity of 3 X 10^8 units/µg
when tested using the D10.G4.1 proliferation assay.

Armenian hamsters were immunized with this rIL-1α.
Monoclonal anti-IL-1α antibodies were identified using
solid phase rIL-1α in a direct ELISA. All antibodies
analyzed inhibited completely the costimulator activity of
our recombinant mouse IL-1α, but showed no inhibition of
recombinant IL-1β bioactivity. The antibodies inhibited
approximately 30% of the D10 costimulator activity present
in supernatants of LPS-stimulated peritoneal macrophages.
The residual activity may represent the as yet unchar-
acterized mouse IL-1β activity. In contrast to the results
observed with culture supernatants, when fixed LPS-stimulated peritoneal macrophages were treated with anti-IL-1α

mAb, the membrane associated bioactivity was completely
inhibited. This indicates that in the mouse, as has been
suggested in man, all membrane IL-1 bioactivity is
immunochemically related to IL-1α. We suggest that this
differential expression of functional IL-1α on the cell
surface to produce membrane IL-1 bioactivity provides the
genetic selection that continues to maintain two functional
interleukin 1 loci.

ACKNOWLEDGEMENT

This work was supported by grants from the NIH, the
National Foundation/March of Dimes, and the Monsanto
Company.

REFERENCES

Auron PW, Webb AC, Rossenwasser LJ, Mucci SE, Rich A,
   Wolff SM, Dinarello CA (1984). Nucleotide sequence of
   human monocyte interleukin 1 precursor cDNA. Proc Natl
   Acad Sci USA 81:7907-7911.
D'Eustachio P, Jadidi S, Fuhlbrigge RC, Gray PW, Chaplin DD
   (1987). Interleukin-1 α and β genes: linkage on chromosome 2 in the mouse. Immunogenetics 26:339-343.
Durum SK, Schmidt JA, Oppenheim JJ (1985). Interleukin-1:
   an immunological perspective. Ann Rev Immunol 3:263-287.
Fuhlbrigge RC, Chaplin DD, Kiely J-M, Unanue ER (1987).
   Regulation of interleukin-1 gene expression by adherence
   and lipopolysaccharide. J Immunol 138:3799-3802.
Germino J, Bastia D (1984). Rapid purification of a cloned
   gene product by genetic fusion and site-specific proteolysis. Proc Natl Acad Sci USA 81:4692-4696.
March CJ, Mosley B, Larsen A, Cerretti DP, Braedt G, Price
   V, Gillis S, Henney CS, Kronheim SR, Grabstein K, Conlon
   PJ, Hopp TP, Cosman D (1985). Cloning, sequence, and
   expression of two distinct human interleukin-1 complementary DNAs. Nature 315:641-647.
Mizel SB (1979). Physicochemical characterization of lymphocyte-activating factor (LAF). J Immunol 122:2167-
   2172.

Monokines and Other Non-Lymphocytic Cytokines, pages 47–53

CHARACTERIZATION OF CIS AND TRANS ACTING ELEMENTS INVOLVED IN HUMAN proIL-1 BETA GENE EXPRESSION

Burton D. Clark[1], Matthew J. Fenton[1], Homero L. Rey[1],
Andrew C. Webb[2], and Philip E. Auron[1]

Division of Health Sciences and Technology[1],
Massachusetts Institute of Technology, Cambridge, MA 02139;
Department of Biological Sciences[2], Wellesley College,
Wellesley, MA 02181

Introduction

Human interleukin 1β is an important monokine with a broad range of biological actions. We have previously described the differential expression of the proIL-1β gene following induction of human monocytic cells with lipopolysaccaride (LPS) or phorbol myristic acetate (PMA) [1, 2]. These studies showed that IL-1β message was rapidly and transiently expressed in several different monocytic cell lines (THP-1, HL60) and in *in vitro*-aged human peripheral blood monocytes when stimulated with LPS. Expression was found to be non-transient when stimulated with PMA.

These data have suggested to us a model for regulation that invokes a transcriptional activator during the induction of the gene followed by the action of a transcriptional repressor to partially down-regulate transcription. To better understand the expression of the proIL-1β gene, we have begun to investigate what *cis* and *trans*-acting elements may be involved in the regulation of the gene.

We have used two approaches to analyze DNA sequences upstream of the transcriptional initiation site of the proIL-1β gene. The first approach makes use of chimeric plasmids containing proIL-1β DNA sequences fused to the bacterial chloramphenicol acetyl transferase (CAT) gene. The insertion of the proIL-1β promoter in front of the promoter-less CAT gene allows for promoter testing by the expression of CAT in a transfected host cell. Using this technique, we have identified regions of the proIL-1β gene necessary for expression of the gene. The second approach involves electrophoretic gel mobility shift assays to identify sequences to which *trans*-acting factors can bind. This method provides additional information on the regions identified by the CAT functional analysis by determining if nuclear factors bind to important *cis*-acting sequences. By using an electrophoretic gel mobility shift (band-shift) assay with nuclear extracts isolated from cells at various stages of induction, we have located regions of the proIL-1β upstream sequence which bind distinct *trans*-acting factors. These include a factor that binds to an 'OCTA' sequence [3] and a putative repressor factor.

Transcriptional Analysis Using CAT Vectors

Homology analysis of the sequenced IL-1 genes [4, 5, 6]reveals two regions, designated R_1 and R_2, which share strong homology among the three genes. Figure 1 shows only the sequences that are homologous among these three genes. Overall, there is very little upstream sequence similarity. Therefore, the clear relatedness within regions R_1 and R_2 could suggest that they have important regulatory functions.

Various upstream DNA fragments of the proIL-1β gene were inserted into promoter-less CAT expression vectors. Figure 2 shows a schematic representation of proIL-1β gene putative regulatory regions and the sequences tested in the CAT transfection assay system. These constructs contain successively smaller fragments of the proIL-1β upstream sequence generated by progressive cleavage at specific endonuclease sites. The 3' terminus for clones PT, AT, DT, NT, and HT are at position +12 (*Taq* I site) relative to the transcriptional initiation site of the proIL-1β gene. Clones PX, HX, and PXΔN have a 3' terminus at position +313 (*Xba* I site) and contain regions of intron 1 with sequences that may be important for transcription [4].

R1 Region

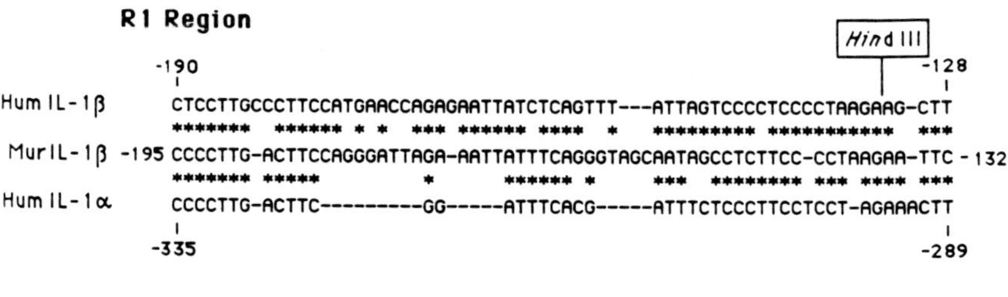

R2 Region

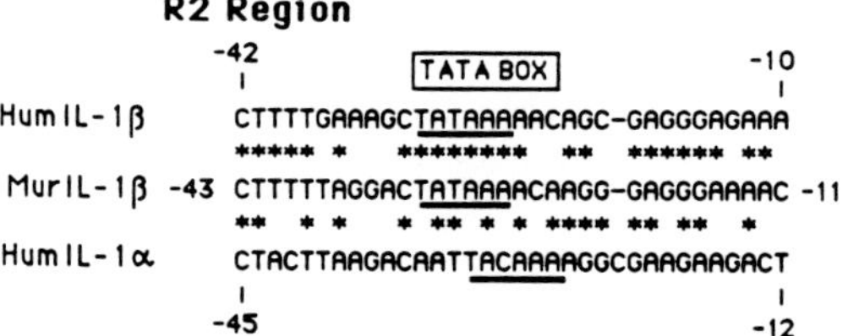

Figure 1. proIL-1 gene upstream homology regions.

Human cell lines, THP-1, U937, Colo/16, and HeLa were transfected with the various IL-1β-CAT chimeric plasmids. After transient expression, cell lysates were assayed for CAT activity by thin layer chromatography. The conversion of chloramphenicol to 1,acetyl or 3,acetyl-chloramphenicol indicates the presence of CAT in the cell lysates. Figure 3 shows representative thin layer chromatograms for CAT assays from THP-1 and HeLa cell lysates. These data show that the proIL-1β upstream sequences alone are only able to direct CAT expression in monocytic THP-1 cells and not in non-monocytic HeLa cells. Furthermore, the IL-1β-CAT plasmid, HT, with 132 bp of upstream sequence, poorly directs CAT expression whereas the presence of a larger upstream IL-1β fragment in the CAT construct (AT or PT) improves CAT expression. Chromatograms for CAT assays from Colo/16 were the same as seen for HeLa cell lysates and U937 was similar to THP-1 (data not shown). Figure 3 also shows the results of CAT transfection studies in which an SV40 enhancer region is inserted within the vector as a control. A summary of the CAT transfection studies is seen in Table 1.

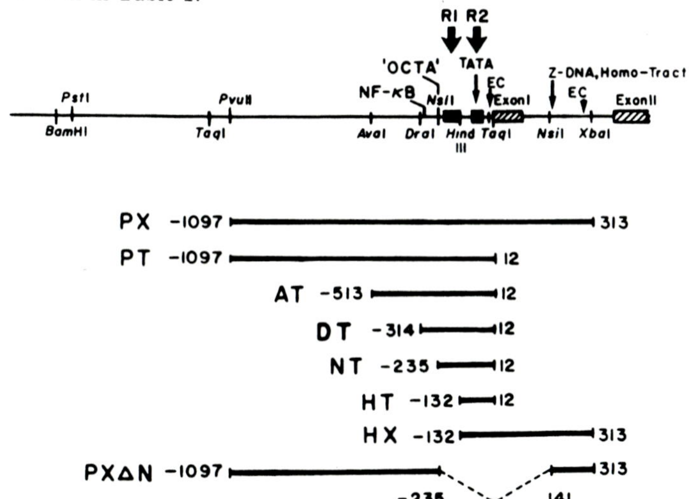

Figure 2 Schematic representation of IL-1β putative regulatory regions and sequences tested in the CAT transfection assay system.

Electrophoretic Band Shift Assays

Band-shift assays were performed to determine if portions of the proIL-1β upstream region, identified as being important for expression of the gene in the CAT assays described above, also bound specific nuclear factors. Figure 4A shows the location of the two upstream regions which were used as radiolabeled probes. The *Dra* I-*Hind* III and *Hind* III-*Taq* I fragments contain, respectively, the R_1 and R_2 homology regions. These fragments were incubated with nuclear extracts from unstimulated or LPS stimulated (1 or 5 hr.) THP-1 cells. Portions of the binding reactions were analyzed on polyacrylamide gels and visualized by autoradiography as shown in Figure 4B. These data show that the 145 bp probe generates two discrete complexes (arrows) using nuclear extracts from resting and 1 hr LPS-stimulated THP-1 cells, while an additional complex was observed using nuclear extracts from 5 hr LPS-stimulated THP-1 cells. The 181 bp probe generated a single complex which was observed in reactions using all three nuclear extracts. The complexes were specific since the addition of a 100-fold molar excess of the same DNA as unlabeled competitor, and not non-specific competitor DNA, abolished most of the complex formation.

HeLa Cells

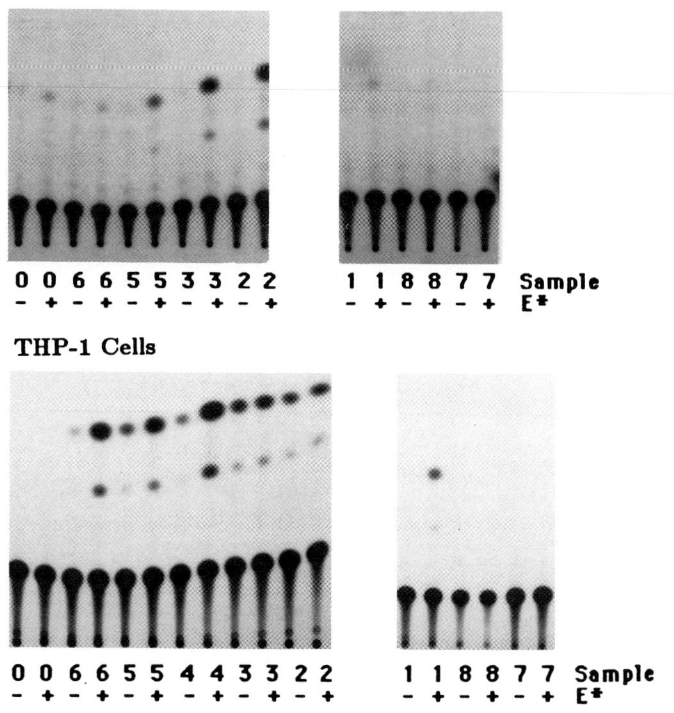

THP-1 Cells

Figure 3. Representative CAT assay data for IL-1β-CAT transfections in HeLa and THP-1 cells. Sample designations correspond to those indicated in Table 1. E* with + or - refer to the presence or absence of the SV40 enhancer sequence.

Table 1. Summary of CAT transfection studies.

#	DNA Insert	HeLa Cells		Colo/16 Cells		THP-1 Cells		U937 Cells	
		+E*	−E*	+E	−E	+E	−E	+E	−E
1	PX	+	−	++	−	++++	−	+++	−
2	PT	+++++	−	+++++	−	+++++	+++	+++++	+
3	AT	++++	−	++++	−	++++	++++	+++++	++
4	DT	n.d.	n.d.	n.d.	n.d.	+++++	+++	+++++	+
5	NT	+++	−	++	−	+++++	+++	+++++	+++
6	HT	+	−	+	−	+++++	+	+++++	+
7	HX	−	−	−	−	+	−	+	−
8	PXΔN	−	−	−	−	−	−	−	−
0	None	+	−	±	−	−	−	+++++	−

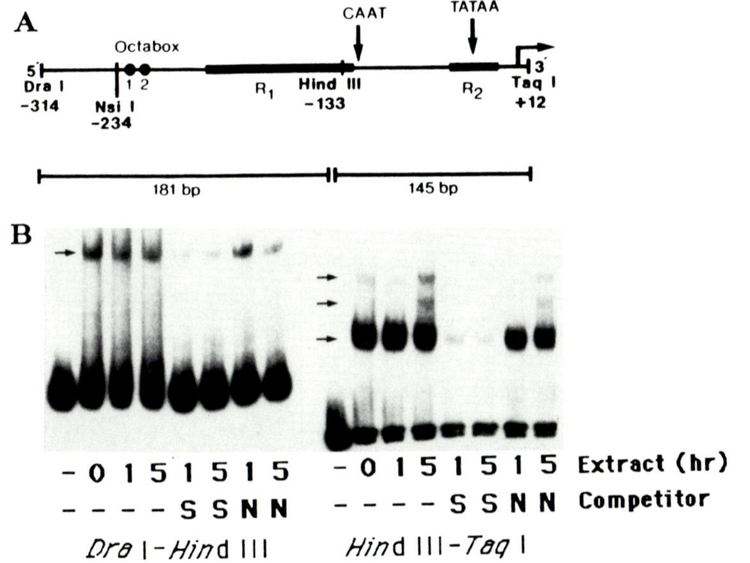

Figure 4. IL-1β band-shift analysis for THP-1 cell nuclear extracts. A. The upstream region of the proIL-1β gene used to generate labeled DNA fragments is shown. Sequences homologous to those reported for other genes are indicated ('OCTA' box, CAAT, TATAA). R$_1$ and R$_2$ denote upstream regions conserved among IL-1 genes; B. Electrophoretic gel shift assays for the two α-^{32}P dATP labeled probes. Binding reactions contained DNA alone (first lane in each panel), or extracts from 0, 1, or 5 hr. LPS treated cells. Specific (S) or non-specific (N) DNA was used as competitor.

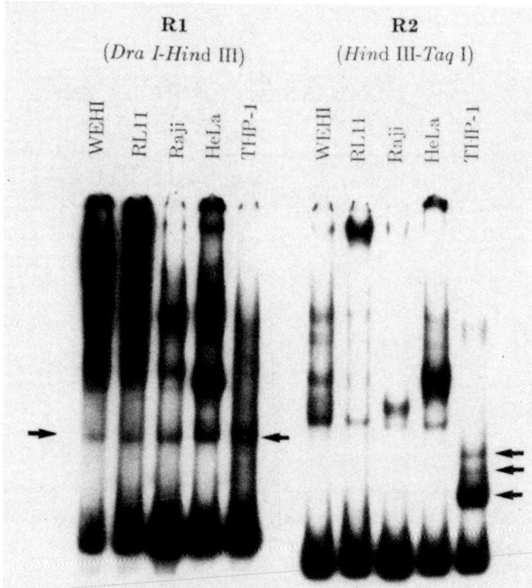

Figure 5. Non-monocytic cells do not contain nuclear factors which recognize proIL-1β promoter sequences. The 181 and 145 bp probe fragments were tested in an electrophoretic gel shift assay using nuclear extracts from THP-1 and several non-monocytic cells. Arrows denote the specific DNA-protein complexes observed in monocytic nuclear extracts.

Summary

The CAT assay data described above shows that the proIL-1β upstream sequences were able to direct CAT expression and that this expression was cell-type specific (THP-1 and U937). This tissue specific expression is in agreement with IL-1β mRNA expression (data not shown). Even the keratinocyte cell line, Colo/16, which is a low-level, constitutive producer of ETAF (IL-1-like), does not have the tissue specificity to express CAT. Furthermore, IL-1β-CAT constructs containing the SV40 enhancer can direct CAT expression in all cell types tested, but in the absence of the enhancer, only monocytic cell lines (THP-1 and U937) can express CAT.

In THP-1 cells, the DNA fragment containing the R_2 homology region is required to direct CAT expression. This expression is increased in the presence of additional upstream DNA sequences extending into, and beyond the R_1 region. Clones AT and PT with 513 and 1097 bp of upstream IL-1β sequence respectively, direct CAT expression with nearly equal efficiency, with or without the SV40 enhancer, whereas clone DT with 314 bp of upstream IL-1β sequence does not. This suggests that DNA sequences between positions -513 and -314 may possess enhancer-like activity.

Electrophoretic band shift assays have identified specific regions of the proIL-1β upstream sequence that bind nuclear factors. These nuclear factors may mediate proIL-1β gene expression. A factor present maximally in 5 hr. extracts, and specific for THP-1 cells, binds to the *Hind* III-*Taq* I fragment with a kinetic profile reflecting that previously proposed for a transcriptional repressor that down-regulates IL-1β transcription (Figure 5) [2].

Acknowledgements

This work was supported by Cistron Biotechnology Inc. BDC is an Arthritis Foundation Postdoctoral Fellow.

References

1. Fenton, M.J., Clark, B.D., Collins, K.L., Webb, A.C., Rich, A., and Auron, P.E. (1987) J.Immunol. 138, 3972-3979.
2. Fenton, M.J., Clark, B.D., Alexander, S.J., Webb, A.C., and Auron, P.E. (1988)in Mechanisms of control of gene expression, Cullen, B., Gage, L.P., Siddiqui, M.A.Q., Skalka, A.M., and Weissbach, H., Ed., pp. 125-135, Alan R. Liss, New York.
3. Singh, H., Sen, R., Baltimore, D., and Sharp, P.A. (1986) Nature 319, 154-158.
4. Clark, B.D., Collins, K.L., Gandy, M.S., Webb, A.C., and Auron, P.E. (1986) Nucl. Acids Res. 14, 7897-7914.
5. Telford, J.L., Macchia, G., Massone, A., Carinci, V., and Melli, M. (1986) Nuc. Acids Res. 14, 9955-9963.
6. Furutani, Y., Notake, M., Fukui, T., Ohue, M., Nomura, H., Yamada, M., and Nakamura, S. (1986) Nucl. Acids Res. 14, 3167-3179.

Monokines and Other Non-Lymphocytic Cytokines, pages 55–60
© 1988 Alan R. Liss, Inc.

CONTROL OF LPS INDUCED INTERLEUKIN-1 AND TUMOR NECROSIS
FACTOR mRNAs EXPRESSION BY INHIBITORS OF SECOND MESSENGER
PATHWAYS IN MURINE MACROPHAGES

Elizabeth J. Kovacs, Danuta Radzioch, Howard A.
Young and Luigi Varesio

Department of Anatomy (E.J.K.), Loyola University
Stritch School of Medicine, Maywood, IL 60153 and
Program Resources, Inc. (D.R.) and Laboratory of
Molecular Immunoregulation (H.A.Y., L.V.), BRMP,
National Cancer Institute, Frederick Cancer
Research Facility, Frederick, MD 21701

INTRODUCTION

A number of macrophage functions are ascribed to their
ability to produce cytokines including interleukin-1 (IL-1)
α, IL-1 β, and tumor necrosis factor (TNF) α (Degliatoni et
al, 1985; Oppenheim et al, 1986; Rubin et al, 1986; Beutler
and Cerami, 1986). Unstimulated macrophages do not produce
appreciable levels of these mediators, but after
stimulation with a variety of agents including lipopolysaccaride (LPS), macrophages can be induced to express IL-1
α, IL-1 β, and TNF-α genes (Gery et al, 1972; Beutler et
al, 1986; Kornbluth and Eddington 1986; Gifford and
Lohmann-Matthes, 1986).

While the molecular activation of macrophages
following their interaction with LPS remains unresolved
(Morrison and Rudbach, 1981; Jacobs, 1984), a number of
activities of LPS-treated macrophages are identical to
those initiated by phorbol myristate acetate, suggesting
that some LPS induced functions are mediated by protein
kinase c (PKc). However, recent studies have shown that
the activation of PKc alone is not sufficient to account
for the complete functional response of macrophages to LPS
(Sommers et al, 1986). In view of this heterogeneity of
the effect of LPS, we investigated the nature of the
pathway(s) by which LPS induces gene expression for IL-1

and TNF-α. Here, we report on the differential regulation of IL-1α , IL-1 β, and TNF-α mRNA expression in murine macrophages and the second messenger pathways involved in this control.

MATERIALS AND METHODS

Peritoneal macrophages were obtained from C57BL/6N male mice (Division of Research Services, NIH) 4 days after injection of 1% thioglycolate medium (BBL Microbiology Systems, Cockeysville, MD) as described elsewhere (Radzioch et al, 1986). Following adherence to plastic, macrophages were cultured in medium (RPMI 1640 with 10% fetal bovine serum) in the presence or absence of LPS (1 ug/ml; Difco Laboratories, Detroit, MI) with or without an inhibitor of PKc (1-(5-isoquinolinyl-sulfonyl)-2-methylpiperazine; H7) or an inhibitor of Calcium/Calmodulin (CaM) kinase (N-(6-amino-hexyl)-5-chloro-1-napthalene-sulfonamide; W7) (Sigma Chemical Co, St. Louis, MO).

Cells were harvested and total cellular RNA was isolated by guanidine-isothiocyanate extraction (Chirgwin et al, 1979) followed by cesium chloride density gradient centrifugation (Glisin et al, 1974). Northern blot analysis was performed as described by (Radzioch et al, 1986). The cDNA probe for human IL-1 α was obtained from Dr. M Yamada (Dainippon Pharmaceuticals, Osaka, Japan); human IL-1 β cDNA from Dr. D Carter (The Upjohn Co, Kalamazoo, MI); human TNF-α genomic DNA from Dr. A Oliff (Merck, Sharp and Dohme, West Point, PA); and chicken β -actin cDNA from Dr. DW Cleveland (Johns Hopkins University, Baltimore, MD).

RESULTS

The expression of IL-1 α, IL-1 β and TNF-α mRNAs was assessed in freshly isolated murine peritoneal macrophages. In the absence of stimulation macrophages did not express detectable levels of the cytokine mRNAs. However, after stimulation with LPS, mRNAs for TNF-α and both IL-1 genes were expressed (Figure 1). All three cytokine mRNAs exhibited dose dependent inhibition of LPS induced cytokine mRNA expression following treatment with the PKc inhibitor, H7. In contrast, the expression of IL-1 α and IL-1 β mRNAs

differed from TNF-α mRNA in their sensitivity to the CaM
kinase inhibitor, W7. The LPS induced levels of IL-1 α and
IL-1 β mRNAs, but not TNF-α mRNA, were blocked by treatment
with W7. Like TNF-α mRNA expression, the production of

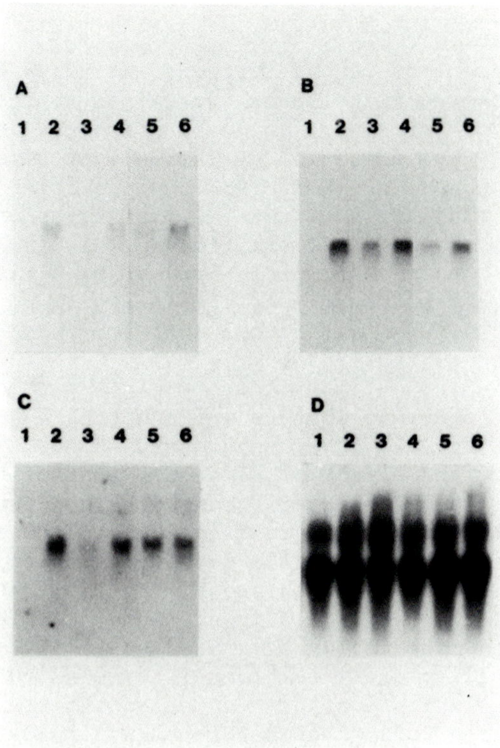

Figure 1. Effect of inhibitors of PKc and CaM kinase on
monokine mRNA expression. Northern blot analysis was
performed with 15 ug RNA from murine peritoneal macrophages
cultured for 6 hours in the absence (lane 1) or presence
(lane 2) of LPS. In addition, macrophages were incubated
with LPS and H7 (25 uM (lane 3) or 4 uM (lanes 4)) or LPS
and W7 (25 uM (lane 5) or 4 uM (lanes 6)). The same blot
was hybridized with a probe for IL-1 α (Panel A), stripped
and rehybridized with IL-1 β (Panel B), then TNF-α (Panel
C) and, finally, actin (Panel D).

biologically active TNF-α following LPS treatment was blocked by H7, but not by W7 (data not shown). The levels of actin mRNA were unchanged by treatment with LPS or the inhibitors.

DISCUSSION

The involvement of second messenger pathways in the control of macrophage function is not unique to the expression of cytokine genes. A number of early activation events, including the secretion of metabolites of arachidonic acid (Adams and Hamilton, 1987), phosphorylation of proteins (Weiel et al, 1986), and the expression of early genes such as c-fos and c-myc (Radzioch et al, 1986; Introna et al, 1986) are inducible by phorbol myristate acetate, presumably mediated by PKc. In addition, the induction of macrophage tumoricidal activity is calcium dependent (Wright et al, 1985).

As with any other inhibitors we cannot rule out that alterations of biochemical pathways other than PKc or CaM may contribute to the effect of H7 or W7, respectively. The levels of H7 and W7 used to block cytokine gene expression in these studies were identical to those reported to inhibit PKc inducible c-fos expression in murine macrophages (D. Radzioch and L. Varesio, unpublished observation) and they were much lower than the doses of H7 at which protein kinase A may be inhibited (Hidaka et al, 1984). The inability of W7 to block TNF-α mRNA induction provides a clear indication that CaM dependent kinases are not involved in the induction of TNF-α mRNA expression by LPS. Moreover, it confirms the lack of cellular cytotoxicity of the inhibitor W7 used in these experiments.

An additional observation concerns the steady state levels of IL-1α and IL-1β mRNAs in murine macrophages. Unlike peptone elicited peritoneal exudate cells from CBA/J mice reported by Fuhlbrigge et al (1987), we find that thioglycolate elicited macrophages from C57BL/6N mice do not express IL-1α or IL-1β mRNAs in response to adherence to tissue culture plastic. This difference could easily be explained by the different forms of elicitation of cells or the strains of mice used in the studies.

The results of these studies have both immediate

practical and long term value. Agents like W7 can be used
to block the production of IL-1 but not TNF-α This will
allow us not only to selectively suppress a subset of the
functions of differentiated macrophages which may be
beneficial clinically, but also to further expand our
knowledge of the signals controlling the expression of
these pluripotent mediators.

ACKNOWLEDGEMENTS

We thank Dr. Joost J. Oppenheim for his critical
comments and thoughtful suggestions and Judy Maples for
typing the manuscript.

REFERENCES

Adams, DO, TA Hamilton (1987). Molecular transduction
    mechanisms by which IFN-gamma and other signals
    regulate macrophage development. Immunol Rev 97:5.
Beutler, B, A Cerami (1986). Cachetin and tumor necrosis
    factor: two sides of the same coin. Nature 320:584.
Beutler, B, N Krochin, IW Milsark, C Luedke, A Cerami
    (1986). Control of cachectin (tumor necrosis factor)
    synthesis: Mechanisms of endotoxin resistance.
    Science 232:977.
Chirgwin, JM, AE Przybyla, RJ McDonald, WJ Rattner (1979).
    Isolation of biologically active ribonucleic acid from
    sources rich in ribonuclease. Biochemistry 18:5294.
Degaliatoni, G, M Murphy, M Kobayashi, MK Francis, B
    Perussia, G Trinchieri (1985). Natural killer cell-
    derived hematopoietic colony-inhibiting factor:
    relationship with tumor necrosis factor and synergism
    with immune interferon. J Exp Med 162:1512.
Fuhlbrigge, RC, DD Chaplin, J-M Kiely, ER Unanue (1987).
    Regulation of interleukin 1 gene expression by
    adherence and lipopolysaccharide. J Immunol 138:3799.
Gery, I, RK Gershon, BH Waksman (1972). Potentiation of
    the thymocyte response to mitogens. J Exp Med 136:128.
Gifford, GE, M-L Lohmann-Matthes (1986). The requirement
    for the continual presence of LPS for the production of
    TNF-α by thioglycolate induced peritoneal murine
    macrophages. Int J Cancer 38:135.
Glisin, V, R Crvenjqakav, C Byus (1974). Ribonucleic
    acid isolation by cesium chloride centrifugation.

Biochemistry 13:2633.

Hidaka, H, M Inagaki, S Kawamato, Y Sasaki (1984).
Isoquinolinesulfonamides, novel and potent inhibitors
of cyclic nucleotide dependent protein kinase and
protein kinase C. Biochemistry 236:5036.

Introna, M, TA Hamilton, RE Kaufman, DO Adams, RC Bast, Jr
(1986). Treatment of murine peritoneal macrophages with
bacterial lipopolysaccharide alters expression of c-fos
and c-myc oncogenes. J Immunol 137:2711.

Jacobs, DM (1984). Structural features of binding of
lipopolysaccharide to murine lymphocytes. Rev Inf Dis
6:501.

Kornbluth, RS, TS Eddington (1986). Tumor necrosis factor
production by human monocytes is a regulated event:
induction of TNF-α-mediated cellular cytotoxicity by
endotoxin. J Immunol 137:2585.

Morrison, DC, JA Rudbach (1981). Endotoxin-cell membrane
interactions leading to transmembrane signalling. Cont
Top Mol Immunol 8:187.

Oppenheim, JJ, EJ Kovacs, K Matsushima, SK Durum (1986).
There's more than one interleukin-1. Immunol Today
7:45.

Radzioch, D, B Bottazzi, L Varesio (1986). Augmentation of
c-fos mRNA expression by activators of protein kinase C
in fresh, terminally differentiated resting macrophages.
Molec and Cell Biol 7:595.

Rubin, BY, SL Anderson, SA Sullivan, BD Williamson, EA
Carswell, LJ Old (1986). Nonhematopoietic cells
selected for resistance to tumor necrosis factor produce
tumor necrosis factor. J Exp Med 164:1350.

Sommers, SD, JE Weiel, TA Hamilton, DO Adams (1986).
Biochemical mechanisms of macrophage activation:
Phorbol esters and calcium ionophore act synergistically
to prime macrophages for tumor cell destruction. J
Immunol 136:4199.

Weiel, JE, TA Hamilton, DO Adams (1986). LPS induces
altered phosphate labelling of proteins in murine
peritoneal macrophages. J Immunol 136:3012.

Wright, B, I Zeidman, R Greig, G Poste (1985). Inhibition
of macrophage activation by calcium channel blockers and
calmodulin antagonists. Cellular Immunology 95:46.

DYNAMICS AND REGULATION OF MACROPHAGE TUMOR NECROSIS
FACTOR-α (TNF), INTERLEUKIN-1-α (IL-1α), AND INTERLEUKIN-
1-β (IL-1β) GENE EXPRESSION BY ARACHIDONATE METABOLITES

Steven L. Kunkel, Wendy E. Scales, Robert
Spengler, Mary Spengler, and Jim Larrick
Department of Pathology, University of Michigan
Medical School, Box 0602, Ann Arbor, Michigan,
48109 (S.L.K.,W.S.,R.S. and M.S.), and Depart-
ment of Immunology, Cetus Corp., Palo Alto,
California (J.L.)

INTRODUCTION

Macrophage derived TNF and IL-1 are increasingly
being recognized as important communication signals that
are active in both physiologic and immunologic events.
The central role of TNF and IL-1 in these systems occurs
via their pleomorphic effector functions that are essential to the orchestration of many normal and immunopatho-
logical processes. Historically, the biologic effects of
IL-1 and TNF centered around their lymphocyte activity and
tumor necrosing activities, respectively. The effector
activities of IL-1 and TNF have subsequently been expanded
and include an ever growing list of important biological
properties. For example, these monokines have many
related and overlapping effects on various cell systems
including: fibroblasts, neutrophils, endothelial cells,
osteoclasts, granulocytes, and lymphoid cells (1). It is
now evident that the full spectrum of cellular responses
induced by TNF and/or IL-1 have yet to be fully
elucidated.

Many studies have demonstrated that TNF and IL-1 have
potent effector cell activity, yet few investigations have
addressed the signals involved in regulating the production and gene expression of these monokines. Recent
investigations using elicited murine peritoneal macrophages have demonstrated that the production and gene
expression of TNF and IL-1 can be "up-regulated" by gamma
interferon and super-induced by cyclohexamide (2). In
addition to gamma interferon; endotoxin, phorbol esters,

various viruses, and poly I:C all can induce transcription
of IL-1 and TNF genes in various macrophage populations
(3) and macrophage cell lines (3). Conversely, glucocorticoids (dexamethosone, prednisone, and hydrocortisone)
can suppress the transcription of macrophage IL-1 and TNF.
The reports of positive signals for monokine gene expression appear to be more evident than the number of reported
negative signals.

Recent studies in our laboratory have focused on
exploring the suppression of TNFα, IL-1α, and IL-1β gene
expression via endogenous mediators. Treatment of macrophages with LPS can induce a concomitant increase in IL-1,
TNF, and prostaglandin E_2 (PGE_2) levels (4,5). A kinetic
analysis demonstrated a rapid rise in monokine production
followed by an accelerated, linear increase in PGE_2
levels. Plateau levels of IL-1 and TNF were found to
occur coincident with the accumulation of elevated concentrations of PGE_2 in macrophage supernatants. Further
analysis using exogenous PGE_2 demonstrated a suppressive
effect on the production of biologically active TNF and
IL-1 (4,5). This evidence suggests that PGE_2 may serve as
a potent modulator of macrophage-peptide production. In
the following study, we present data that addresses the
cellular regulation of IL-1 and TNF and the molecular
regulation of IL-1α, IL-1β, and TNF-α.

RESULTS

A unique attribute of monocyte/macrophages is their
potential to synthesize large amounts of arachidonic acid
metabolites (such as PGE_2 and PGI_2) that may potentially
regulate monokine products in an autocrine manner. As
shown in Table 1, PGE_2 dramatically suppresses the production of extracellular IL-1, as assessed by the thymocyte co-proliferation assay, in a dose dependent manner.
Treatment of LPS-stimulated macrophages with 10^{-6} or 10^{-8} M
PGE_2 reduced supernatant IL-1 by 75% and 60%, respectively; while the production of cell-associated IL-1 was
not significantly altered.

	IL-1 (Units/10^6 cells)					
	Supernatant			Lysates		
Time (hours)	LPS	LPS + PGE$_2$ 10^{-6}M	LPS+ PGE$_2$ 10^{-8}M	LPS	LPS + PGE$_2$ 10^{-6}M	LPS + PGE$_2$ 10^{-8}M
1.5	50	–	–	50	75	75
3	70	25	50	125	275	325
6	600	50	300	500	650	700
16	800	200	300	650	750	800

Table 1. Comparative effects of PGE$_2$ on the kinetics of IL-1 bioactivity found in the cellular supernatants or lysates.

Time (min) PGE$_2$ added after LPS	% Inhibition* of TNF (1 μg/ml LPS)	% Inhibition of TNF (10 ng/ml LPS)
0	32.8±6.6	75.7±8.8
30	38.2±7.5	75.2±8.3
60	37.0±3.6	76.2±6.7
90	18.8±9.1	41.8±10.5
120	0	50.1±19.9
150	0	39.8±6.0
180	0	52.8±4.1
No PGE$_2$	0	0.0

* Based on TNF activity 4 hr. post LPS addition.
Values represent mean ± SEM (N=4-11).

Table 2. Ability of PGE$_2$ to suppress LPS-dependent TNF production when added at timed intervals post LPS challenge.

Previous studies from our laboratory have demonstrated that cyclooxygenase inhibitors can dose-dependently reduce LPS-stimulated PGE_2 levels, while TNF production was concomitantly increased (5). Further investigations showed that exogenous PGE_2 could dramatically suppress the production of biologically active TNF (5). In the former study LPS-induced TNF levels were dose-dependently reduced over a wide concentration of PGE_2. In an extension of these studies we have examined the ability of PGE_2 to regulate the production of TNF when added after the LPS challenge. As shown in Table 2, PGE_2 ($1\mu M$) was efficacious in reducing LPS-dependent TNF production when added up to 90 min. post LPS. The suppression of TNF was not significantly different when PGE_2 was added concomitantly, 30 min, or 60 after LPS stimulation. The ability of subsequent PGE_2 addition to regulate LPS-dependent TNF production was more dramatic when 10 ng/ml LPS served as the initial stimulus. PGE_2 addition 3 hours post LPS (10 ng/ml) stimulation still demonstrated a 50% reduction in TNF activity. Nevertheless, the production of TNF in response to higher concentration of LPS (1 µg/ml) was also susceptible to PGE_2-induced regulation.

The above observations demonstrating differential regulation of monokines by PGE_2 led to an investigation of the molecular hit mechanism. Using Northern blot analysis, we have demonstrated that the kinetics of LPS-induced mRNA accumulation for IL-1α and IL-1β are very similar, with both monokines demonstrating a peak in mRNA levels 6 hours post LPS challenge. Levels of mRNA for these two monokines persisted for 16 hours. The expression of TNF mRNA in response to LPS occurred more rapidly and peaked in approximately 2.5 hours, with a more accelerated degradation. These data suggest that mRNA for TNF is rapidly "up-regulated" and rapidly degraded, compared to IL-1α and IL-1β. The ability of PGE_2 to modulate mRNA accumulation for IL-1α, IL-1β, and TNF was studied by adding LPS + PGE_2 and harvesting mRNA at 6 hours and 2.5 hours for IL-1α/IL-1β and TNF, respectively. As shown in Figure 1, PGE_2 suppressed LPS-induced TNF mRNA accumulation, but did not affect the levels of either IL-1α or IL-1β mRNA. The difference in PGE_2 regulation of mRNA for these monokines in response to LPS is reflected in the different levels of assayable TNF and IL-1. Apparently, TNF is under strict regulation by PGE, at both the cellular and molecular levels. On the contrary, IL-1α

and IL-1β mRNA accumulation is not under as stringent
regulation.

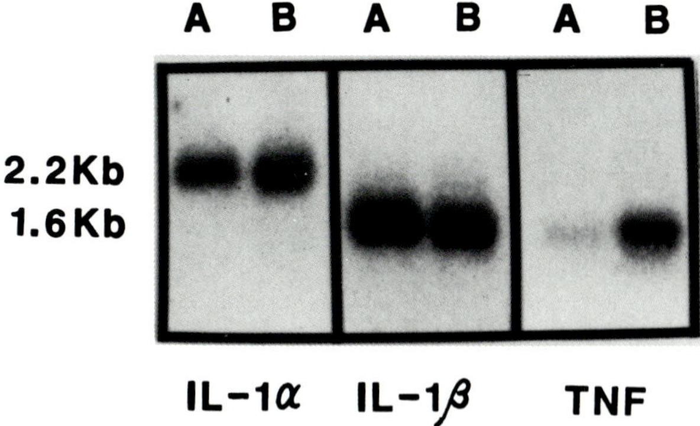

Figure 1:   Northern blot analysis of IL-1α, IL-1β and
TNF-α mRNA production by macrophages in the presence of
LPS (1 ug/ml) + 10^{-6}M PGE$_2$ (A) or LPS (1 ug/ml) alone (B).
Messenger RNA was extracted from stimulated macrophages at
2.5 and 6 hours for TNF and IL-1α/IL-1β, respectively.
LPS + PGE$_2$ were added concomitantly to macrophages for
TNF analysis and -1 hour for IL-1α/IL-1β analysis.   The
blots were hybridized with either ^{32}P labeled cDNA or ^{32}P
labeled oligonucleotides.

DISCUSSION

We have demonstrated that the gene expression (mRNA
accumulation) for TNF is suppressed by PGE$_2$, while mRNA
levels for IL-1α and IL-1β are not altered. Interestingly, extracellular IL-1 and TNF were significantly reduced by
PGE$_2$ treatment; yet, cell associated IL-1 was not
affected. These studies suggest that PGE$_2$ may have
important transcriptional and post-transcriptional regulatory mechanisms that dictate the synthesis of IL-1 and TNF
during inflammation.
The ability of arachidonate metabolites, such as PGE$_2$
to serve as an autocoid and modulate the release of TNF
and IL-1 may have important implications regarding the
localization of an immune response. Upon specific stimulation, not only are macrophage-derived TNF and IL-1
up-regulated to act as cell-to-cell communication signals,

but the concomitant production of PGE_2 by the same macrophage can act as an endogenous mediator to initiate the modulation of TNF and IL-1 production. Although PGE_2 can regulate de novo TNF and IL-1 production, the molecular hit mechanism leading to a regulated state appears to be different. The involvement of TNF in pathophysiologic responses may dictate that this monokine is under strict regulatory control. On the contrary, IL-1 appears to be involved in many immunologic and normal physiologic responses and its regulation is not as strongly controlled. These differences may have important consequences with regard to the pathophysiology of these mediators in disease states.

ACKNOWLEDGEMENTS

The authors wish to acknowledge the expert secretarial help of Ms. Peggy Weber. This research was supported in part by National Institutes of Health grants HL31237, HL31963, HL35276. Dr. Kunkel is an Established Investigator of the American Heart Association.

REFERENCES

1.   Le J, Vileck J (1987) Tumor necrosis factor and interleukin-1: cytokines with multiple overlapping biological activities. Lab Invest 56:234-248.
2.   Collart MA, Belin D, Vassalli J, Kossodo S, Vassalli P (1986) γ-interferon enhances macrophage transcription of the tumor necrosis factor/cachectin, interleukin-1, and urokinase genes, which are controlled by short-lived responses. J Exp Med 164:2113-2118.
3.   Larrick J, Kunkel SL (1988) The role of tumor necrosis factor and interleukin-1 in the immuno-inflammatory response. Pharmaceutical Res (in press).
4.   Kunkel SL, Chensue CH, Phan SH (1986) Prostaglandins as endogenous mediators of interleukin-1 production. J Immunol 136:186-194.
5.   Kunkel SL, Wiggins RC, Chensue SW, Larrick J (1986) Regulation of tumor necrosis factor production by prostaglandin E_2. Biochem Biophys Res Comm 137:404-410.

Monokines and Other Non-Lymphocytic Cytokines, pages 67–72
© 1988 Alan R. Liss, Inc.

REGULATION OF TNF GENE EXPRESSION BY LIPOPOLYSACCHARIDE,
CYCLIC AMP AND INTERFERON.

Steven M. Taffet

Departments of Microbiology/Immunology and
Biochemistry/Molecular Biology, SUNY Health Science
Center at Syracuse, Syracuse, New York 13210

INTRODUCTION

Tumor necrosis factor-α (TNF-α) has been associated with
the induction of macrophage tumoricidal activity and has been
implicated as a mediator of tumoricidal activity in some
cases (Feinman et al., 1987). TNF-α is induced by bacterial
lipopolysaccharide, LPS (Beutler et al., 1986) and its
synthesis is inhibited by prostaglandin E_2, PGE_2 (Kunkel et
al., 1986). In previous studies, macrophage tumoricidal
activity was induced by LPS, and inhibited by prostaglandin
E_2. Prostaglandin E_2 appears to inhibit tumoricidal activity
by a cAMP dependent mechanism (Taffet and Russell, 1981).
Interferon-gamma (IFN-γ) which does not induce tumoricidal
activity, does increase the sensitivity of macrophages for
LPS (Pace et al., 1983). The inhibitory effect of PGE_2 on
tumoricidal activity was blocked by IFN-γ treatment (Pace and
Russell, 1985) . In this study, we have determined some of
the parameters of TNF-α induction in macrophages, in order to
determine if TNF-α is regulated in a manner consistent with
the regulation of tumoricidal activity.

METHODS

Recombinant rat interferon-gamma was purchased from
Amgem. 8-bromo cAMP and LPS 0111:B4 (phenol extracted, and
chromatographically purified) were purchased from Sigma (St.
Louis, MO). All cells were grown in Dulbecco's modification
of Eagle's Medium (DMEM, GIBCO) supplemented with fetal
bovine serum (FBS, Hyclone; Logan, UT). All media and

reagents were free of detectable endotoxin, determined by
using the Limulus amebocyte lysate assay.

Confluent monolayers of RAW264 cells plated in 100 mm-
diameter tissue culture dishes were serum starved for 24
hours prior to assay for TNF-α mRNA. Bone marrow-derived
(BM) macrophages were grown in medium containing 10% FBS, 5%
horse serum and 10% L-cell conditioned medium. 10-14 days
after plating, these cells were nearly confluent and were
shifted to DMEM containing 5% FBS for 24 hour before TNF-α
mRNA determination. Cytoplasmic RNA was isolated using
vanadyl ribonucleoside complex as an inhibitor of RNAase.
TNF-α mRNA levels were determined by dot hybridization to a
^{32}P-labeled cDNA probe kindly provided by Dr. B. Beutler
(Beutler et al., 1986). Nuclear transcription run-off was
used as a determination of transcription rate. Both of these
techniques have been described in detail (Shurtleff et al.,
1988). Resulting autoradiographs were quantitated using a
scanning densitometer and the results are presented as
relative densimetric units.

RESULTS

Bacterial LPS induced a rapid increase in the rate of
transcription of TNF-α mRNA in the RAW264 macrophage-like
cell line (Figure 1). Transcription rates increased within
15 minutes after LPS stimulation and were maximal 30 to 60
minutes after LPS addition (Taffet et al. in preparation).
The increase in transcription resulted in a rapid accumulation of TNF-α mRNA peaking by 60 minutes after stimulation. A similar increase in TNF-α mRNA was induced in BM
macrophages with maximal levels induced 60 minutes after LPS
treatment. In both RAW264 cells and BM macrophages, TNF-α
mRNA levels decreased slightly by 90 minutes after treatment.
TNF-α mRNA levels of 80% of the maximal induction were then
maintained in excess of 5 hours.

Previous studies have shown that PGE$_2$ reduces the
synthesis of TNF-α mRNA (Kunkel et al., 1986). In this
study, we used cAMP analogues in order to determine the
effect of elevated cAMP on TNF expression. Increases in 8-
bromo cAMP caused a concentration dependent decrease in TNF-α
mRNA. Analogues that decreased LPS-induced TNF-α mRNA levels
in order of potency were 8-thioethyl cAMP > 8-bromo cAMP >

8(6-aminohexyl)amino cAMP > N^6, 2-0-dibutyryl cAMP > N^6-benzoyl cAMP > cAMP. This order of potency indicates that there is a potential role for the Type II cAMP-dependent protein kinase in the down regulation of TNF-α mRNA. The down regulation was not a general inhibition of mRNA syn-

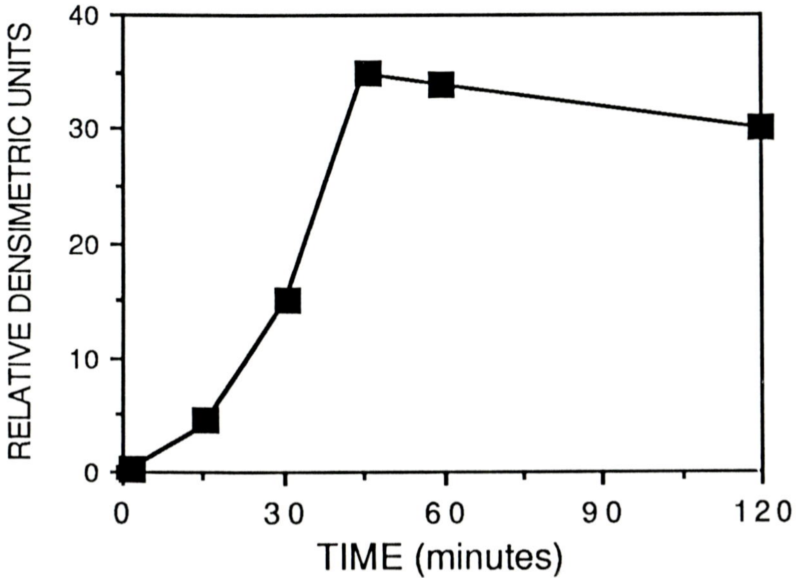

Figure 1. Induction of TNF mRNA after LPS treatment. RAW264 cells were serum starved for 24 hours and treated with LPS (1μg/ml) for various times before cell lysis. Cells were harvested by scraping, RNA extracted, dotted onto nitrocellulose and hybridized with nick translated cDNA probe.

thesis as the expression of at least one other gene, ornithine decarboxylase (ODC), was enhanced by cAMP treatment.

Utilizing the nuclear transcription run-off assay we were able to determine that the effect of cyclic AMP on TNF-α mRNA was at the level of transcription. Table 1 is the results of one such experiment. When RAW264 cells were treated with 1 μg/ml LPS there was a 5 fold increase in TNF-α mRNA transcription. The addition of 1 mM 8-bromo cAMP reduced the TNF-α mRNA transcription rate to the unstimulated level. As a control, ODC transcription rate was also determined. LPS treatment resulted in a 6 fold increase in ODC

transcription and 8-bromo cAMP treatment further enhanced
this expression 2 fold.

Table 1. Transcription runoff assay

Cell Treatment[a]	RDU[b]	
	ODC	TNF
Control	43.9	45.8
LPS[c]	277.5	235.5
LPS + 8-br cAMP[d]	559.1	54.4

[a] Cells were treated for 2 hours before nuclei isolation
[b] Relative densimetric units read from a densitometer
[c] Lipopolysaccharide, 1µg/ml
[d] 8-bromo cAMP, 1mM

Treatment with recombinant rat interferon gamma did not
induce TNF-α mRNA in RAW264 cells or in BM macrophage cultures. IFN-γ did act synergistically with LPS to induce TNF-
α mRNA. There was no effect of interferon when cells were
treated for less than 4 hours prior to LPS addition. Treatment for 8 or more hours increased had maximal effect of
subsequent LPS treatment. The optimal concentration of
interferon for the induction of TNF by LPS was 10 units per
ml in bone marrow cultures and greater than 100 units per ml
when using RAW264 cells. All additional studies were done
using bone-marrow derived macrophages. Figure 2. demonstrates the effect of IFN-γ on LPS induction of TNF-α mRNA.
When no LPS was added IFN-γ had no effect on TNF-α mRNA. When
LPS was present at levels greater than 0.1 ng/ml interferon
could potentiate the LPS induced increase in TNF-α mRNA. The
effect of IFN-γ was generally greatest between 1 and 10 ng/ml
LPS.

IFN-γ also had a profound effect on the inhibition of
TNF-α mRNA induced by 8-bromo cAMP. As seen in table 2 when
IFN was added in addition to LPS, the inhibition due to 8-
bromo cAMP was prevented at some concentrations of cAMP.
Higher concentrations of 8-bromo cAMP were still inhibitory.

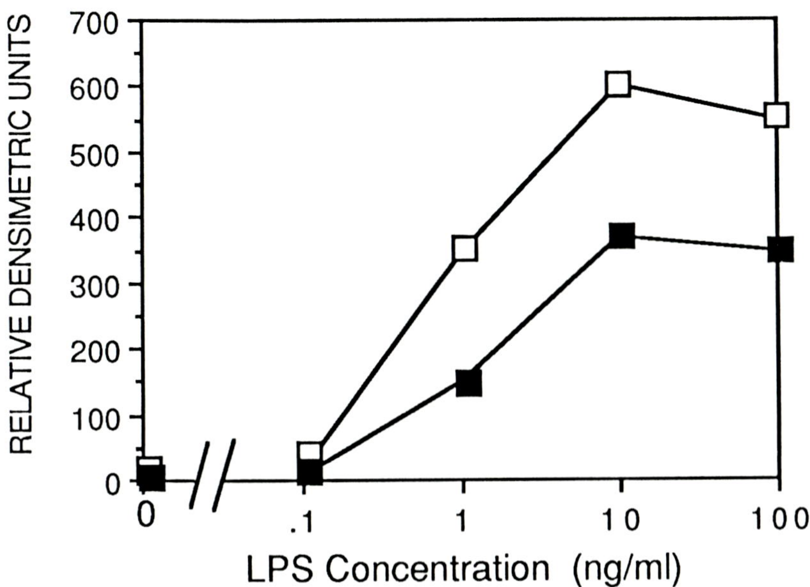

Figure 2. <u>Interferon effects on TNF-α mRNA.</u> Cultures of bone marrow derived-macrophages were incubated in medium containing 5% FBS for 24 hours. The cells were treated with 10 units/ml of rIFN-γ for 12 hours followed by LPS at various concentrations for 1 hour. RNA was then isolated and hybridized to a ^{32}P-labeled cDNA probe.   (■) no IFN, (□) IFN.

Table 2.   Effect of interferon-gamma on cAMP inhibition.

cAMP[a] (μM)	RDU[b]	
	− IFN	+ IFN[c]
100	184	252
300	30	264
1000	45	68

[a] Cells were treated with 1 μg/ml LPS and 8-bromo cAMP for 1 hour before RNA isolation
[b] Relative densimetric units read from a densitometer
[c] rIFN-γ , 10 units per ml, 12 hr

CONCLUSIONS

1. LPS induces a rapid increase in TNF-α mRNA.
2. The induction of TNF-α mRNA by LPS is due to a rapid increase in transcription.
3. cAMP analogues prevent the increase in TNF-α mRNA transcription.
4. IFN-γ could not induce TNF-α mRNA, but could enhance the response to LPS.
5. IFN-γ blocks the inhibition of TNF-α mRNA synthesis caused by cAMP.

(The author wishes to acknowledge Sheila Shurtleff, Ali Yashruti, and Christine McElwain for their work on this project. This work was supported by N.I.H. grant #AI24236)

REFERENCES:

Beutler, B., Krochin, N., Milsark, I.W., Leudke, C. and Cerami, A. (1986). Control of cachectin (tumor necrosis factor) synthesis :mechanisms of endotoxin resistance. Science 232: 977-980.

Feinman, R., Henriksen-DeStefano, D., Tsujimoto, M. and Vilcek, J.(1987) Tumor necrosis factor is an important mediator of tumor cell killing by human monocytes. J. Immunol. 138:635-640.

Kunkel S.L., Wiggins, R.C., Chensue, S.W., and Larrick, J. (1986). Regulation of macrophage tumor necrosis factor production by PGE_2. Biochemical and Biophysical Research Communications 137:404-410.

Pace, J.L., Russell, S.W., Torres, B. and Johnson, H.M. (1983). Recombinant mouse gamma interferon induces the priming step in macrophage activation for tumor cell killing. J. Immunol. 130:2011-2013.

Pace, J.L. and Russell, S.W. (1984). Gamma interferon interferes with the negative regulation of macrophage activation by prostaglandin E2. Mol. Immunol. 21:249-254.

Shurtleff, S.A., McElwain, C.M. and Taffet, S.M.(1988). Rapid expression of ornithine decarboxylase mRNA in a macrophage-like cell line: Cyclic AMP repression of the requirement for protein synthesis. J. Cell Physiology, In Press.

Taffet, S.M., and S.W. Russell.(1981). Macrophage-mediated tumor cell killing: regulation of expression of cytolytic activity by prostaglandin E. J. Immunol. 126:424-427.

CLONING OF THE cDNAs FOR RAT INTERLEUKIN-1α AND β.

Tsutomu Nishida, Tohru Hirato, Naoki Nishino,
Keiko Mizuno, Yasuyo Sekiguchi, Masaaki Takano,
Kazuyoshi Kawai, Satoru Nakai and Yoshikatsu
Hirai

Laboratories of Celluar Technology, Otsuka
Pharmaceutical Co.,Ltd., 463-10 Kagasuno
Kawauchi-cho, Tokushima, 771-01, Japan

INTRODUCTION

Interleukin-1(IL-1) is a cytokine released from
various cell types (Oppenheim et al., 1986). The cDNAs for
both human IL-1α and β have been cloned (Auron et al.,
1984; March et al., 1985; Furutani et al., 1985; Nishida et
al., 1987) and the availability of their recombinant
products has contributed to clarify the biological
activities of IL-1 (Dinarello, 1986; Hirai et al., in
press). It has become evident that IL-1 has multipotential
activities which are involved in the regulation of immune,
inflammatory, endocrine and central nervous system
(Dinarello, 1986). Therefore the utilization of the animal
model will facilitate to elucidate the role of IL-1 in
vivo. Rat is considered to be appropriate as an animal
model, but rat IL-1 cDNA has not been isolated. We report
here the molecular cloning of rat IL-1α and β cDNAs.

METHODS

Isolation of rat IL-1β cDNA clones
Sprague-Dawley rats were injected i.v. with 100µg/kg
of E.coli lipopolysaccharide (LPS). After 6 hours,
poly(A)$^+$RNA was prepared from the brain of the rats.
Poly(A)$^+$RNA was used to construct of the cDNA library in
λgt10 vector. 3 X 10^5 plaques of the cDNA library were
screened with the ^{32}P-labeled human IL-1β cDNA insert
(HindIII-AccI fragment 525bp). Five hybridizing clones
were isolated. Four of five clones hybridized with a probe
prepared from the 5' end of the human IL-1β cDNA insert

(PstI-HindIII, 463bp). One of them, λRIL-5, was chosen
for the analysis of the nucleotide sequence of cDNA insert.

<u>Isolation of rat IL-1α cDNA clones</u>
    Sprague-Dawley rats were infused i.p. with 30ml of
10%(w/v) proteose peptone. After 4 days, peritoneal
exudate cells(PEC) were harvested. Washed cells were
resuspended at 2 X 10^6 cells/ml in RPMI-1640 medium
supplemented with 10% FCS, 10µg/ml of LPS and 0.1µg/ml
indomethacin, and plated on plastic petri dishes and
incubated for 13.5 hours. Poly(A)$^+$ RNA was prepared from
adherent cells and the cDNA library was constructed with
poly(A)$^+$ RNA by using the pcDV-1 vector-primer and the pL1
linker fragment according to the procedure of Okayama and
Berg (Okayama and Berg, 1983). The 5' end of the human
IL-1α cDNA insert (BalI-MvaI fragment, 285bp) radiolabeled
with ^{32}P was used to screen 6.8 X 10^4 colonies of the cDNA
library. Two clones were isolated and one of them,
pcD-RT-IL-1α(6), was chosen for the analysis of the
nucleotide sequence of cDNA insert.

<u>Transfection into monkey COS-1 cells</u>
    Plasmid DNA was transfected into monkey COS-1 cells
as described previously (Nishida et al.,1987).

<u>Biological assays for rat IL-1</u>
    The assay for growth inhibitory factor (GIF) against
human melanoma cell line A375 has been described (Nishida
et al., 1987; Hirai et al., in press). The lymphocytes
activating factor (LAF) measured the incorporation of
^{3}H-thymidine into BALB/c mouse thymocytes in the presence
of phytohemagglutinin (PHA) as previously described
(Oppenheim et al., 1976). One LAF unit is half value of
maximum uptake of ^{3}H-thymidine with human recombinant IL-1β
(Kikumoto et al., 1987).

RESULTS AND DISCUSSIONS

    When LPS was injected into rats, Northern blot
analysis showed that rat mRNA homologous to human IL-1β
cDNA was induced in the brain. Therefore the cDNA library
was constructed by using mRNA derived from the brain of
LPS-injected rats. We isolated four cDNA clones
hybridizing with human IL-1β cDNA probes and clone λRIL-5
was chosen for the analysis of the nucleotide sequence of

the cDNA insert. The cDNA insert is 1327bp in length and encodes a protein of 268 amino acid residues. The nucleotide sequence of the coding regions of this cDNA and human IL-1β cDNA is 77% homologous. (Nishida et al., submitted). The amino acid sequence deduced from this cDNA sequence is shown in Figure 1 and is homologous to human IL-1β (68%) and murine IL-1β (89%). Therefore these data suggest that this cDNA corresponds to rat IL-1β cDNA although we have not confirmed the biological activities of the protein encoded in this cDNA.

```
Rat      MATVPELNCEIAAFDS-EENDLFFEADRPQKIKDCFQALDLGCPDESIQL    49
Murine   **********MPP***-D*******V*G***M*G***TF**********    49
Human    **E****AS*MM*YY*GN*D*******G*KQM*CS**D***CPL*GG***    50

Rat      QISQQHLDKSFRKAVSLIVAVEKLWQLPMSCPWSFQDEDPSTFFSFIFEE    99
Murine   ******IN****Q***************V*F**T*****M**********    99
Human    R**DH*YS*G**Q*A*VV**MD**RKMLVP**QT**EN*L****P*****   100

Rat      EPVLCDSWDDDD-LLVCDVPIRQLHCRLRDEQQKCLVLSDPCELKALHLN   148
Murine   **I********N**************Y********S************H*   149
Human    **IFF*T*-*NE-AY*H*A*V*S*N*T***S***S**M*G*Y*******Q   148

Rat      GQNISQQVVFSMSFVQGETSNDKIPVALGLKGKNLYLSCVMKDGTPTLQL   198
Murine   ****N***I*******P********************************   199
Human    **DME**************E*************E*******L**DK*****   198

Rat      ESVDPKQYPKKKMEKRFVFNKIEVKTKVEFESAQFPNWYISTSQAEHRPV   248
Murine   *************************S*******E*************K**   249
Human    ******N******************INN*L****************NM**   248

Rat      FLGNSNG-RDIVDFTMEPVSS                               268
Murine   ****NS*-Q**I*****S***                               269
Human    ***GTK*GQ**T****QF***                               269
```

Figure 1. Amino acid sequence of rat IL-1β compared with IL-1β sequences from murine (Gray et al., 1986) and human (Auron et al., 1984; March et al., 1985; Nishida et al., 1987). The letters represent the single-letter abbreviations for amino acids. The asterisk represents an amino acid residue that is identical to the residue shown for rat IL-1β. Gaps (-) have been inserted to achieve maximum homology.

As for rat IL-1α cDNA, we failed to isolate rat IL-1α cDNA clones from the rat brain cDNA library. Another cDNA library was constructed from mRNA derived from LPS-stimulated rat peritoneal macrophages by using Okayama-Berg cDNA expression vector and was screened with human IL-1α cDNA probe. Two clones were isolated and clone pcD-RT-IL-1α(6) was chosen for the analysis of the

nucleotide sequence. This cDNA insert is 1992bp (except
poly A) in length and encodes a protein of 270 amino acid
residues. The nucleotide sequence of the coding regions of
this cDNA and human IL-1α cDNA is 73% homologous. (Nishida
et al., submitted). The amino acid sequence deduced from
this cDNA sequence is shown in Figure 2 and is homologous
to human IL-1α (65%), rabbit IL-1α (64%) and murine IL-1α
(83%), respectively.

```
Rat      MAKVPDLFEDLKNCYSENEEYSSAIDHLSLNQKSFYDASYGSLHENCTDK    50
Murine   ****************D***********************T***Q          50
Rabbit   ***************F********************EP***D*MN*         50
Human    ******M************D**S***********HV***P***G*M*Q       50

Rat      FVSLRTSETSKMSTFTFKESRVVVSATSNKGKILKKRRLSFNQPFTEDDL   100
Murine   *************N********T*****SN***********SET******   100
Rabbit   V***S*****VSPNL**Q*NV*A*T*---S***********L***I*DV**    97
Human    S***SI*****T*KL*****M***AT---N**V********LS*SI*D***    97

Rat      EAIAHDLEE-TIQPRSAPHSFQNNLRYKLIRIVKQEFIMNDSLNQNIYVD   149
Murine   QS*T*****-*********YTY*SD*****MKL*R*K*V********T**Q*   149
Rabbit   *TNVS*P**GI*K***V*YT**R*M***YL**I****TL**A***SLVR*   147
Human    ****N*S**EI*K*****F**LS*VK*NFM**I*Y***L**A***S*IR-   146

Rat      MDRIHLKAASLNDLQLEVKFDMYAYSSGG-DDSKYPVTLKVSNTQLFVSA   198
Murine   V*KHY*STTW*****Q***********-**********I*DS******   198
Rabbit   TSDQY*Q**P*QN*GDA*****GV*-MTS-E**IL****RI*Q*P*****   195
Human    ANDQY*T**A*HN*DEA*****G**-KSSK**A*IT*I*RI*K***Y*T*   195

Rat      QGEDKPVLLKEIPETPKLITGSETDLIFFWEKINSKNYFTSAAFPELLIA   248
Murine   ****Q*******L*******************KS***********Y***F**   248
Rabbit   *N**E******M****RI**D**S*IL****TQGN****K***N*Q*F**   245
Human    *D**Q******M**I**T******N*L****THGT******V*H*N*F**   245

Rat      TKEQSQVHLARGLPSMIDFQIS                               270
Murine   *****R***********T*****                              270
Rabbit   **PEHL**M********T*****                              267
Human    **QDYW*C**G*P**IT****LENQA                           271
```

Figure 2. Amino acid sequence of rat IL-1α compared with
IL-1α sequences from murine (Lomedico et al., 1984), rabbit
(Furutani et al., 1985) and human (March et al., 1985;
Furutani et al.,1985; Nishida et al., 1987). The letters,
the asterisk and the gap (-) are those explained in the
legend to Figure 1.

The protein encoded in this cDNA exhibited the GIF
activity and LAF activity as shown in Table 1. These data
confirm that this cDNA encodes rat IL-1α. The fact that
human recombinant IL-1α and β (Hirai et al., in press),
and also rat recombinant IL-1α exhibit the growth inhibitory
function against human melanoma cell line A375 suggests that
GIF activity is common to IL-1 derived from various species.

Table 1.   Expression of recombinant rat IL-1α in COS cells.

clone	GIF(u/ml)	LAF(u/ml)
pcD-RT-IL-1α(6)	46.9	8
mock	0	0

The amino acid sequence of IL-1α or IL-1β among species is homologous overall and Figure 2 and 3 show the difference of the conserved region between IL-1α and β. In IL-1α, N-terminal region (Met^1-Arg^{114}) of rat IL-1α is much more homologous to human IL-1α (74%), rabbit IL-1α (71%), and murine IL-1α (89%), respectively. In contrast to IL-1α, C-terminal region (Val^{117}-Ser^{268}) of rat IL-1β is much more homologous to human IL-1β (78%) and murine IL-1β (90%), respectively. We have no idea of the significance of the difference of the conserved region. Recently it has been shown that both precursor form and mature form of human IL-1α bind to the IL-1 receptor and precursor form of IL-1β does not bind (Mosley et al., 1987), and membrane-associated, biologically active, IL-1 is α type (Conlon et al., 1987). These functions of IL-1α might relate to the conservation of N-terminal region in IL-1α.

REFERENCES

Auron PE, Webb AC, Rosenwasser LJ, Mucci SF, Rich A, Wolff SM, Dinarello CA(1984). Nucleotide sequence of human monocyte interleukin 1 precursor cDNA. Proc Natl Acad Sci USA 81: 7907-7911.
Conlon PJ, Grabstein KH, Alpert A, Prickett KS, Hopp TP, Gillis S(1987). Localization of human mononuclear cell interleukin 1. J Immunol 139: 98-102.
Dinarello CA (1986). Multiple biological properties of recombinant human interleukin 1 (beta). Immunobiol 172:301-315.
Furutani Y, Notake M, Yamayoshi M, Yamagishi J, Nomura H, Ohue M, Furuta R, Fukui T, Yamada M, Nakamura S (1985). Cloning and charactarization of the cDNAs for human and rabbit interleukin-1 precursor. Nucleic Acid Res 13:5869-5882.

Gray PW, Glaister D, Chen E, Goeddel DV, Pennica D (1986). Two interleukin 1 genes in the mouse: Cloning and expression of the cDNA for murine interleukin 1β. J Immunol 137:3644-3648

Hirai Y, Masui Y, Nakai S, Kikumoto Y, Nishida T, Hong Y-M (in press). Interleukin 1 : cDNA cloning, production and biological activities of human interleukin 1. In Gann Monograph on Cancer Research : Cellular and Molecular Mechanisms of Tumor Immunity, Japan Scientific Societies Press.

Kikumoto Y, Hong Y-M, Nishida T, Nakai S, Masui Y, Hirai Y (1987). Purification and characterization of recombinant human interleukin-1β produced in Escherichia coli. Biochem Biophys Res Commun 147:315-321

Lomedico PT, Gubler V, Hellmann CP, Dukovich M, Giri JG, Pan Y-CE, Collier K, Semionow R, Chua AO, Mizel SB (1984). Cloning and expression of murine interleukin-1 cDNA in Escherichia coli. Nature 312:458-461

March CJ, Mosley B, Larsen A, Cerretti DP, Braedt G, Price V, Gillis S, Henney CS, Kronheim SR, Grabstein K, Conlon PJ, Hopp TP, Cosman D (1985). Cloning, sequence and expression of two distinct human interleukin-1 complementary DNAs. Nature 315:641-647.

Mosley B, Urdal DL, Prikett KS, Larsen A, Cosman D, Conlon PJ, Gillis S, Dower SK (1987). The interleukin-1 receptor binds the human interleukin-1α precursor but not the interleukin-1β precursor. J Biol Chem 262: 2941-2944.

Nishida T, Nishino N, Takano M, Kawai K, Bando K, Masui Y, Nakai S, Hirai Y (1987). cDNA cloning of IL-1α and IL-1β from mRNA of U937 cell line. Biochem Biophys Res Commun 143:345-352

Okayama H, Berg P (1983). A cDNA cloning vector that permits expression of cDNA inserts in mammalian cells. Mol Cell Biol 3:280-289.

Oppenheim JJ, Shneyour A, Kook AI (1976). Enhancement of DNA synthesis and cAMP content of mouse thymocytes by mediator(s) derived from adherent cells. J Immunol 116:1466-1472.

Oppenheim JJ, Kovacs EJ, Matsushima K, Durum SK (1986). There is more than one interleukin 1. Immunol Today 7:45-56.

Monokines and Other Non-Lymphocytic Cytokines, pages 79–82
© 1988 Alan R. Liss, Inc.

QUANTITATIVE ANALYSIS OF IL-1α AND ß mRNA IN HUMAN
MONOCYTES AND MACROPHAGES

Michael F. Smith, Jr.[*], Friedrich R. Kueppers[*],
Peter R. Young[+], and John C. Lee[#]
[*]Department of Microbiology and Immunology,
Temple Univ. School of Medicine, Philadelphia, PA
19140 and Departments of [+]Molecular Genetics and
[#]Immunology, Smith Kline and French Labs,
Philadelphia, PA 19101

INTRODUCTION

Interleukin-1 (IL-1), originally described as a
cytokine produced primarily by monocyte/macrophages which
promotes the proliferation of T lymphocytes (Gery et al.
1972), has now been demonstrated to be produced by a
variety of cell types and to have many diverse biological
activities <u>in</u> <u>vitro</u> and <u>in</u> <u>vivo</u> (Oppenheim et al. 1986).
Complementary DNAs (cDNAs) for two distinct human IL-1
molecules have been cloned and expressed in <u>E</u>. <u>coli</u> (March
et al. 1985). These two forms (termed α and ß) differ
in isoelectric point (pI 5 and 7 respectively) and amino
acid sequence and yet bind the same cell surface receptor
(Killian et al. 1986) and have a similar spectrum of
biological activities (Rupp et al. 1986).
Although a considerable amount of information has
accumulated on the biological activities mediated by these
two molecules, relatively little is known about the
regulation of IL-1 expression at the transcriptional
level. A number of studies have suggested that stimulated
human monocytes express IL-1ß at a level significantly
higher than IL-1α (March et al. 1985, Fuhlbrigge et al.
1987). However, in all cases there has been a general
lack of good accurate quantitation of the relative levels
of the two IL-1 forms at either the mRNA or protein level.
As a first step to explore the mechanisms that control
the expression of the two IL-1 species, we have used a
quantitative RNA dot blot assay to examine the expression
of IL-1α and ß in human peripheral blood monocytes,
alveolar macrophages, and cultured monocytes. We now

present quantitative evidence of the differential
expression of the two forms of IL-1 at the transcriptional
level.

RESULTS AND DISCUSSION

We used the SP6 _in_ _vitro_ transcription system (Promega
Biotec) to provide reference RNAs specific for IL-1α and
IL-1ß. These reference RNAs were then used as standards
in RNA dot blot assays to permit an exact determination of
the amount of IL-1α or ß specific mRNA within each RNA
sample. Duplicate blots were made and hybridized to either
the IL-1α or ß [^{32}P]-labeled cDNA. Specific hybridization was then quantitated and the amount of IL-1 specific
message in each RNA sample was determined by comparison
with a standard curve derived from the reference RNAs.
To determine if the relative levels of IL-1α and
IL-1ß mRNA are consistent throughout the cells of the
monocyte/macrophage lineage we analyzed RNA purified from
unstimulated and LPS stimulated (100 ng/ml for 4 hours)
peripheral blood monocytes (PBM), alveolar macrophages
(AM), and macrophages derived from _in_ _vitro_ culture (7
days) of PBM. Figure 1 shows two identical dot blots.
One was probed with IL-1α cDNA (left) and the other with
IL-1ß cDNA (right).
When specific hybridization for each sample is
quantitated relative to the standards we can demonstrate
distinct differences in the patterns of IL-1 expression in
the three cell types (Table 1). LPS stimulated or
unstimulated PBM express approximately 10-fold more IL-1ß
mRNA than α. Similarly treated AM however express only
2-3-fold more IL-1ß than α. In contrast, cultured
monocytes express almost exclusively IL-1ß at levels at
least 20-fold greater than IL-1α.
The striking difference in ß:α ratios observed in
alveolar macrophages and cultured monocytes (3.5 and 21
respectively) suggests that the latter cell type is not
analogous to the tissue macrophage. Therefore, caution
should be exercised in the interpretation of studies
regarding _in_ _vitro_ cultured monocytes relative to tissue
macrophages.
Interestingly, the levels of IL-1α in AM are
consistently equal to or greater than the levels in
similarly treated PBM. This would suggest that perhaps
there is a greater need for this form of IL-1 than there

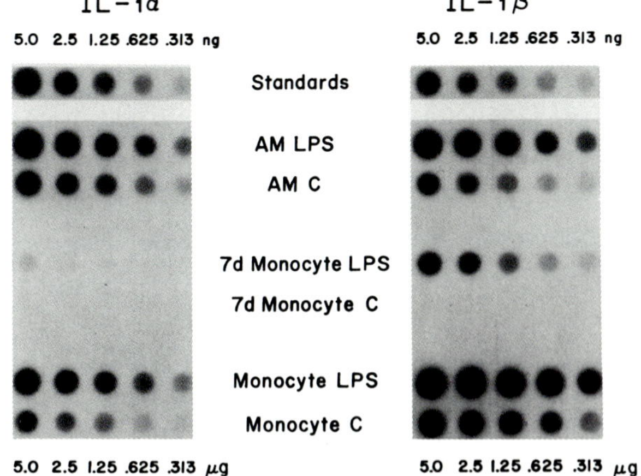

FIGURE 1.   RNA dot blot analysis of AM, PBM, and aged monocytes for IL-1α (left) and IL-1ß (right) mRNA. C=control; LPS=100 ng/ml LPS for 4 hours.

TABLE 1.   IL-1 mRNA Quantitation in unstimulated (C) or LPS stimulated (LPS) PBM, AM, and 7 day aged monocytes.

Cell Type	%IL-1α	%IL-1ß	Ratio ß:α
Monocyte C	0.027	0.276	13.0
Monocyte LPS	0.096	0.71	9.6
AM C	0.056	0.12	2.3
AM LPS	0.123	0.332	3.5
7d Monocyte C	<0.002	0.006	--
7d Monocyte LPS	0.006	0.082	21.0

is for IL-1ß within the milieu of the alveoli. If, as has been suggested by Kurt-Jones et al. (1987), IL-1α is the predominant form expressed on the cell surface thereby restricting its effects to the immediate vicinity of the macrophage, then expression of this IL-1 species may be important in the lung where a systemic inflammatory effect would be undesirable. In the periphery, the effects of

IL-1 may need to be of a more systemic nature thus IL-1ß, being the predominant secreted form, may be of greater importance.

These results suggest that there may be separate mechanisms regulating the expression of the two IL-1 genes depending on the microenvironment in which the various IL-1 producing cell types reside. This differential expression may provide some insight into the specific physiological roles of the two IL-1 species.

REFERENCES

Fuhlbrigge RC, Chaplin DD, Kiely J-M, Unanue ER (1987). Regulation of interleukin 1 gene expression by adherence and lipopolysaccharide. J. Immunol. 138:3799-3802.
Gery I, Gershon RK, Waksman BH (1972). Potentiation of cultured mouse thymocyte responses by factors released by peripheral blood leukocytes. J. Immunol. 107:1778-1780.
Killian PL, Kafka KL, Stern AS, Woehle D, Benjamin WR, Dechiara TM, Gubler U, Farrar JJ, Mizel SB, Lomedico PT (1986). Interleukin 1α and interleukin 1ß bind to the same receptor on T cells. J. Immunol. 136:4509-4514.
Kurt-Jones EA, Fiers W, Pober JS (1987). Membrane interleukin 1 induction on human endothelial cells and dermal fibroblasts. J. Immunol. 139:2317-2324.
March CJ, Mosely B, Larsen A, Cerretti DP, Braedt G, Price V, Gillis S, Henney CS, Kronheim SR, Grabstein K, Conlon PJ, Hopp TP, Cosman D (1985). Cloning, sequence, and expression of two distinct human interleukin 1 complementary DNAs. Nature 315:641-647.
Oppenheim JJ, Kovacs EA, Matsushima K, Durum SK (1986). There is more than one interleukin 1. Immunol. Today 7:45-56.
Rupp EA, Cameron PM, Ranawat CS, Schmidt JA, Bayne EK (1986). Specific bioactivities of monocyte-derived interleukin 1α and interleukin 1ß are similar to each other on cultured murine thymocytes and on cultured human connective tissue. J. Clin. Invest. 78:836-839.

Monokines and Other Non-Lymphocytic Cytokines, pages 83–88

TRANSCRIPTION AND TRANSLATION OF IL-1α AND IL-1β GENES IN THE PRESENCE OF THE GLUCOCORTICOID HORMONE DEXAMETHASONE.

Peter R. Young, Daria. J. Hazuda, Janice R. Connor, and Barbara J. Dalton.
Departments of Molecular Genetics and Immunology, Smith Kline & French Laboratories, King of Prussia, Pa. 19406-0939.

INTRODUCTION.

Glucocorticoid hormones have significant immunosuppressive and anti-inflammatory properties, a finding which has led to wide clinical use (Cupps and Fauci, 1982, Fahey et. al., 1981). Until recently, the molecular basis for this activity was not fully appreciated. However, it has now been shown that the production of a number of T cell derived lymphokines, including IL-2, IL-3, GM-CSF and IFN-γ, are suppressed by the synthetic glucocorticoid analogue dexamethasone (Gillis et. al., 1979, Culpepper and Lee, 1987). In common with many other glucocorticoid effects, this inhibition is manifested at the mRNA level (Culpepper and Lee, 1987).

Given its apparently central role in stimulating immune and inflammatory responses (Dinarello, 1984, Oppenheim et. al., 1986), it would be logical if interleukin-1 (IL-1) production were also inhibited by glucocorticoids. Indeed, Snyder and Unanue (1982) found that glucocorticoids reduced the amount of IL-1 activity secreted from activated mouse macrophages. We wished to examine if this was true for human monocytes, and if so, at what molecular level this regulation occurred. This is of particular interest because of the recent finding that TNFα, another macrophage product, is inhibited at both the transcriptional and translational levels (Beutler et. al., 1986).

MATERIALS AND METHODS.

Human peripheral blood monocytes were prepared from Red Cross buffy coats by centrifugation through Ficoll and Percoll gradients, and attachment to plastic culture dishes. Attached cells, cultured in RPMI1640 and 1% human AB serum, were pretreated 2h with or without dexamethasone before activation with 10ng/ml E. coli LPS in the continued presence or absence of dexamethasone. RNA and protein samples were prepared and analyzed via standard methods (Maniatis et. al., 1982; Griswold et. al., 1986) using cDNAs and polyclonal rabbit antisera specific for IL-1α and IL-1β. IL-1 activity was determined in an EL-4 thymoma cell assay (Simon et. al., 1985).

RESULTS.

When human peripheral blood monocytes are activated with LPS, IL-1 synthesis and secretion are induced. As shown in Table 1, addition of increasing amounts of dexamethasone resulted in a dose-dependent suppression of IL-1 activity in monocyte supernatants sampled 18h after activation.

TABLE I:
EFFECT OF DEXAMETHASONE ON SECRETED IL-1 ACTIVITY.

Treatment		IL-1 activity	
10ng/ml LPS	dexamethasone	units/ml	% control
-	-	1	0
+	-	769	100
+	10^{-9}M	580	75
+	10^{-7}M	530	69
+	10^{-5}M	215	28

Pulse-chase studies with ^{35}S methionine show that IL-1β, the most abundant form of IL-1 secreted from monocytes (Oppenheim et. al, 1986), is synthesized as a 31kd intracellular precursor and secreted as a mixture of the precursor and the mature, active 17kd form (Figure 1). Treatment with dexamethasone reduces the amount of

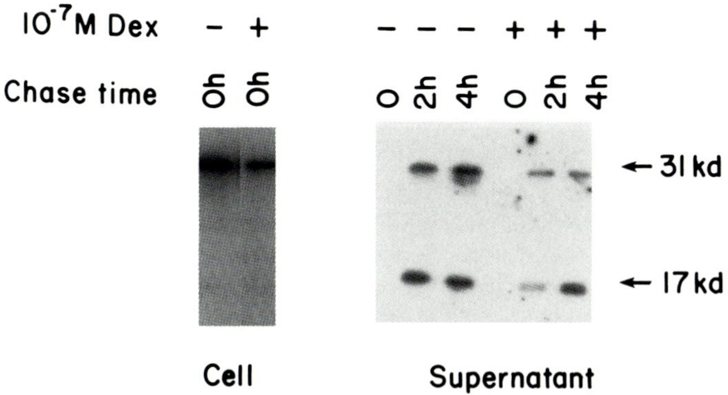

Figure 1. Kinetics of IL-1 synthesis, secretion and processing. Human monocytes were activated with 10 ng/ml LPS for 2h in the presence or absence of dex, pulse labelled with ^{35}S methionine for 1h (t = 0h), then chased with non-radioactive amino acids for the times indicated. IL-1β was detected in cells and supernatants via immunoprecipitation and SDS-PAGE.

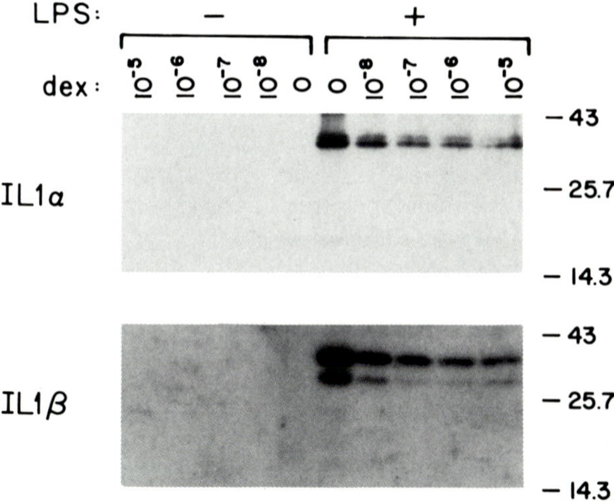

Figure 2. Intracellular accumulation of IL-1. Western blot of cell lysates from human monocytes incubated 20h with (+) or without (−) 10 ng/ml LPS and various concentrations of dexamethasone.

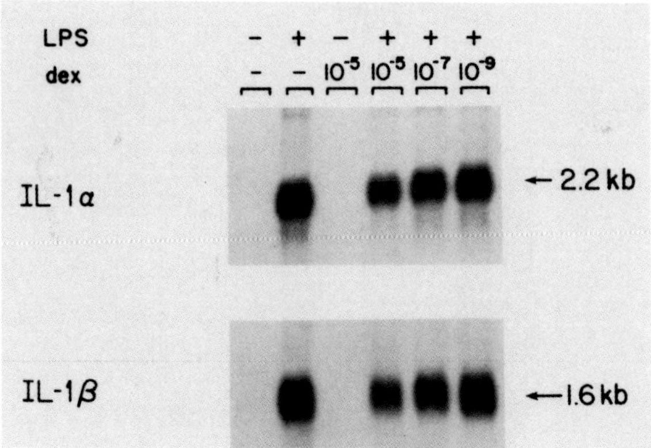

Figure 3.   Northern blot of total RNA isolated from human
monocytes incubated 4h with (+) or without (-) 10 ng/ml
LPS and various concentrations of dexamethasone.

intracellular IL-1β made, with no additional effect on
processing or secretion. Analysis of the effect of
increasing dexamethasone concentration on both
intracellular IL-1 protein accumulation and mRNA levels
shows clearly that the reduction of secreted IL-1
activity is mediated solely by changes in mRNA levels
(Figures 2 and 3). This is true for both IL-1α and
IL-1β. Time course studies indicated that this
inhibition was observed throughout the first 18h of
activation (data not shown).

     To understand whether the reduction in IL-1 activity
was due to a generalized reduction in synthesis by all
cells or a reduction in the number of secreting cells, we
examined activated human monocytes via indirect
immunofluorescence with antiserum to rIL-1β (see Hazuda
et. al., this volume). Quantitation of the stained cells
in several different fields of view shows that the
percentage of fluorescing cells decreases approximately 3
fold upon treatment with dexamethasone (Table II). Thus,
dexamethasone reduces the number of IL-1 synthesizing
cells.

TABLE II:
Quantitation of IL-1β expression in activated monocytes

Dexamethasone Concentration	% cells stained*
no	56.0% ± 13.8%
10^{-7}M	19.4% ± 1.0%
10^{-6}M	19.5% ± 1.0%

*Indirect immunofluorescent detection of IL-1β was
achieved using polyclonal anti-rIL-1β rabbit antisera
followed by FITC labelled goat anti-rabbit IgG.

DISCUSSION.

We have shown that physiological concentrations of
dexamethasone inhibit IL-1 production via a 2-3 fold
inhibition at the mRNA level. This is due, at least in
part, to a reduction in the number of IL-1 synthesizing
cells, which in turn is probably due to regulation of
transcription, since the induction of IL-1 by LPS is
mediated at this level (Fenton et. al., 1987). This
would also match the observations with TNFα (Beutler et.
al., 1986). Whether this suppression occurs directly at
the level of the IL-1 genes or through some intermediate
activating factor(s) is an issue for further study.
Unlike TNFα, we find no evidence of additional
translational regulation of IL-1 by dexamethasone
(Beutler et. al., 1986). This inhibition of IL-1, along
with the inhibition of other lymphokines, helps us to
understand the anti-inflammatory action of
glucocorticoids.

REFERENCES

Beutler, B., Krochin, N., Milsark, I.W., Luedke, C.,
    Cerami, A. (1986). Control of Cachetin (Tumor
    Necrosis Factor) Synthesis: Mechanisms of Endotoxin
    Resistance. Science 232:977-980.
Culpepper J., and Lee, F. (1987). Glucocorticoid
    Regulation of Lymphokine Production by Murine T

lymphocytes. Lymphokines 13:275-289.
Cupps T.R., and Fauci, A.S. (1982).
    Corticosteroid-Mediated Immunoregulation in Man.
    Immunological Rev. 65:133.
Dinarello, C.A. (1984). Interleukin-1. Rev. Infect.
    Diseas. 6:51-95.
Fahey, J.V., Guyre, P.M., and Munck, A. (1981).
    Mechanisms of Antiinflammatory Actions of
    Glucocorticoids. Adv. Inflammation Res. 2:21-51.
Fenton, M.J., Clark, B.D., Collins, K.L., Webb, A.C.,
    Rich, A., and Auron, P.E. (1987). Transcriptional
    Regulation of the Human Prointerleukin-1β gene. J.
    Immun. 138:3972-3979.
Gillis, S., Crabtree, G.R., and Smith, K.A. (1979).
    Glucocorticoid-induced inhibition of T cell growth
    factor production. J. Immun. 123:1624-1631.
Griswold, D.E., Hillegas, L., Antell, L., Shatzman, A.
    and Hanna, N. (1986). Quantitative Western blot
    assay for measurement of the murine acute phase
    reactant, serum amgloid P component. J. Immun. Meth.
    91:163-168.
Maniatis, T., Fritsch, E.F., and Sambrook, J. (1982).
    Molecular Cloning, A Laboratory Manual. Cold Spring
    Harbor Laboratory, 1-545.
Oppenheim, J.J., Kovacs, E., Matsushima, K., and Durum,
    S.K. (1986). There is more than one Interleukin 1.
    Immun. Today. 7:45-56.
Simon, P.L., Laydon, J.T., and Lee, J.C. (1985). A
    modified assay for Interleukin-1 (IL-1). J. Immun.
    Meth. 84: 85-94.
Snyder, D.S. and Unanue, E.R. 1982. Corticosteroids
    inhibit Murine Macrophage Ia expression and
    Interleukin 1 Production. J. Immun. 129:1803-1805.

Monokines and Other Non-Lymphocytic Cytokines, pages 89–93
© 1988 Alan R. Liss, Inc.

DETECTION OF IL-1 GENE EXPRESSION BY IN-SITU HYBRIDIZATION
HYSTOCHEMISTRY:TISSUE LOCALIZATION OF IL-1 mRNA   IN THE
NORMAL C57BL/6 MOUSE

Laszlo Takacs[1], Elizabeth J. Kovacs[1,3], Mark R.
Smith[2], Howard A. Young[1] and Scott K. Durum[1]

[1]Laboratory of Molecular Immunoregulation,
National Cancer Institute, [2]Program Resources
Inc., Frederick MD., [3]present address:Loyola
University, Chicago IL.

INTRODUCTION
     Interleukin-1 (IL-1) is a cytokine with many
activities, including induction of prostaglandins,
proteolytic enzymes and procoagulant activities. Accordingly
the target cells of IL-1 actions are heterogeneous and
include T cells, B cells, fibroblasts, muscle cells,
osteoclasts, epithelial cells, and hematopoietic stem cells
(see reviews 1,2). Molecular cloning of human, murine and
rabbit IL-1 genes (2-6) supported the previous observation
that IL-1 exists in two forms: IL-1 alpha (pI:5) and IL-1
beta (pI:7) are encoded by different genes.
        Most of the knowledge of IL-1 production and IL-1
action is derived from in vitro studies. Given the powerful
inflammatory and immunological effects of IL-1 and
considering the many cell types that can produce IL-1 in
vitro, it is important to determine which cells if any,
produce IL-1 in vivo, and under which circumstances.
Therefore we examined the tissue distribution of cells
expressing IL-1 mRNAs in different organs of the C57BL/6
mouse, kept under pathogen free but otherwise normal
conditions. IL-1 mRNA producing cells were directly
visualized by in-situ hybridization in tissue sections.

MATERIALS AND METHODS
     Tissue sections: C57BL/6 mice were bred in our
disease-free colony.Following carbon dioxide asphyxiation,
different organs were removed and frozen in liquid nitrogen.

Frozen tissues were kept at -70° C. Tissue sections
(7 micron) were cut in a Slee cryostat, placed on microscope
slides and immediately fixed (see below).

Cell suspensions: Cells were attached to poly-L-lysine
coated slides as described previously (7) and further
processed in a similar way to tissue sections.

Fixation storage and rehydration: Methods were adapted
from Lawrence and Singer (1985). Sections were fixed 5 min.
in 4% paraformaldehyde/5mM $MgCl_2$/PBS/pH:7.4. Slides were
stored up to two weeks in 70% ethanol at 4°C. Rehydration
consisted of three sequential ten minute baths consisting
of: 1.) 5mM $MgCl_2$/PBS   2.) 0.1 M glycine /0.2 M TRIS-HCL
(pH:7.4) 3.) 50% formamide/5x SSC. Slides were than
prehybridized and hybridized as described below.

Probes: A 1.2 Kb cDNA probe for human IL-1 alpha and a
1.1 Kb cDNA probe for human IL-1 beta or a control 2.7 Kb
PUC plasmid, were ^{32}P labelled by random oligonucleotide
priming using an Oligolabelling kit (Pharmacia).

In situ hybridization: Slides were prehybridized for
four hours at 37° C using ten μl of the following solution
under a glass coverslip: 50% formamide /0.02% (ficoll,
polyvinylpyrollidone, BSA) /1% glycine /5xSSC/50 mM $NaPO_4$
(pH:6.5) /0.5 mg/ml tRNA. Slides were rinsed in the third
rehydration buffer. A probe mixture was added consisting of
the probe (200,000 cpm/slide), salmon sperm DNA (70 ug/ml),
E.coli tRNA (250 ug/ml), formamide (50%) and SSC
(3x). After boiling 10 min, Denhart's solution (1x) was
added and while still hot, 10 μl of the probe mixture was
added to the section under a glass coverslip. Hybridization
proceeded for 4 hours at 37^0 C. Slides were washed in three
sequential 30 min baths at 25°C: 1.) 1x SSC, 2.) 50%
formamide/ 1x SSC, 3.) 1xSSC. Sections were prepared for
autoradiography using NT-B2 emulsion (Kodak), developed
after 4 days and stained with hematoxylin-eosin.

RESULTS AND DISCUSSION

This in-situ hybridization technique proved useful to
readily visualize single cells hybridizing with IL-1 probes.
The hybridization reaction was sufficienly intense to result
in 10-100 silver grains deposited over single cells
(compared to controls). The hybridization was specific because the PUC probe showed no binding to the sections and the
hybridization of the IL-1 probes could be specifically inhibited by 200x excess of unlabelled probes.

The analysis of a variety of tissues is summarized in the table. In general ; IL-1 alpha and beta showed a similar pattern of hybridization in all cases except the skin where epidermal cell labelling was observed with the IL-1 alpha probe but not IL-1 beta probe. Based on these obsevations it is likely that the cells which produce IL-1 alpha produce IL-1 beta as well. However, since double hybridization was not possible, this point remains unproven.

Many organs contained IL-1 mRNA positive cells, but the largest number of IL-1 mRNA positive cells were found in the lymphoid organs. The distribution and localization of these cells suggests that they are tissue macrophages. IL-1 mRNA positive cells were present in organs that are exposed to enviromental antigens and microbial products (lymph nodes, liver, intestine, lung, uterus), suggesting that IL-1 might be involved in local inflammatory or immune responses in vivo. The presence of IL-1 in the thymus and in the bone marrow suggests that IL-1 has a physiological role in heamatopoietic and T cell differentiation. In the future the ability to detect IL-1 mRNA by in-situ hybridization will be useful in understanding the pathogenesis of certain diseases, and as a diagnostic tool.

TABLE

Tissues	Reactions
Lymphoid tissues	
Thymus	+ cortico/medullary border,medulla
Spleen	+ scattered in the red pulp,very few cells in the white pulp, positive cells in the white pulp are located in the periarteriolar lymphatic sheat
Lymph nodes	+ sinuses, paracortical areas
Peyer's patches	+ interfollicular areas
Bone marrow	+ scattered large cells,stromal cells?

(table continued)
Non lymphoid tissues

Brain	-	(only IL-1 alpha mRNA was examined)
Lung	+	few scattered cells
Heart	-	
Large blood vessels	-	
Endothelium	-	
Liver	+	scattered cells in the sinusoids, Kupffer cells?
Digestive tract	+	scattered cells in stroma of intestinal villi
Kidney	+	very few cells in the medullary area no positive cells were found in the glomeruli
Testis	-	
Ovary	-	
Uterus	+	high level of IL-1 mRNA, positive cells are in the highly cellular subepithelial connective tissue of the endometrium
Pancreas	-	
Suprarenal gland	-	
Thyroid gland	-	
Skin	+	few cells in the epidermal layer, scattered cells in the dermal layer.
Skeletal muscle	-	
Smooth muscle	-	
Cartilage	-	
Immature bone	+	few cells in the cartilage resorption zone of chondrogeneous ossification

REFERENCES

1. Durum,S.K., J.A.Schmidt. and J.J.Oppenheim.1985.
Interleukin 1: an immunological perspective. Ann.Rev.
Immunol. 3:263.

2. Oppenheim,J.J., E.J.Kovacs, K.Matsushima. and
S.K.Durum.1986. There is more than one Interleukin 1.
Immunology Today 7:45.

3. Lodmedico,P.T., U.Gubler, C.P.Hellmann, M.Dukovich,
J.G.Giri, Y.C.E.Pan, K.Collier, R.Seminow, A.O.Chua and
S.B.Mizel 1984. Cloning and expression of interleukin-1 cDNA
in Eschrichia coli. Nature 312:18.

4. Auron,P.E., A.C.Webb, L.J.Rosenwasser, S.F.Mucci,
A.Rich, S.M.Wolff. and C.A.Dinarello.1984. Nucleotide
sequence of human monocyte interleukin-1 precursor
cDNA.Proc.Natl.Acad.Sci.USA 81:7907

5. March.C.J., B.Mosley, A.Larsen, D.P.Ceretti, G.Braedt,
V.Price, S.Gillis, C.S.Henney , S.R.Kronheim, K.Grabstein,
P.J.Conton, T.P.Hopp and D.Cosman.1985. Cloning, sequence
and expression of two distinct human interleukin-1
complementary DNAs. Nature 315:641.

6. Furutani,Y., M.Notake, M.Yamayoshi, J.Yamagishi,
H.Nomura, M.Ohue, R.Furuta, T.Fukui, M.Yamada and S.Nakamura
1985. Cloning and characterisation of cDNAs for human and
rabbit interleukin-1 precursor
Nucleic Acids Res., 13:5869.

7. Tartakovsky,B., E.J.Kovacs, L.Takacs, and S.K.Durum
1986. T cell clone producing an IL-1 like activity following
stimulation by antigen-presenting B cells. J.Immunol.
137:160.

Section III. Regulation of Synthesis/Release of Cytokines

Monokines and Other Non-Lymphocytic Cytokines, pages 97–100
© 1988 Alan R. Liss, Inc.

THE KINETICS OF IL1 SECRETION FROM ACTIVATED MONOCYTES - DIFFERENCES BETWEEN IL1α AND IL1β

Daria Hazuda, John Lee and Peter Young

Departments of Molecular Genetics and Immunology
and Anti-infectives Therapy, Smith Kline &
French Laboratories, King of Prussia, PA 19406

INTRODUCTION

Upon activation with lipopolysaccharide (LPS),
monocytes synthesize and secrete large amounts of
interleukin 1 (IL1). Two separate genes for IL1 have
been cloned and shown to encode the two known pI species
of IL1, α and β, pI 5 and 7 respectively (March, 1985;
Auron, 1984; Furutani, 1985; Lomedico, 1984).

Both IL1's are synthesized as larger precursor
proteins of 31 kD which are processed to the mature 17 kD
form (Giri, 1985; Limjuco, 1986). Precursor IL1α is
biologically active, whereas precursor IL1β is not
(Moseley, 1987). Neither IL1 encodes a classic
hydrophobic signal sequence for secretion (Oppenheim,
1986). We have undertaken pulse-chase experiments on
LPS-activated monocytes to investigate the processing and
secretion of IL1α and β.

METHODS

Human peripheral blood monocytes were prepared from
Red Cross buffy coats. Attached cells were activated
with 10 ng/ml E. coli LPS in 1% fetal bovine serum for 2
h prior to metabolic labelling with 200 μCi
^{35}S-methionine and 100 μCi ^{35}S-cysteine (Amersham)
for 1 h. Cells were washed and then chased in
non-radioactive medium. Cell lysates and supernatants
were analyzed by immunoprecipitation with polyclonal

rabbit antisera specific for IL1α or IL1β.

RESULTS AND DISCUSSION

Polyclonal antisera generated against either
recombinant IL1α or β could distinguish the two
isoelectric forms in immunoprecipitations of
LPS-activated monocyte lysates and supernatants. As
shown in Fig. 1A and B, no processed IL1 (α or β) is
detected in cell lysates. Both the 31 and 17 kD forms of
IL1β are present, however, in the media (Fig. 1C and D),
indicating that processing is not required for
secretion.

No precursor-product relationship is apparent between
the secreted 31 and 17 kD forms of IL1β; the kinetics of
their appearance and accumulation in the media are nearly
identical (Fig. 2A). The relative amounts of the 17 and
31 kD forms remain constant throughout each experiment
(Fig. 2b). In addition, 31 kD IL1β added to monocyte
cultures is not processed (data not shown). Processing
and secretion are, therefore, intimately coordinated.

The kinetics of IL1 secretion is unique in comparison
with other secreted proteins; release of IL1 is delayed.
As demonstrated by immunofluorescence, large pools of IL1
accumulate intracellularly (Fig. 3). The intracellular
half-lives of IL1α and IL1β are 15 and 2.5 h,
respectively. The discrepancy in the half-lives is a
reflection of the different kinetics with which IL1α and
β are secreted. IL1β is released continuously beginning
2 h after synthesis (Fig. 1D), whereas the secretion of
IL1α is delayed for an additional 10 h (Fig. 1C). The
unique kinetics of secretion demonstrated for IL1α and β
suggests that the release of each pI series is controlled
by a selective mechanism(s), which is distinct from the
classical signal directed pathway via the endoplasmic
reticulum. The observation that greater than 50% of the
IL1β synthesized is released (Fig. 2A), demonstrates that
secretion of IL1 is a relatively efficient process
incompatible with leakage due to compromised cell
viability.

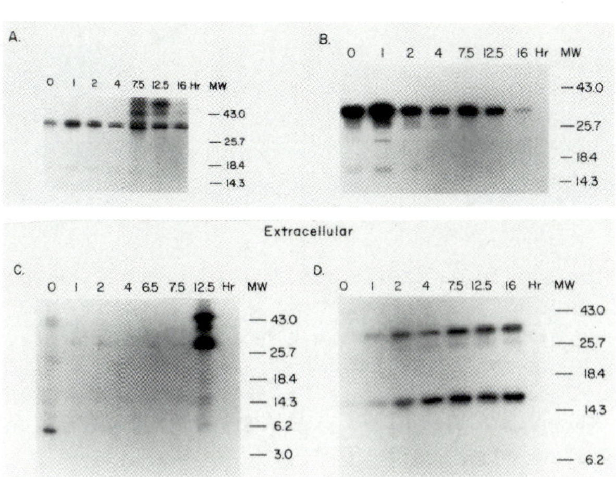

Fig. 1: Pulse Chase of Intracellular and Extracellular
IL1α and β.
Monocytes were pulse-labelled and then chased with
non-radioactive media for the times indicated. Cell
lysates (A and B) and supernatants (C and D) were
analyzed by immunoprecipitation with antisera specific
for either IL1α (A and C) or IL1β (B and D).

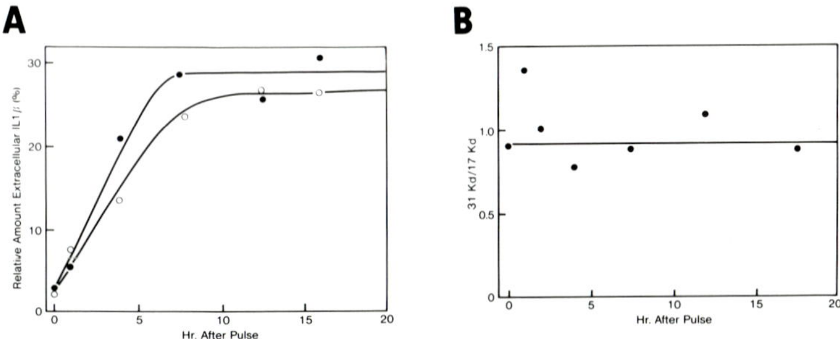

Fig. 2: Quantitation of Secreted 31 and 17 kD IL1β.
Autoradiograms of the secreted 31 kD (o--o) and 17 kD
(●--●) IL1β as in Fig. 1D were quantitated by
densitometry and then expressed as a mol percent of the
IL1β present in the cell at the 1 h chase time (maximal
incorporation). The relative amount of each IL1β (Fig.
2A) or the ratio of the two forms (Fig. 2B) is graphed as
a function of chase-time.

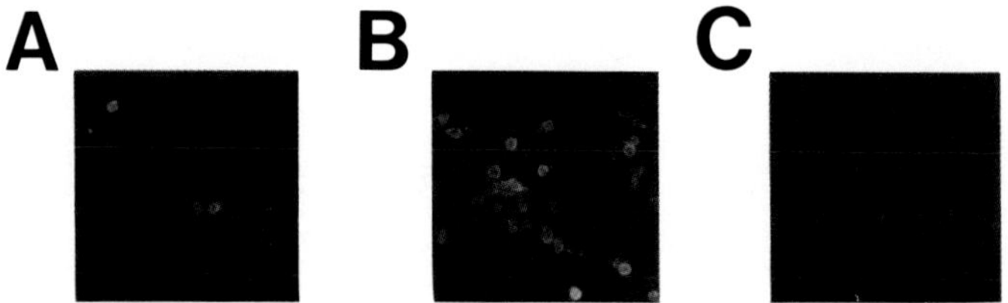

Fig. 3: Immunofluorescence of IL1β in Monocytes.
Indirect immunofluorescence of IL1β was performed using
polyclonal anti-rIL1β rabbit antisera, followed by
FITC-labelled goat - anti-rabbit IgG. Fig. 3A, monocytes
prior to LPS-activation; 3B, after LPS-activation; 3C,
same as in 3B except that anti-rIL1β antisera was
pre-incubated with 2 µg of rIL1β.

REFERENCES

Auron PE, Webb AC, Rosenwasser LJ, Mucci SF, Rich A, Wolff
    SM, Dinarello CA (1984). Proc Natl Acad Sci 81:
    7907-7911.
Furutani Y, Notake M, Yamayoshi M, Yamagishi JI, Nomura H,
    Ohue M, Ruruta R, Fukui Y, Yamada M, Nakamura S
    (1985). Nucl Acids Res 13: 5869-5882.
Giri JG, Lomedico PT, Mizel SB (1985). J Immun 134:
    343-349.
Limjuco G, Galuska S, Chin J, Cameron P, Boger J, Schmidt
    JA (1986). Proc Natl Acad Sci 83: 3972-3976.
Lomedico PT, Gubler U, Hellman CP, Dukovich M, Giri JG,
    Pan Y-CE, Collier K, Semionow R, Chua AO, Mizel S
    (1984). Nature 312: 458-462.
March CJ, Mosley B, Larsen A, Cerretti DP, Braedt G,
    Price V, Guillis S, Henney CS, Kronheim SR, Grabstein
    K, Conlon PJ, Hopp TP, Cosman D (1985). Nature 315:
    641-647.
Moseley B, Urdal DL, Prickett KS, Larsen A, Cosman D,
    Conlon PJ, Gillis S, Dower SK (1987). J Biol Chem 262:
    2941-2944.
Oppenheim JJ, Kovacs E, Matsushima K, Durum SK (1986).
    Immun Today 8: 46-51.

Monokines and Other Non-Lymphocytic Cytokines, pages 101–107
© 1988 Alan R. Liss, Inc.

A PLASMA MEMBRANE ANCHORING MECHANISM FOR IL-1

Dan T. Brody and Scott K. Durum

Biological Carcinogenesis Development
Program, Program Resources, Inc., and
Laboratory of Molecular Immunoregulation, BRMP,
NCI-Frederick Cancer Research Facility,
Frederick, MD 21701

INTRODUCTION

In the macrophage, LPS stimulation results in the
initial appeearence of pro-IL-1 in the cytoplasm (Giri et
al., 1985). A plasma membrane-associated biological
activity (membrane IL-1) can be detected (Kurt-Jones et
al., 1985) in close temporal association with the
accumulation of intracellular pro-IL-1. IL-1 then appears
extracellularly, first as pro-IL-1, and then later as the
mature 17 kDa molecule. However, the export of IL-1 is
never fully complete, since a significant portion of the
IL-1 biological activity always remains associated with the
cell (both plasma membrane and cytoplasm). This subcellular
distribution is unusual for a released protein. Most
cellular proteins destined for export follow the
conventional pathway established for secreted proteins,
they are synthesized on bound ribosomes and enter the
endoplasmic reticulum via their signal sequence, moving
through the golgi apparatus to secretory vesicles. IL-1 is
anomolous in this respect, since it lacks a signal
sequence, does not appear to associate with the endoplasmic
reticulum, and is yet released from the cell. The existence
of a plasma membrane-associated form of IL-1 is also
puzzling, since the cDNA deduced amino acid sequence does
not predict a membrane-spanning hydrophobic region
(Lomedico et al., 1984) (see figure 1).

Membrane IL-1 was first described as an IL-1 biological activity associated with intact stimulated mouse macrophages that had been lightly fixed in paraformaldehyde, and with purified plasma membrane preparations (Kurt-Jones et al., 1985). Since this initial observation, membrane IL-1 has been demonstrated as an IL-1 biological activity released from intact stimulated human macrophages by trypsin proteolysis (Matsushima et al., 1986), and recently by immunoflouresence using an anti-IL-1 alpha antisera (Conlon, 1987). Beuscher et al. recently identified murine membrane IL-1 as pro-IL-1 alpha, based on cell-surface iodination and immunoprecipitation (Beuscher et al., 1987).

Little is known about the biochemical mechanism involved in the anchoring of IL-1 to the plasma membrane. Although IL-1 behaves as an integral membrane protein by some criteria (failure to elute in high salt, failure to elute at low pH, and dissociation from the plasma membrane by mild detergent or proteolysis) it is difficult to postulate a mechanism wherein such a highly hydrophilic molecule could actually integrate into the lipid bilayer of the plasma membrane. One possible mechanism that has been suggested is that IL-1 might be anchored through a glycolipid linkage, like Thy-1 and decay accelerating factor (DAF). However, recent studies indicate that the attachment of a glycolipid anchor to these membrane proteins occurs in the RER after the removal of a conventional C-terminal transmembrane region (Cross, 1987). Pro-IL-1 does not appear to be associated with the RER (Bakouche et al., 1987), (as predicted by its lack of a signal peptide), and does not have a membrane-integrating region within its sequence. This argues against a glycolipid anchoring mechanism for membrane IL-1. Another possible mechanism that has been explored is that pro-IL-1 might somehow have an affinity for the plasma membrane, and spontaneously associate with it. Alternatively, it might associate first with a carrier protein that integrates into the plasma membrane. Bakouche et al. showed that lysates from stimulated human monocytes (a potent source of intracellular pro-IL-1) contain a biological activity that can associate with liposomes (Bakouche et al., 1987), lending support to such hypotheses.

IL-1 biological activity has been found (in a biologically latent form activated by trypsin) in

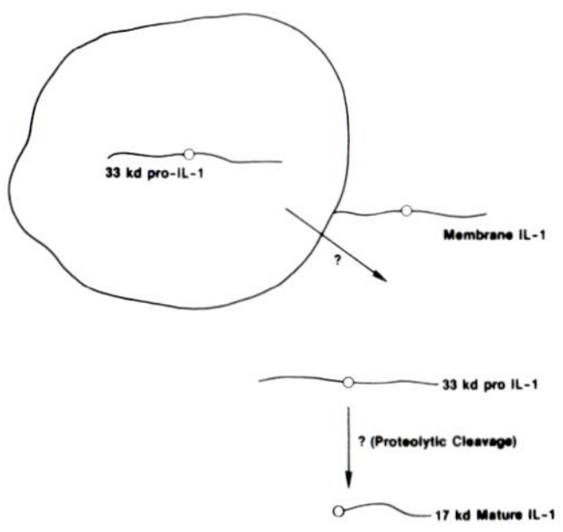

FIGURE 1. Schematic of IL-1 alpha synthesis showing the intracellular, membrane, and soluble forms of IL-1 alpha.

FIGURE 2. Proposed anchoring of glycosylated pro-IL-1 alpha to the plasma membrane via a lectin -like interaction with a carrier molecule.

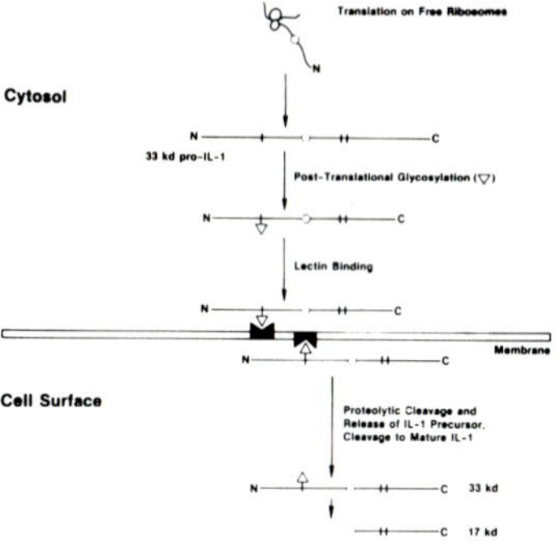

association with lysosomes (Bakouche et al., 1987). It is well known that nascent proteins destined for the lysosomes are sorted by virtue of a high-mannose oligosaccharide marker that is recognized by a mannose-specific, lectin-like receptor (Sly and Fischer, 1982). These mannosylated proteins are segregated to the lysosomes. Perhaps pro-IL-1, like these lysosomal proteins, is glycosylated and recognized by a membrane-bound lectin-like receptor. This lectin-like association would thus provide both an IL-1 release pathway and a membrane anchoring mechanism (see figure 2).

RESULTS

If pro-IL-1 is associated with the plasma membrane by
a lectin-like interaction, it should be possible to elute
IL-1 from intact stimulated macrophages with the
appropriate carbohydrate. Table 1 shows the results of
incubating LPS-stimulated macrophages with the
monosaccharides D-mannose or D-fucose at 4° C in PBS.
Trypsin and PBS were included as positive and negative
controls, respectively. The resulting supernatants were
dialyzed free of carbohydrate, and the IL-1 content
measured by the thymocyte co-mitogenicity assay. It is
clear that mannose, and not fucose, liberates IL-1
biological activity from intact LPS-stimulated macrophages.
To demonstrate that the eluted material was derived from
the plasma membrane, LPS-stimulated macrophages were
treated with D-mannose or D-fucose, fixed in 1%
paraformaldehyde, and assayed for membrane IL-1 biological
activity. As shown in table 1, mannose depletes the
stimulated macrophage of membrane IL-1, whereas fucose does
not.

TABLE 1. Elution of Membrane IL-1 Activity by D-mannose.

macrophage treatment	released IL-1	membrane IL-1
none	3,376(622)	N.D.
0.5 M mannose	20,782(4,084)	13,130(1022)
0.5 M fucose	6,153(188)	33,177(1619)
trypsin	17,834(4,291)	N.D.

If the export of IL-1 is mediated by a lectin-like
receptor that binds a glycosylated form of pro-IL-1,
inhibiting glycosylation should likewise inhibit IL-1
release from the stimulated macrophage. Table 2 shows the
results of incubating resident mouse macrophages with LPS
and increasing concentrations of the glycosylation
inhibitor 2-deoxyglucose. After treatment, the samples were
dialyzed to remove the inhibitor, and the IL-1 content was
measured by the D10 assay. In the presence of inhibitor,
the level of cell-associated IL-1 activity increases in a
dose-dependent manner. The IL-1 activity released into the
supernatant decreased in response to the inhibitor,
demonstrating that IL-1 release is impaired if
glycosylation is inhibited.

TABLE 2. Effect of 2-deoxyglucose on IL-1 Release.

	IL-1 activity	
inhibitor	cell-associated	released
none	14,747(488)	19,533(940)
1 ug/ml	20,184(956)	16,702(1,810)
10 ug/ml	28,635(2,849)	14,633(2,105)
100 ug/ml	29,850(7,828)	9,213(1,921)

The biochemical nature of membrane IL-1 was characterized by briefly trypsinizing intact LPS-stimulated macrophages and subjecting the supernatant to immunoprecipitation with an anti-mouse IL-1 alpha antiserum (a gift from Dr. W. Benjamin of Hoffman-LaRoche, Nutley, NJ). The macrophages were shown to be completely viable by trypan blue exclusion following the trypsinization procedure. As shown in figure 3, panel A, trypsinization results in the release of a 33 kDa pro-IL-1 (lane 4). In an analogous experiment, LPS-stimulated macrophages were incubated at 4°C in D-mannose, a procedure that results in the release of biologically active IL-1 into the supernatant. The supernatant was subjected to immunoprecipitation as above. As show in figure 3, panel B, mannose also released a 33 kDa pro-IL-1 from intact macrophages (lane 4).

The above experiments suggested that pro-IL-1 alpha is glycosylated in the mouse macrophage. To examine this possibility, LPS-stimulated macrophages were biosynthetically labeled with D-[^{14}C]mannose, and the lysates subjected to immunoprecipitation with anti-mouse IL-1 alpha antiserum. The resulting autoradiogram (figure 4) reveals a doublet around 33 kDa (lane 3), indicating that at least some pro-IL-1 alpha is glycosylated in the mouse macrophage.

In conclusion, we have shown that 1) Membrane IL-1 biological activity is specifically released from intact stimulated macrophages by treatment with mannose, 2) an inhibitor of glycosylation inhibits the release of biologically active IL-1, 3) brief trypsinization releases 33 kDa pro-IL-1 alpha from intact macrophages, 4) a 33 kDa pro-IL-1 alpha is specifically eluted from macrophages by mannose treatment, and 5) pro-IL-1 alpha is glycosylated in

A.

B.

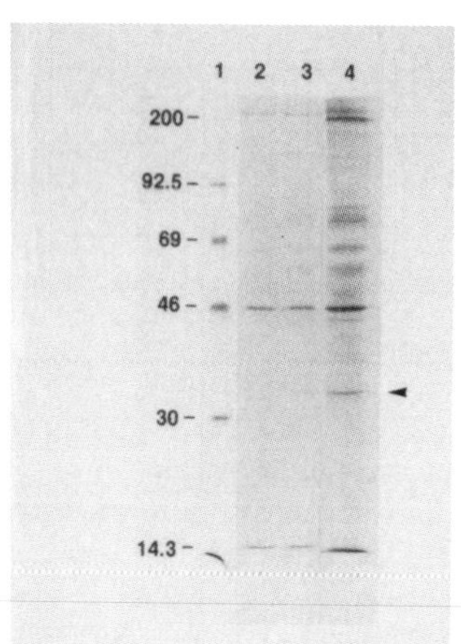

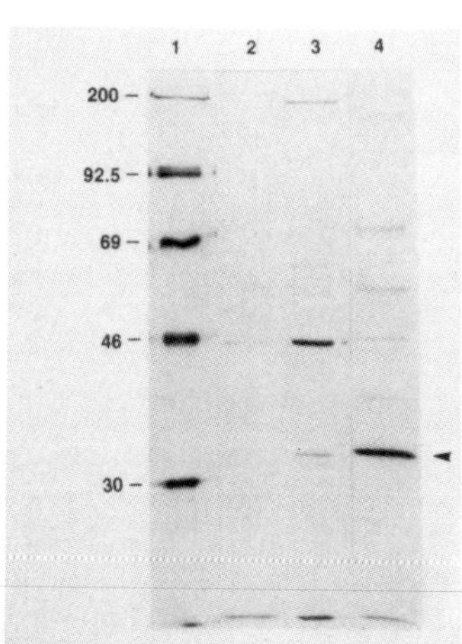

FIGURE 3. Panel A. Brief trypsinization releases a 33 kDa pro-IL-1 alpha (arrow) from LPS-stimulated murine macrophages. Molecular weight markers (lane 1), nonspecific binding control (lane 2), immunoprecipitate of a lysate of LPS-stimulated macrophages (lane 3), and immunoprecipitate of a supernatant generated by the trypsinization of intact LPS-stimulated macrophages (lane 4). Panel B. Mannose elutes a 33 kDa pro-IL-1 alpha (arrow)from intact LPS-stimulated macrophages. Lanes 1,2, and 3 are as in panel A

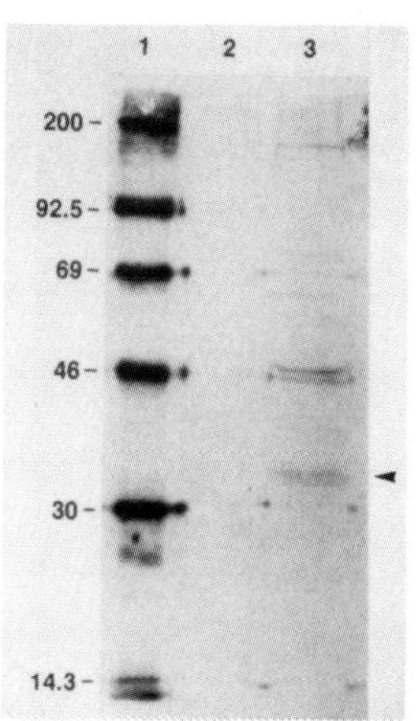

Lane 4 shows the immunoprecipitate of a supernatant generated by treating intact LPS-stimulated macrophages with 0.5 M D-mannose in PBS at 4 °C.

FIGURE 4. Glycosylation of pro-IL-1 alpha in murine macrophages. Nonspecific binding control (lane 2), immunoprecipitate of D-[^{14}C]mannose-labeled 33 kDa pro-IL-1 alpha (arrow) from a lysate of LPS-stimulated macrophages (lane 3).

the LPS-stimulated mouse macrophage. These conclusions
support the hypothesis that membrane IL-1 alpha is anchored
to the plasma membrane via a lectin-like interaction that
is dissociable by mannose.

ACKNOWLEDGEMENTS

Research sponsored, at least in part, by the National
Cancer Institute, DHHS, under contract NO1-CO-74102 with
Program Resources, Incorporated.

REFERENCES

Bakouche O, Brown DC, Lachman, LB (1987). Subcellular
    localization of human monocyte interleukin 1:evidence for
    an inactive precursor molecule and a possible mechanism
    for IL-1 release. J Immunol 138:4249-4255.
Bakouche O, Brown DC, Lachman LB (1987) Liposomes
    expressing IL-1 biological activity. J Immunol 138:4256
    -4262.
Beuscher HU, Fallon RJ, Colten HR (1987). Macrophage
    membrane interleukin 1 regulates the expression of acute
    phase proteins in human hepatoma Hep 3B cells. J Immunol
    139:1896-1901.
Conlon PJ, Grabstein KH, Alpert A, Prickett KS, Hopp TS,
    Gillis S (1987). Localization of human mononuclear cell
    interleukin 1. J Immunol 139:98-102.
Giri JG, Lomedico PT, Mizel SB (1985). Studies on the
    synthesis and secretion of interleukin 1: I. A 33,000
    molecular weight precursor for interleukin 1. J Immunol
    134:343-349.
Kurt-Jones EA, Beller DI, Mizel SB, Unanue ER (1985).
    Identification of a membrane-associated interleukin 1 in
    macrophages. Proc Natl Acad Sci USA 82:1204-1208.
Lomedico PT, Gubler U, Hellman CP, Dukovich M, Giri JG, Pan
    YE, Collier K, Semionow R, Chua AO, Mizel SB (1984).
    Cloning and expression of murine interleukin-1 cDNA in
    Escherichia coli. Nature 312:458-462.
Matsushima K, Taguchi M, Kovacs EJ, Young HA, Oppenheim
    JJ (1986). Intracellular localization of human monocyte
    associated interleukin 1 (IL-1) activity and release of
    biologically active IL-1 from monocytes by trypsin and
    plasmin. J Immunol 136: 2883-2891.
Sly WS, Fischer HD (1982). The phosphomannosyl recognition
    system for intracellular and intercellular transport of
    lysosomal enzymes. J Cell Biochem 18:67-85.

Monokines and Other Non-Lymphocytic Cytokines, pages 109–112
© **1988 Alan R. Liss, Inc.**

AUTOREGULATION OF IL1 PROTEIN PRODUCTION

Jean C Manson, Julian A Symons, Francesco S di Giovine, Stephen Poole*, Gordon W Duff.

University of Edinburgh Dept Medicine, Rheumatic Diseases Unit, Northern General Hospital, Edinburgh, UK. and *NIBSC, Potters Bar, Herts, UK

INTRODUCTION

Interleukin 1 (IL1) is a primary mediator of host response to infection and injury through its ability to regulate proliferation, maturation and function of many cell types. Abnormal regulation of IL1 could therefore lead to pathological states and increasing evidence suggests that IL1 may contribute to the pathogenesis of many autoimmune diseases.

IL1 is the product of at least two genes, IL1 alpha and beta (March et al., 1985). Messenger RNA for IL1 is absent from unstimulated cells but its production is induced by various stimuli such as bacterial endotoxin, urate crystals and other cytokines (Dinarello et al., 1986). Recent reports have also shown that IL1 can induce its own synthesis (Dinarello et al., 1987) which may be important for the potentiation of immune and inflammatory responses. Much less is known about down-regulation of IL1 synthesis but hyperthermia, prostaglandin E and factors from antigen-desensitized guinea pigs have all been shown to reduce IL1 production.

METHODS

We have been studying the autoregulation of IL1 production in human mononuclear cells (HMNC) prepared from healthy individuals by standard procedures. The cells were cultured with either human recombinant (Hr) IL1 alpha or

beta for up to 20hrs. Following incubation, cells and
supernatants were separated and the level of endogenous IL1
beta was assessed by (a) immunoblot analysis (Manson et al.,
1986) (b) radio-immunoassay using a commercially available
kit (Cistron, Biotechnology, Pine Brook, NJ). IL1
bioactivity was measured using EL4/CTLL conversion assay
(Gearing et al., 1987).

RESULTS

      HMNC cultured in the presence of HrIL1 alpha
(0.05-10ng/ml) showed a biphasic response in the production
of endogenous IL1 beta. Immunoblot analysis showed (Figure
1) a stimulation of cell associated IL1 beta at
concentrations of 0.05-0.2ng/ml (HrIL1 alpha) but as the
concentration was increased to 0.5ng/ml an inhibition in the
production of endogenous IL1 beta was observed. As the
concentration of exogenous HrIL1 alpha was further increased
to 1-10ng/ml, a stimulation of cell associated IL1 beta
polypeptides was again observed. A similar biphasic response
was obtained when exogenous HrIL1 beta was added to the
medium although the inhibition of endogenous IL1 beta
production occurred over a wider concentration range
(0.5-5ng/ml).

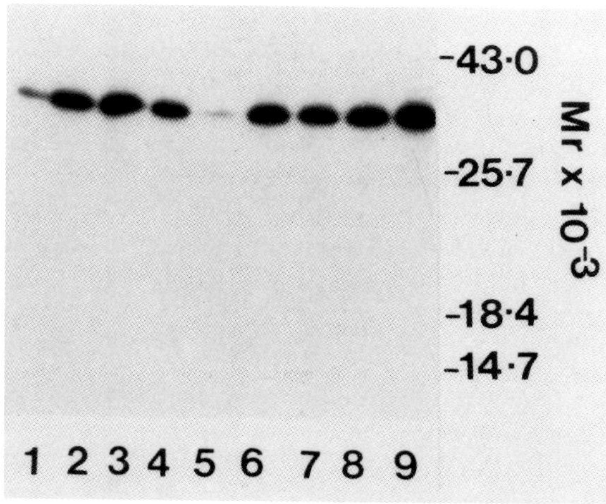

Figure 1   IL1 beta synthesis in response to HrIL1 alpha.
(1) medium alone; (2-9) HrIL1 alpha (0.05, 0.1,
0.2, 0.5, 1.0, 2.0, 5.0, and 10.0ng/ml).

To confirm the immunoblot analysis, ILl alpha and beta were measured by radioimmunoassay (Figure 2) and ILl bioactivity was measured by EL4/CTLL assay (Table 1). These results showed a biphasic response of both ILl alpha and beta production with increasing concentrations of either exogenous HrILl alpha or beta.

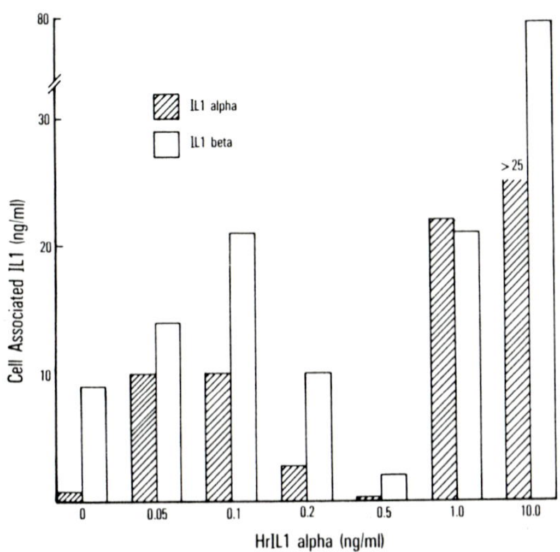

Figure 2   Cell associated ILl alpha and beta measured by radioimmunoassay in HMNC and incubated for 20hrs with HrILl alpha (0.05-10ng/ml)

Measurement of ILl in the supernatants by EL4/CTLL bioassay (not shown) and ILl beta radioimmunoassay (Table 1) confirmed that the decrease in cell associated ILl was not due to extracellular release.

Table 1
Cell associated and extracellular ILl beta (ng/ml) measured by radioimmunoassay in HMNC incubated for 20hrs with HrILl alpha (0.1-10ng/ml)

Exogenous HrILl alpha	Cell Associated ILl beta	Extracellular ILl beta
0	9.0	0.25
0.1	21.2	1.6
0.5	1.7	<0.25
1.0	21.8	1.3
10.0	61.9	3.5

Experiments using specific neutralising antisera established that the stimulation of endogenous IL1 production was due to the recombinant proteins (not shown). To assess the involvement of prostaglandins in the inhibition of endogenous IL1 production, PGE_2 levels were measured in the supernatants by radioimmunoassay (Seragen Inc. Boston, MA.). No increased level of prostaglandins was detected in supernatants where IL1 production was reduced (data not shown) suggesting that the inhibition of IL1 production is not due to increased prostaglandin synthesis. We are presently investigating whether the biphasic response to IL1 production is a property of a single cell population or a result of the interaction of the different populations present in the HMNC preparations. The molecular basis of the down regulation of IL1 production and the involvement of other cytokines in this phenomenon is under study.

REFERENCES

Dinarello CA, Cannon JG, Wolff SM, Bernheim HA, Beutler B, Cerami A, Figari IS, Palladino MA, O'Connor JV. (1986) Tumor necrosis factor (cachectin) is an endogenous pyrogen and induces the production of interleukin 1. J. Exp. Med., 163: 1433-1450.
Dinarello CA, Ikejima T, Warner SJ, Orencole SF, Lonnemann G, Cannon JG, Libby P. (1987). Interleukin 1 induces interleukin 1. J. Immunol. 139: 1902-1910.
Gearing AJH, Bird CR, Bristow A, Poole S, Thorpe R. (1987) A simple bioassay for interleukin 1 which is unresponsive to interleukin 2. J. Immunol. Methods, 99, 7-11.
Manson JC, Liddell AD, Leaver CJ, Murray K. (1986) A protein specific to mitochondria from S-type male sterile cytoplasm of maize is encoded by an episomal DNA. EMBO J. 5: 2775-2780.
March CJ, Mosley B, Larsen A, Cerretti DP, Braedt G, Price V, Gillis S, Henney C, Kronheim SR, Grabstein K, Colon PJ, Hopp TP, Cosman D. (1985). Cloning, sequence and expression of two distinct human interleukin complementary DNAs. Nature 315: 641-647.

Monokines and Other Non-Lymphocytic Cytokines, pages 113–118

MECHANISMS OF INTERFERON-γ AND CYCLOHEXIMIDE ENHANCEMENT OF INTERLEUKIN 1 PRODUCTION IN CULTURED HUMAN MONOCYTES

William P. Arend, Fenneke G. Joslin, Shahid Jameel and Donald B. Carter
Div. of Rheumatology, Dept. of Medicine, Univ. of Colorado Health Sciences Ctr. (W.P.A., F.G.J., S.J.), Denver, CO 80262; Upjohn Company (D.B.C.), Kalamazoo, MI 49001.

INTRODUCTION

Interferon-γ (IFN-γ) alone, in the absence of contaminating bacterial lipopolysaccharides (LPS), does not induce interleukin 1 (IL 1) production in human monocytes. However, IFN-γ augments the stimulatory properties of sub-optimal levels of LPS (Arenzana-Seisdedos et al., 1985). Freshly-isolated human monocytes cultured in vitro for one day or longer display a progressive loss in the ability to produce IL 1 in response to LPS stimulation. The addition of IFN-γ during this culture of monocytes maintains the ability of the cells to produce IL 1 after LPS induction (Arend et al., 1985; Arenzana-Seisdedos et al., 1985). The objective of these studies was to examine the mechanisms whereby IFN-γ maintains LPS-responsiveness for IL 1 production in cultured human monocytes and to assess the possible role of new protein synthesis in regulation of IL 1 production.

MATERIALS AND METHODS

Human mononuclear leukocytes (MNL) were isolated from the EDTA-anticoagulated blood of normal donors and adherent monocytes obtained, as recently described (Arend et al., 1987). In some experiments the MNL were further separated by Percoll gradients before adherence. The adherent cells were cultured in RPMI 1640 medium with 2% low-endotoxin FCS for 24 hr at 37°C in the presence or absence of varying concentrations of IFN-γ or cycloheximide (Cx). To remove the Cx, the cells were washed and soaked three times in RPMI for 40 min each time at 37°C. The adherent cells then were incubated for a further 24 hr in RPMI with 2% FCS and 2 ng/ml LPS. The cell supernatants and lysates were harvested and assayed for IL 1 activity in the murine thymocyte assay, as described (Arend et al., 1987). In some experiments IL 1 protein was measured using a radioimmunoassay kit (Cistron, Pine Brook, NJ). Total cellular RNA was extracted from monocytes cultured under various conditions using standard techniques with guanidine isothiocyanate lysis and cesium chloride gradient centrifugation. Northern blot or slot blot analyses were performed on extracted RNA by in vitro hybridization with specific cDNA probes for human IL 1β and β_2M mRNA or for 28S ribosomal RNA. Transcriptional rate analysis was performed by nuclear run-on techniques and mRNA half-life was determined after stopping transcription by treatment with 5 µg/ml actinomycin D.

RESULTS AND DISCUSSION

IFN-γ and Cycloheximide Effects on IL 1 Production

Monocytes cultured in LPS-free medium for one day exhibited a marked decrease in IL 1 production after a second 24 hr culture with 2 ng/ml LPS. The presence of 100 U/ml IFN-γ during the first day's culture led to a partial to full maintenance of IL 1 production during a second day culture with LPS. The results of preliminary studies indicated that the decrease in LPS-responsiveness of monocytes cultured in medium was not due to any alteration in LPS binding to the cells. Furthermore, neither this change nor the effects of IFN-γ were mediated by arachidonic acid metabolites. No evidence could be found for the production of an IL 1 inhibitor by the cultured monocytes during the preincubation in medium.

The possibility next was considered that during culture of monocytes in medium, synthesis of an intracellular protein occurred that blocked some step in subsequent LPS-induced IL 1 production. The results of early experiments indicated that after a 24 hr incubation of adherent monocytes in 0.125-1.0 µg/ml Cx and a 2 hr wash-out period, LPS-induced total protein synthesis was nearly intact. The effects of a 24 hr preincubation in Cx, in the absence or presence of IFN-γ, on subsequent LPS-stimulated IL 1 pro-

duction was determined. The results indicated that preincubation in 0.125-1.0 µg/ml Cx alone led to an enhancement in
IL 1 production over a second day culture in LPS (Figure
1). Furthermore, a marked enhancement in IL 1 production
was observed after preincubation in IFN-γ and Cx.

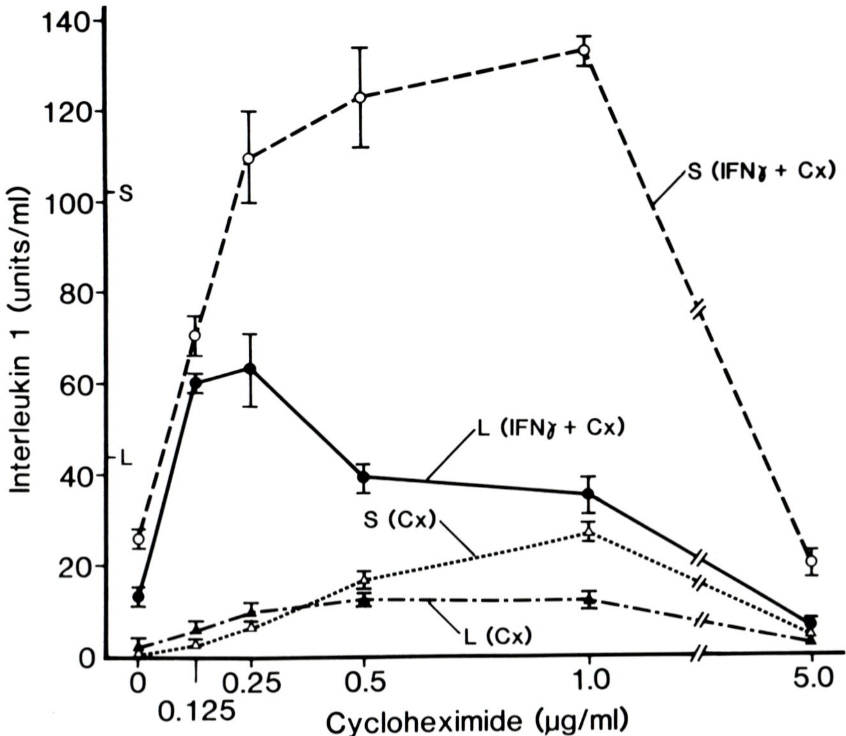

Figure 1:   Effects of preincubation in IFN-γ and Cx on subsequent LPS-induced IL 1 production. Adherent human
monocytes were preincubated for 24 hr in medium with or
without Cx, then were washed extensively before a second
24 hr culture with 2 ng/ml LPS. The concentrations of Cx
are expressed on the abscissa and IL 1 activity in the cell
supernatants (Δ---Δ) and lysates (▲·--·▲) on the ordinate. An
identical experiment was performed with monocytes preincubated in 100 U/ml IFN-γ with or without Cx before a second 24 hr culture with 2 ng/ml LPS (O---O, supernatants;
●—●, lysates). Monocytes incubated with 2 ng/ml LPS

These results indicate that preincubation of monocytes with IFN-γ, Cx or both agents leads to a marked increase in subsequent LPS-induced IL 1 production. Experiments were next performed to determine at what intracellular level in IL 1 production these effects were being mediated.

IL 1β mRNA, Activity and Protein Levels in Human Monocytes

Total cellular RNA was extracted from monocytes with levels measured over 48 hr after LPS stimulation using specific cDNA probes. IL 1β mRNA levels rose rapidly to a peak at 2-3 hr, then declined slightly and were maintained at a plateau through 48 hr. β$_2$M mRNA levels were high in unstimulated cells then slowly decreased while 28S mRNA levels remained constant over the 48 hr time period. Northern blot analyses on freshly-isolated monocytes or on cells cultured for one day in medium, IFN-γ, Cx or both agents, revealed 1.7 kb IL 1β mRNA of near equal levels at 3 hr after LPS stimulation. IL 1β mRNA levels next were determined by scanning densitometry of slot blots on RNA obtained 3 and 24 hr after LPS stimulation. 100 ng of total cellular RNA was applied to each slot. These results indicated that the monocytes preincubated in medium for one day exhibited a decrease in IL 1β mRNA levels between 3 and 24 hr after subsequent LPS stimulation (Table 1). However, preincubation in IFN-γ, Cx, or both reagents led to a partial or complete restoration of IL 1β mRNA levels at 24 hr after LPS stimulation. IL 1β activity and protein were determined (total lysates and supernatants) after the second 24 hr culture in LPS. The cells preincubated in medium alone displayed a marked decrease in subsequent LPS-induced IL 1 production. However, there was not a good correlation between the effects of preincubation in IFN-γ and/or Cx on IL 1β mRNA levels and IL 1 production. For instance, cells incubated for one day in both IFN-γ and Cx contained baseline levels of IL 1β mRNA at 3 and 24 hr after LPS stimulation but IL 1β activity or protein levels

---

during the first 24 hr culture showed 102.1 ± 6.5 and 44.6 ± 9.4 U/ml of IL 1 production in supernatants and lysates, respectively, as indicated on the ordinate. The data are expressed as the mean ± SD based upon triplicate determinations from one experiment. Similar results were obtained in two additional experiments.

Table 1:   IL 1β mRNA levels, IL 1 activity and IL 1 protein

Cells	mRNA levels* (scanning units)		IL 1 activity[+] (U/ml)	IL 1β protein[+] (ng/ml)
	3 hr	24 hr		
Freshly-isolated	19.6	29.9	125.4	11.0
Aged 1 d in: medium	19.4	9.6	15.2	1.0
100 U/ml IFN-γ	18.2	14.3	36.0	2.0
0.25 µg/ml Cx	24.8	19.3	48.0	2.9
IFN-γ and Cx	21.7	22.2	77.3	5.8

* mRNA levels 3 or 24 hr after subsequent stimulation with
100 ng/ml LPS.

[+] IL 1 activity and protein in 1 d-aged cells determined
over a second 24 hr culture with LPS.

The decrease in IL 1β mRNA levels observed 24 hr
after LPS stimulation of monocytes preincubated in medium
could be secondary to decreased transcription, increased
mRNA degradation or to both mechanisms. The preliminary
results of nuclear run-on experiments indicated that IL 1β
transcriptional rate was decreased only slightly in medium-
aged cells when measured 24 hr after subsequent LPS stimulation. However, preincubation in IFN-γ and Cx appeared to
restore the transcriptional rate to normal levels. Furthermore, the half-life of total cellular IL 1β mRNA appeared to
be slightly accelerated in medium-aged cells and to be prolonged two-fold by preincubation in cycloheximide and
IFN-γ. These alterations in IL 1β mRNA stability were sufficient to fully account for the observed changes in steady-
state mRNA levels. However, the alterations in IL 1 production in aged monocytes were more marked than could be
explained by changes in transcription and mRNA stability.
Further studies are necessary to determine whether IFN-γ
and Cx are acting independently through different mechanisms, whether IL 1β mRNA from monocytes aged under various conditions is capable of inducing translation in vitro,
and whether similar changes are observed with cytoplasmic
mRNA. The possibility remains that the major defect in
IL 1 production in aged monocytes and macrophages lies in

---

were only restored to 50-60% of those observed with freshly-isolated cells. However, there was variation between
donors in the degree of maintenance of LPS-induced IL 1
production seen after preincubation of monocytes in IFN-γ
and Cx.

initiation and completion of translation or in post-translational events.

SUMMARY

Monocytes preincubated in medium exhibited a decrease in subsequent LPS-induced IL 1 production. Preincubation in IFN-γ, Cx or both agents led to a partial to complete maintenance of subsequent LPS-induced IL 1 production. IL 1β mRNA levels 3 hr after LPS stimulation were the same in freshly-isolated monocytes or in cells preincubated for 24 hr in IFN-γ, Cx or both agents. However, monocytes preincubated for 24 hr in medium exhibited a decreased IL 1β mRNA level after a second 24 hr culture in LPS. Cells preincubated in both Cx and IFN-γ exhibited restoration of IL 1β mRNA to baseline levels when measured at 24 hr after LPS. However, the changes in IL 1β activity or protein levels appeared to be greater than could be explained by IL 1β mRNA levels alone. The results of preliminary experiments indicated that alterations in transcriptional rates and in IL 1β mRNA stability were not sufficient to explain the changes in IL 1 production. The major mechanism of decreased IL 1 production in cultured monocytes and macrophages may involve translational or post-translational events.

REFERENCES

Arend WP, Ammons JT, Kotzin BL (1987). Lipopolysaccharide and interleukin 1 inhibit interferon-γ-induced Fc receptor expression on human monocytes. J Immunol 139: 1873-1879.

Arend WP, D'Angelo S, Massoni RJ, Joslin FG (1985). Interleukin 1 production by human monocytes: Effects of different stimuli. In Kluger MJ, Oppenheim JJ, Powanda MC (eds): "The Physiologic, Metabolic and Immunologic Actions of Interleukin 1": New York, Alan R Liss, pp 399-407.

Arenzana-Seisdedos F, Virelizier JL, Fiers W (1985). Interferons as macrophage-activating factors. III. Preferential effects of interferon-γ on the interleukin 1 secretory potential of fresh or aged human monocytes. J Immunol 134:2444-2448.

Monokines and Other Non-Lymphocytic Cytokines, pages 119–123
© 1988 Alan R. Liss, Inc.

DIFFERENTIAL EFFECTS ON HUMAN MONOKINE TRANSCRIPTION AND
TRANSLATION FOLLOWING STIMULATION WITH LPS PLUS γ-INTERFERON

Mary W. Vermeulen and Heinz G. Remold

Department of Rheumatology and Immunology,
Brigham and Women's Hospital, and Havard
Medical School, Boston, MA   02115

Many different stimuli, such as γ-IFN, LPS, MDP, and
GM-CSF are known to activate macrophages. We have been
studying the effects of these activators at the level of
monokine RNA expression. We have previously demonstrated
that cultured human monocytes respond specifically to
activating stimuli (Vermeulen et al., 1987). In extending
our studies to examine interactions between stimulators, we
have obtained some unexpected results concerning monokine
gene expression at the transcriptional and translational
levels.

Our studies were conducted with human peripheral blood
monocytes, collected by leukapheresis. Mononuclear
leukocytes were obtained by sedimentation over
ficoll-hypaque. Monocytes were purified by overnight
adherence. Cells were matured in culture for a period of 5
to 7 days prior to stimulation, and were at least 96%
monocytes at this time, as judged by esterase staining
(Kaplow, 1981). Culture conditions were as pyrogen-free as
possible: routine monitoring of media with the chromogenic
Limulus lysate assay (MA Bioproducts) always indicated that
LPS levels were less than the sensitivity limit of the
assay, which is 10 pg/ml.

At the beginning of each experiment, media were replaced
and stimulators added, either alone or in combination.
Incubation intervals of 2 to 72 hours were followed by
removal of supernatants, lysis of cells in 4M guanidinium
thiocyanate, and isolation of total RNA (Chirgwin et al.,
1979). RNA was either separated by electrophoresis on

formaldehyde-agarose gels for Northern blots (Maniatis et
al., 1982), or applied directly to nylon membranes for
dot-blots (Kafatos et al., 1979). cDNA probes for HLA-DR
(Korman et al., 1982), IL-1β (Auron et al., 1984), and TNF
(Wang et al., 1985) were radiolabeled by nick translation.

First we examined RNA levels for HLA-DR in stimulated
and control cultured monocytes. We have previously shown
that within 2.5 hours, stimulation with 100 U/ml of γ-IFN
resulted in a significant increase in the level of DR RNA.
LPS had no ability to raise DR RNA levels above the
constitutive expression seen in unstimulated cells.
Interestingly, stimulation with the combination of 10 ng/ml
of LPS and 100 U/ml of γ-IFN prevented the enhancement seen
with γ-IFN alone (Vermeulen et al., 1987). This finding is
consistent with two studies using murine cells in which LPS
reduced the γ-IFN-mediated enhancement of Ia mRNA (Koerner
et al., 1987) and protein (Steeg et al., 1982) expression.

Next, we looked at levels of IL-1β RNA (Table 1). Here
we found that 10 ng/ml of LPS induced IL-1β RNA much more
effectively than did 100 U/ml of γ-IFN. The combination
yielded significantly less IL-1β RNA than did LPS alone. We
saw a similar effect with RNA for TNF (Table 2). LPS
induction of TNF RNA was decreased by the inclusion of γ-IFN
in the media.

Table 1: IL-1β RNA levels observed in cultured monocytes
after 2 or 24 hour incubations with LPS (100 ng/ml), γ-IFN
(100 U/ml), or both. Quantities deduced from relative
radiolabeled cDNA probe signal strengths on autoradiographs.

Condition	2 hr	24 hr
unstimulated control	--	--
LPS	++++	++
γ-IFN	+	--
LPS + γ-IFN	++	+

Table 2: TNF RNA levels observed after 2 and 24 hour
incubations.   Stimulator concentrations as in Table 1.

Condition	2 hr	24 hr
unstimulated control	--	--
LPS	++	+
γ-IFN	--	--
LPS + γ-IFN	$\pm$	--

In additional experiments, we studied the effects of a
second lymphokine, GM-CSF. At 100 U/ml, GM-CSF also
dramatically reduced the expression of TNF RNA induced by 10
ng/ml of LPS. Interestingly, costimulation with the same
doses of GM-CSF and LPS resulted in greater TNF protein
production than with LPS alone (Table 3).

Table 3: Mean TNF protein levels, in U/ml ($\pm$ s.e.m.) in
supernatants of cultured monocytes after 6, 24, and 72 hour
incubations with GM-CSF (100 U/ml), LPS (100ng/ml), or both.
Assayed by L929 cytotoxicity.

Condition	6 hr	24 hr	72 hr
unstimulated control	<10	<10	<10
GM-CSF	<10	<10	<10
LPS	50.3 + 9.2	40.3 + 9.0	<10
GM-CSF + LPS	58.6 + 23	91.7 + 24	<10

An increase in monokine protein levels under conditions
which down-regulate monokine RNA levels was also observed by
others. Both IL-1 (Philip and Epstein, 1986; Okusawa et
al., 1987) and TNF (Beutler et al., 1986; Sayers et al.,
1987) protein levels are synergistically increased by the
combination of LPS and γ-IFN, relative to stimulation with
LPS alone.

One explanation for the up-regulation of monokine
protein expression concurrent with RNA level down-regulation
is that γ-IFN might be serving two functions in these
cultures. It is known that 10 U/ml γ-IFN can completely
inhibit LPS-induced PGE_2 release from monocytes (Browning
and Ribolini, 1987). In this way, γ-IFN could prevent the
normal PGE_2-mediated inhibition of LPS-induced monokine
production (Kunkel et al., 1986), probably at the levels of

translation and/or secretion. Our RNA data would suggest
that γ-IFN may also supply another form of down-regulation,
acting at the transcriptional level, since the combination
of γ-IFN plus LPS results in monokine RNA levels lower than
those observed with LPS alone. This could be due to
decreased synthesis or increased instability of RNA, or
both.

In summary, we have found expression of monokine RNA
which differs from protein-level expression under the same
conditions. These data suggest that LPS-induced gene
expression of monokines is subject to controls at more than
one level. Further studies on this topic are in progress.

REFERENCES

Auron PE, Webb AC, Rosenwasser LJ, Mucci SF, Rich A, Wolff
    SM, Dinarello CA (1984). Nucleotide sequence of human
    monocyte interleukin 1 precursor cDNA. Proc Natl Acad Sci
    USA 81:7907-7911.
Beutler B, Tkacenko V, Milsark I, Krochin N, Cerami A
    (1986). Effect of γ-interferon on cachectin expression by
    mononuclear phagocytes. J Exp Med 164:1791-1796.
Browning JL, Ribolini A (1987). Interferon blocks
    interleukin 1-induced prostaglandin release from human
    peripheral monocytes. J Immunol 138:2857-2863.
Chirgwin JM, Przybyla AE, MacDonald RJ, Rutter WJ (1979).
    Isolation of biologically active ribonucleic acid from
    sources enriched in ribonuclease. Biochemistry
    18:5294-5299.
Kafatos FC, Jones CW, Efstratiadis A (1979). Determination
    of nucleic acid sequence homologies and relative
    concentrations by a dot hybridization procedure. Nucleic
    Acids Res 7:1541-1547.
Kaplow LS (1981). Cytochemical identification of mononuclear
    macrophages. In Manual of Macrophage Methodology.
    Herscowitz HB, Holden HT, Bellanti JA, Ghaffar A, eds.
    Marcel Dekker, New York. pp 199-207.
Koerner TJ, Hamilton TA, Adams DO (1987). Suppressed
    expression of surface Ia on macrophages by LPS: evidence
    for regulation at the level of accumulation of mRNA.
    J Immunol 139:239-243.
Korman AJ, Auffray C, Schamboeck A, Strominger JL (1982).
    The amino acid sequence and gene organization of the heavy
    chain of the HLA-DR antigen: homology to immunoglobulins.
    Proc Natl Acad Sci USA 79:6013-6017.

Kunkel SL, Chensue SW, Phan SH (1986). Prostaglandins as
  endogenous mediators of interleukin 1 production. J
  Immunol 136:186-192.
Maniatis T, Fritsch EF, Sambrook J (1982). <u>Molecular
  Cloning</u>. Cold Spring Harbor, New York.
Okusawa S, Dinarello CA, Yancey KB, Endres S, Lawley TJ,
  Frank MM, Burke JF, Gelfand JA (1987). C5a induction of
  human interleukin 1. Synergistic effect with endotoxin
  or interferon-γ. J Immunol 139:2635-2640.
Philip R, Epstein LB (1986). Tumor necrosis factor as
  immunomodulator and mediator of monocyte cytotoxicity
  by itself, γ-interferon, and interleukin-1. Nature
  323:86-89.
Sayers TJ, Machier I, Chung J, Kugler E (1987). The
  production of TNF by mouse bone marrow-derived macrophages
  in response to bacterial LPS and a chemically synthesized
  monosaccharide precursor. J Immunol 138:2935-2940.
Steeg PS, Johnson HM, Oppenheim JJ (1982). Regulation of
  murine macrophage I-A antigen expression by an immune
  interferon-like lymphokine: inhibitory effect of
  endotoxins. J Immunol 129:2402-2407.
Vermeulen MW, David JR, Remold HG (1987). Differential mRNA
  responses in human monocytes activated by interferon-γ and
  muramyl dipeptide. J Immunol 139:7-9.
Wang AM, Creasy AA, Ladner MB, Lin LS, Strickler J, Van
  Arsdell JN, Yamamoto R, Mark DF (1985). Molecular cloning
  of the cDNA for human tumor necrosis factor. Science
  228:149-154.

Monokines and Other Non-Lymphocytic Cytokines, pages 125–130

β-ENDORPHIN INHIBITS INTERLEUKIN 1β RELEASE BY HUMAN PERIPHERAL BLOOD MONONUCLEAR CELLS

Charles F. Brummitt, M.D., Burt Sharp, M.D. Genya Gekker, William F. Keane, M.D., and Phillip K. Peterson, M.D.
Department of Medicine, Hennepin County Medical Center; and the University of Minnesota Medical School, Minneapolis, MN 55415

INTRODUCTION

Interleukin-1 (IL-1), a key mediator of the immune response, promotes T lymphocyte activation, induces fever, and stimulates an acute-phase response (Dinarello, 1984). β-endorphin (β-END), a pro-opiomelanocortin (POMC) derived peptide co-secreted with ACTH, has receptors on polymorphonuclear leukocytes, lymphocytes and monocytes (Sharp et al, 1987; Wybran et al, 1979; Hazum et al, 1979; Lopker et al, 1980), and induces a variety of functional alterations in these cells. We recently observed that β-END is capable of inhibiting production of interferon-γ (IFN-γ) and lymphocyte proliferation by cultured peripheral blood mononuclear cells (PBMNC) (Peterson et al, 1987). Since IL-1 has an important role in mediating lymphocyte activation, we hypothesized that β-END suppressed lymphocyte activation and IFN-γ production by inhibiting IL-1.

MATERIALS AND METHODS

PBMNC were isolated and cultured as previously reported (Peterson, 1987). Concanavalin A (Con-A, Sigma) at 10 ug/ml, lipopolysaccharide (LPS, List Biological Lab, Inc.) from <u>Salmonella minnesota</u> at 10 ng/ml, and varicella-zoster virus antigen (VZV, Whitaker M.A. Bioproducts) at 1:50 dilution (after UV light inactivation for 1h) were used as stimuli for IL-1β. Human β-END$_{1-31}$ (Peninsula Labs), naloxone hydrochloride (kindly provided by National Institute on Drug Abuse), prostaglandin E_2 (PGE_2, Sigma) and indomethacin (Sigma) were brought to desired final concentration in culture medium.

PBMNC (2 x 10^5 cells) were added to 96-well flat bottom microtiter plates, washed and resuspended in 100 ul of culture medium or culture medium to which inhibitors of IL-1β had been added. Cells were preincubated with β-END for 3h as this time period had been previously established as optimal for suppression of IFN-γ (Peterson, 1987). In experiments with naloxone or indomethacin, cells were exposed for 30 min followed by β-END or culture media for 3h. Stimuli of IL-1β were added for 18h. In experiments comparing IL-1β and IFN-γ release, a 72h incubation was employed as this had previously been established as optimal for the IFN-γ response.

IL-1β was measured by a competitive radioimmunoassay (Cistron Biotechnology). The IL-1β assay was validated by the finding that IL-1β release by PBMNC paralleled previously reported studies (Kunkel et al, 1986). In all experiments, PBMNC were concurrently exposed to culture medium alone and IL-1β levels from unstimulated cells were subtracted from stimulated cells. IFN-γ release into the supernatants of PBMNC cultured for 72h was measured using a radioimmunoassay (Centocor, Malvern PA) as reported previously (Peterson, 1987). Data are expressed as mean $\pm$ S.E.   The differences between means of multiple groups was determined by one-way analysis of variance; comparisons between individual groups were calculated by the method of Bonferoni (Wallenstein et al, 1980). For comparisons between two groups, statistical significance was assessed by Student's t-test. Significance was defined as p<0.05.

RESULTS

A dose response study, using concentrations of β-END that encompass its physiologic range, showed Con A-stimulated PBMNC release 2.75 $\pm$ 0.53 ng/ml of IL-1β. PBMNC exposed to nanomolar or picomolar β-END for 3 h prior to adding Con A resulted in suppression of IL-1β to 50% of Con A-stimulated control cells (Fig. 1A); there was insignificant suppression at lower concentrations tested. PBMNC exposed to β-END alone released levels of IL-1β similar to PBMNC exposed to media alone (data not shown). Pretreatment of PBMNC with equimolar concentration of the opioid antagonist naloxone for 30 min prior to addition of

10^{-12}M β-END (Fig. 1B) blocked the suppressive effect of β-END. These findings suggest that an opioid receptor is involved in the β-END-mediated suppression of IL-1β release from Con A-stimulated cells.

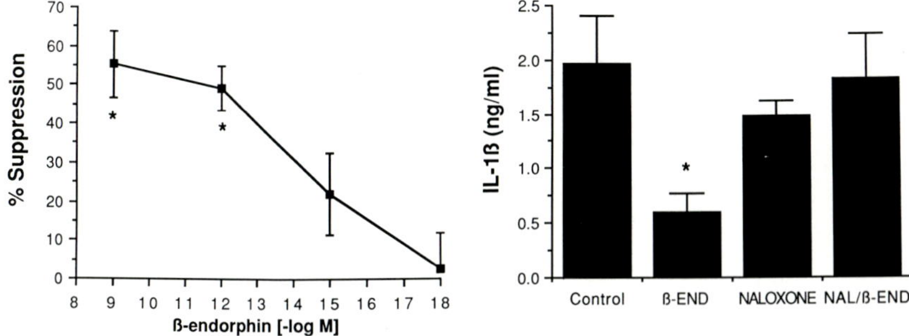

Figure 1. Dose response curve (A) and reversal by naloxone (B) of the effect of β-END on IL-1 β release by PBMNC. n=9 (A) and n=6 (B) donors. * p<0.05 by Bonferoni comparison of multiple groups.

We next examined whether β-END is capable of inhibiting IL-1β induced by other stimuli of IL-1β (Table 1). β-END at 10^{-12}M is capable of significantly inhibiting the IL-1β response to VZV antigen and to Con A but not to LPS.

TABLE 1 Effect of various stimuli on the ability of β-END to suppress PBMNC release of IL-1β.

	IL-1β (ng/ml)		
Stimulus[a]	Control Cells	β-END Exposed Cells	P Value[b]
Con-A	2.24 + .37	.98 + .27	<0.05
VZV	1.46 + .29	.48 + .28	<0.05
LPS	1.65 + .32	1.73+.30	.45

[a] n>5 donors for each stimulus.
[b] Statistical comparison was by student t-test.

Regarding the mechanism of β-END suppression of IL-1β, PGE_2 has been shown to post-transcriptionally inhibit IL-1 production (Knudsen et al, 1986). We had previously shown that β-END is capable of stimulating PGE_2 by PBMNC (Peterson, 1987), and that the suppression of IFN-γ by β-END is inhibited by indomethacin <u>in vitro</u> or <u>in vivo</u>. We asked therefore whether indomethacin would inhibit the suppression of IL-1β induced by β-END. In a concurrent assay both IL-1β and IFN-γ were suppressed by exposure to β-END for 3 h followed by 72 h stimulation with Con-A. This was reversed if PBMNC were first exposed to indomethacin (0.5µM) for 30 min (Fig 2). These findings suggest that a product(s) of the cyclooxygenase pathway of arachidonic acid metabolism is involved in β-END-mediated suppression of IL-1β release.

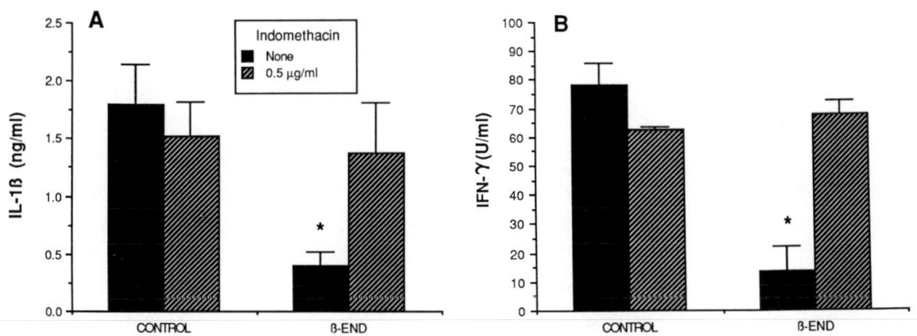

Figure 2.   Effect of indomethacin on β-END-mediated suppression of IL-1β (A) and IFN-γ (B). PBMNC were incubated for 72 h. n = 3. *p<0.05 by student t test.

We next evaluated the effect of exogenous PGE_2 on PBMNC stimulated with LPS and Con-A (Fig. 3). IL-1β release following Con-A stimulation was significantly inhibited by PGE_2 at 10^{-8} and 10^{-6} M. In contrast, LPS stimulation of IL-1β release could only be inhibited by PGE_2 at a concentration of 10^{-6}M.

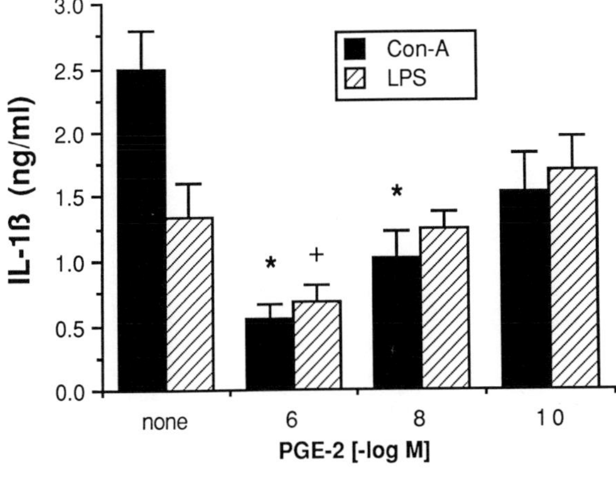

Figure 3. PGE_2 inhibits IL-1β release. Inhibition of Con-A (solid bars) is seen at 10^{-6} and 10^{-8}M PGE_2, but only 10^{-6}M PGE_2 for suppression of LPS. p<0.05 by Bonferoni comparison of multiple groups. n=7.

This differential sensitivity of IL-1β release to PGE_2 could explain, in part, the inability of β-END to suppress IL-1β release induced by LPS as β-END stimulates PGE_2 production by PBMNC yielding concentrations of 10^{-8} M (Peterson, 1987). While this concentration of PGE_2 appears to be adequate to suppress IL-1β release induced by Con-A, it is insufficient to inhibit LPS-induced IL-1 β. Other investigators (Kunkel et al, 1986) have shown that 10^{-8}M PGE_2 is capable of suppressing LPS stimulated IL-1 release, but they employed different cell types (peritoneal macrophages) which may have differing sensitivities to PGE_2.

DISCUSSION

This study demonstrates that physiologic levels of β-END can inhibit the release of IL-1β by PBMNC. This suppression requires interaction of β-END with a naloxone inhibitable opioid receptor, and appears to be mediated by arachidonic acid metabolite(s) such as PGE_2. We found that β-END mediated suppression of IL-1β was achieved following mitogen (Con-A) or antigen (varicella zoster virus) stimulation but not following stimulation by LPS; this may be due to decreased susceptibility of LPS stimulated PBMNC to inhibition by prostaglandins such as PGE_2.

These findings have relevance to an understanding of how the systemic response induced by IL-1 is regulated. IL-1 has been shown to stimulate pituitary derived POMC peptides (Besedovsky, 1986), and to stimulate central nervous system levels of β-END (Murphy et al, 1983). While the exact mechanism of how IL-1 achieves this regulation of pituitary peptides is not clear (reviewed in Lumpkin, 1987), our data demonstrates that a POMC derived peptide, β-END can inhibit <u>in vitro</u> further IL-1β release. Thus one function of β-END may be to provide negative feedback on IL-1β, and participate in a regulatory loop between IL-1β and the hypothalamic-pituitary axis. Further study will also be needed to determine whether POMC gene products derived from splenic lymphocytes and macrophages (Lolait et al, 1986; Westly et al, 1986) have a similar regulatory function.

ACKNOWLEDGEMENTS

The authors would like to thank Kathy McAllen for technical assistance and Rosemary Pellegrini for typing the manuscript.

REFERENCES

Besedovsky HA, del Rey A, Sorkin E, Dinarello CA (1986). Immunoregulatory feedback between IL-1 and glucocorticoid hormones. Science 233:652-654.

Dinarello CA (1984). Interleukin 1. Rev Infect Dis 6:51-96.

Hazum E, Chang K-J, Cuatrecasas P (1979). Specific non-opiate receptors for β-endorphin. Science 205:1033-1035.

Knudsen PJ, Dinarello CA, Strom TB (1986). Prostaglandins post transcriptionally inhibit monocyte expression of interleukin 1 activity by increasing intracellular cyclic adenosine monophosphate. J Immunol 137:3189.

Kunkel SL, Chensue SW, Phan SH (1986). Prostaglandins as endogenous mediators of interleukin 1 production. J Immunol 136:186-192.

Lolait SJ, Clements JA, Markwick AJ, Cheng C, McNally M, Smith AI, Funder JW (1986). Pro-opiomelanocortin messenger ribonucleic acid and posttranslational processing of β-endorphin in splenic macrophages. J Clin Invest 77:1776.

Lopker A, Abood LG, Hoss W, Lionetti FJ (1980). Stereoselective muscarinic acetylcholine and opiate receptors in human phagocytic leukocytes. Biochem Pharmacol 29:1361-1365.

Lumpkin MD (1987). The regulation of ACTH secretion by IL-1. Science 238:452-454.

Murphy MT, Koenig JI, Lipton JM (1983). Changes in central concentration of β-endorphin in fever. Fed Proc 42:1010A.

Peterson PK, Sharp B, Gekker G, Brummitt C, Keane WF (1987). Opioid-mediated suppression of interferon-γ production by cultured peripheral blood mononuclear cells. J Clin Invest 80:824-831.

Sharp BM, Tsukayama DT, Gekker G, Keane WF, Peterson PK (1987). β-endorphin stimulates human polymorphonuclear leukocyte superoxide production via a stereoselective opiate receptor. J Pharm Exp Ther 242:579-582.

Wallenstein SC, Lucker CL, Fleis JL (1980). Some statistical methods useful in circulation research. Circ Res 47:1-9.

Westly HJ, Kleiss AJ, Kelley KW, Wong PKY, Yuen P-H (1986). Newcastle disease virus-infected splenocytes express the pro-opiomelanocortin gene. J Exp Med 163:1589.

Wybran J, Appelbloom T, Famaey J-P, Govaerts A (1979). Suggestive evidence for receptors for morphine and methionine-enkephalin on normal human blood T lymphocytes. J Immunol 123:1068-1070.

Monokines and Other Non-Lymphocytic Cytokines, pages 131–136
© 1988 Alan R. Liss, Inc.

GENERATION OF INTERLEUKIN-1 IN A MACROPHAGE CELL LINE AND ENHNACEMENT OF INTERLEUKIN-1 FIBROBLAST PROLIFERATIVE ACTIVITY BY SUBSTANCE P.

Edward S. Kimball, Jeffry L. Vaught, Francis J. Persico and M. Carolyn Fisher

Department of Biological Research, Janssen Research Foundation, Spring House, PA 19477 USA

INTRODUCTION

Interleukin-1 (IL-1) is a peptide hormone whose wide spectrum of activities include immunoregulation, connective tissue cell activation, and inflammation (Durum et al., 1985; Dinarello, 1984; Dinarello et al., 1986). In the context of connective tissue cell activation, some of the notable inflammatory properties of IL-1 include fibroblast proliferation and secretion of prostaglandins, collagenase and plasminogen activator. IL-1 displays similar activities on synovial fibroblasts which form the lining of articular joints. This connective tissue activating property implicates IL-1 as an important mediator of the pathology associated with rheumatoid arthritis (RA). IL-1 is secreted by infiltrating macrophages and by cells of the synovial lining, and has been detected in synovial fluid of patients with rheumatoid arthritis.

The mechanism of macrophage and synoviocyte activation in the joint may not necessarily be wholly dependent on immune system-derived substances, however. For example, substance P (SP), a neuropeptide responsible for the transmission of pain in afferent nerve fibers is secreted from sensory nerve endings in the joint (Hokfelt et al., 1975) and has been directly implicated in the exacerbation of the arthritic state (Levine et al., 1984). SP has been shown to activate macrophages to secrete prostaglandins (Hartung et al., 1986) and other inflammatory mediators (Hartung and von Toyka, 1983), and was recently reported to activate synoviocytes to secrete PGE_2 and collagenase (Lotz et al., 1987). Because of the involvement of SP

with a variety of non-neuronal somatic cell types found in
the joint we investigated the possibility that some of the
arthritogenic activities of SP may be due to IL-1 induction and interactions on connective tissue cells. We
therefore studied the affect of SP and three related
neuropeptides, SP_{4-11}, neurokinin-A (NK-A) and NK-B, on
production of IL-1 by the P388D1 macrophage cell line
(Mizel et al., 1978). We also examined whether SP influ-
enced IL-1 induced fibroblast proliferation.

MATERIALS AND METHODS
    IL-1 Generation: P388D1 cells were cultured at a den-
sity of 5 x 10^5 cells/well in 24-well cluster plates
(Costar, Cambridge, MA) for four hours in RPMI-1640 supplemented with 1% glutamine and penicillin-streptomycin
and either LPS (0.3 μg/mL), substance P (Boehringer-
Mannheim, Indianapolis, IN), substance P_{4-11} (Peninsula
Research, Belmont, CA), NK-A or NK-B (Peninsula Research).
The cells had been deposited into the plates 24 hours in
advance in RPMI-1640 supplemented with 10% FCS. However,
serum was excluded from the medium used for stimulation
and IL-1 production. The cells were washed extensively
with serum-free medium prior to stimulation. Following
the initial four-hour incubation the media containing LPS,
SP or other stimulants were aspirated and discarded. The
cells were then washed three times with fresh serum-free
RPMI-1640, and the cultures continued for an additional
18 hours in serum-free medium. The 18-hour supernatants
were harvested, centrifuged and then tested for IL-1
activity.

    IL-1 Assays: IL-1 activity in the P388D1 supernatants
was determined according to a method described by Larrick
et al. (1985) that measures the ability of IL-1-containing
samples to induce IL-2 secretion by the LBRM T-cell line.
IL-2 was measured by increased proliferation of the IL-2-
dependent HT-2 cell line. The LBRM/TG6 cells and HT-2
cells were a generous gift from Dr. J. Larrick (Cetus
Corp., Emeryville, CA). Serial dilutions of culture
supernatants were added in triplicate to 96-well culture
plates and incubated 24 hours. Then, hypoxanthine (1 mM)
and azaserine (100 μg/mL) were added to each well, and
after an additional four hours ^{3}H-thymidine (1 μCi/
well) was added for a final four hours. The cells were
harvested for liquid scintillation counting (LSC) of
radioactivity incorporated into the HT-2 cells.

Fibroblast Proliferation was observed using the Balb/3t3 cell line. To 5 x 10^4 cells/well was added serial dilutions of IL-1 with or without SP in DMEM supplemented with insulin-transferrin-selenium and 50 µM indomethacin. Assays were run in triplicate in 96-well plates. After 66 hours cells were pulsed with ^{3}H-thymidine for six more hours and harvested for LSC.

RESULTS
Supernatants from P388D1 cells were examined for secreted IL-1 as a result of treatment with LPS, SP or SP_{4-11}. As shown in Figure 1, SP at 30 ng/mL induced IL-1 secretion to levels above those observed for medium-treated controls. SP was slightly less potent than LPS (300 ng/mL) as an IL-1 inducer. SP and LPS were equipotent in other experiments. However, SP_{4-11} (10 ng/mL), the C-terminal octapeptide fragment of SP with potent agonist activity (Pernow, 1983) was consistently a more potent inducer of IL-1 than SP.

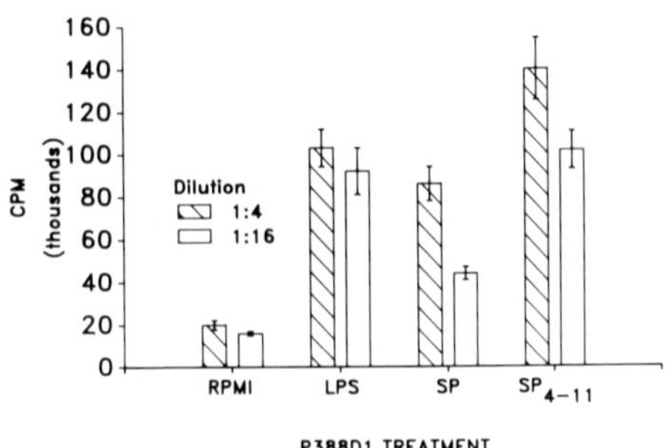

FIGURE 1. Generation of IL-1 by Substance P. Serial dilutions of P388D1 supernatants tested in the LBRM/HT-2 assay. Average cpm of triplicate cultures ± S.E.

These data are consistent with the known rank order of activity for SP and SP_{4-11} in other pharmacological systems. SP is also an inducer of histamine, but SP_{4-11} is not (Pernow, 1983). Therefore, these results preclude a histaminergic mechanism. Doses of SP lower and higher than 30 ng/mL were less active in inducing IL-1 (not shown). The absence of activity at higher doses is typical of some neuropeptide receptor-mediated events and may reflect high-dose down-regulation or tachyphylaxis. In

order to help determine if SP induction of IL-1 was a
receptor-specific process, 30 ng/mL SP was mixed with
100 ng/mL of the SP antagonist D-Pro^2, D-Trp^{7,9}-SP (DPDT)
and then incubated with P388D1 cells. As shown in Figure
2, the SP antagonist strongly inhibited SP-induced IL-1
production. At the dose used, 100 ng/mL, DPDT alone was a
weak promoter of IL-1 secretion, consistent with its' having partial agonist activity (Lundberg et al., 1983). In
contrast to inhibiting IL-1 production by SP, DPDT failed
to affect LPS-induced IL-1 secretion.

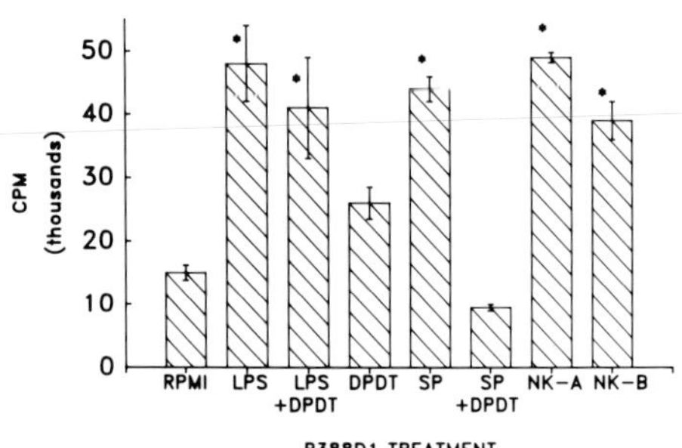

FIGURE 2. IL-1 induction by SP, NK-A and NK-B, and an-
tagonism of SP by DPDT. IL-1 activity in 1:8 dilutions of
P388D1 culture supernatants. Asterisks indicate significant difference (p<0.001) from unstimulated (RPMI) cultures. Average cpm ± S.E.

Two structurally related neuropeptides, NK-A and NK-B,
were also examined for their ability to induce IL-1 secretion. NK-A, at 30 ng/mL was approximately as effective an
IL-1 inducer as 300 ng/mL LPS. NK-B (30 ng/mL) was
slightly less potent than NK-A (Figure 2).

SP has been reported to be a weak fibroblast mitogen
(Nilsson et al., 1985), and also to activate synovial
fibroblasts (Lotz et al., 1987). We therefore decided to
examine SP as an IL-1 potentiating factor. Balb/3t3
fibroblasts proliferate in response to IL-1 (Dower et al.,
1986; Kimball et al., 1987). As shown in Figure 3, this
IL-1-induced proliferation is enhanced approximately two-
fold by the addition of as little as 3 ng/mL SP.

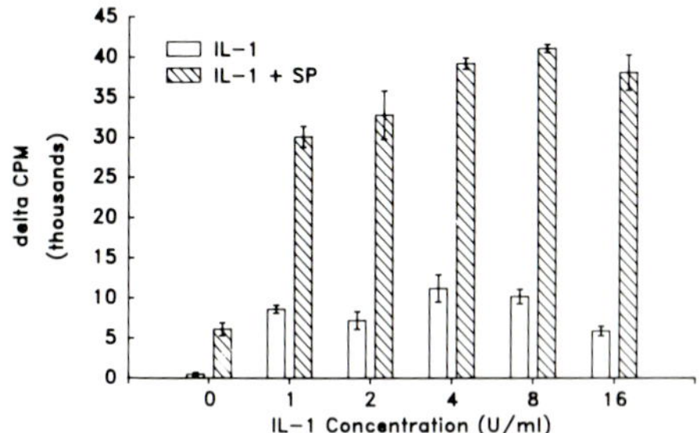

FIGURE 3.   Potentiation of IL-1-Induced Proliferation of
Balb/3t3 Fibroblasts. ^{3}H-thymidine incorporation as a
result of increasing rIL-1$_{alpha}$ concentration with or
without 3 ng/mL SP.   Average cpm ± S.E. of triplicate
cultures.

DISCUSSION

These results support the hypothesis that SP, and possibly other neurokinins, may play a role in the generation
and maintainance of inflammation in rheumatoid arthritis
by promoting IL-1 production and potentiating IL-1 activity on connective tissue cells in the joint. The synovium
and infiltrating macrophages are both potential sources of
IL-1 production, and the synovium is a target for IL-1 activation. The joint is also enervated by SP secretory
sensory nerve endings. As shown, SP at nM levels is capable of activating macrophages to secrete IL-1 and also is
capable of subsequently potentiating the effect of IL-1 on
connective tissue cells. This suggests that a cyclical
mechanism of pain, concomitant IL-1 release and subsequent
additional inflammation and exacerbation of existing inflamed tissue may occur episodically during RA. These
results also imply that the use of neurokinin specific
antagonists may become part of the strategy for allevia-
tion of the symptoms and amelioration of the pathology
observed in inflammatory diseases such as RA.

REFERENCES
Dinarello CA (1984). Interleukin 1: Reviews of Infectious Diseases. 6:51.

Dinarello CA, Cannon JG, Mier JW et al. (1986). Multiple
  biological activites of human recombinant interleukin 1.
  J Clin Invest 77:1734.
Dower SK, Call SM, Gillis S and Urdal DL (1986). Similar-
  ity between the interleukin 1 receptors on a murine T-
  lymphoma cell line and on a murine fibroblast cell line.
  Proc Nat Acad Sci USA 83:1060.
Durum SK, Schmidt JA and Oppenheim JJ (1985). Interleukin
  1: An Immunological Perspective. Ann Rev Immunol 3:263.
Hartung HP and von Toyka K (1983). Activation of macro-
  phages by substance P: induction of oxidative burst and
  thromboxane release. Eur J Pharmacol 89:301.
Hartung HP, Wolters K and von Toyka K (1986). Substance P:
  Binding properties and studies on cellular responses in
  guinea-pig macrophages. J Immunol 136:3856.
Hokfelt T, Kellerth JO, Milsson G and Pernow B (1975).
  Experimental immunohistochemical studies on the localization and distribution of substance P in cat primary
  sensory neurones. Brain Res 100:235.
Kimball ES, Fisher MC and Persico FJ (1987). Potentiation
  of Balb/3t3 fibroblast proliferative response by IL-1
  and EGF. Submitted for Publication.
Larrick JW, Brindley L and Doyle MV (1985). An improved
  assay for the detection of interleukin 1. J Immunol Meth
  79:39.
Levine JD, Clark R, Devor M, et al. (1984). Intraneuronal
  substance P contributes to the severity of experimental
  arthritis. Science 226:547.
Lotz M, Carson DA and Vaughn JH (1987). Substance P activation of rheumatoid synoviocytyes: Neural pathway in
  pathogenesis of arthritis. Science 235:893.
Lundberg JM, Saria A, Brodin E, Rosell S and Folkers K
  (1983). A substance P antagonist inhibits vagally
  induced inflammation and bronchial smooth muscle con-
  traction in the guinea-pig. Proc Nat Acad Sci, USA
  80:1120.
Mizel SB, Oppenheim JJ and Rosenstreich DL (1978).
  Characterization of lymphocyte-activating Factor (LAF)
  produced by the macrophage cell line, P388D1. J Immunol
  120:1504.
Nilsson J, von Euler AM and Dalsgaard CJ (1985).
  Stimulation of connective tissue cell growth by substance P and substance K. Nature 315:61.
Pernow B (1983). Substance P. Pharmacol Rev 35:85.

Monokines and Other Non-Lymphocytic Cytokines, pages 137–140
© 1988 Alan R. Liss, Inc.

INTERLEUKIN-1 SECRETION BY HUMAN PERIPHERAL BLOOD MONONUCLEAR CELLS IN RESPONSE TO INTERLEUKIN-2

Robert P. Numerof, Charles A. Dinarello and
James W. Mier

Department of Medicine, New England Medical
Center, Boston, Massachusetts 02111

INTRODUCTION

The traditional role for interleukin-2 (IL-2) has been
that of a growth factor for T cells (Smith et al., 1979).
However, IL-2 can now be viewed as a multifunctional molecule
which acts on a variety of cell types (Robb, 1984). One of
the first functions outside the realm of T cell proliferation demonstrated for IL-2 was its ability to induce the
secretion of cytokines. These IL-2-inducible secretory
proteins include IFN-γ (from T cells and NK cells) (Handa
et al., 1983; Kasahara et al., 1983), BCGF-1 (from T cells)
(Howard et al., 1983) and TNF-α(from adherent blood
mononuclear cells) (Nedwin et al., 1985).

Interleukin-1 can be detected in the culture supernatants of LPS-stimulated peripheral blood mononuclear cells
(PBMC) by measuring the ability of the supernatants to
induce proliferation of lectin-stimulated murine thymocytes
(Gery et al., 1972) or D10 T cells (Kaye et al., 1982).
However, since IL-2 itself is active in such IL-1 bioassays,
the complete removal or neutralization of IL-2 would be
required to detect IL-1 in the culture supernatants of
IL-2-treated PBMC. The recent development of highly specific
radioimmunoassays for IL-1α (Lonnemann et al., 1987) and
IL-1β (Lisi et al., 1987) has enabled us to measure low
levels of IL-1 in the presence of high concentrations of
IL-2.

We now report that rIL-2 induces the secretion of IL-1α
and IL-1β from PBMC. These results suggest that IL-1

secretion may occur _in vivo_ in patients undergoing IL-2
therapy.   If this proves to be true, IL-1 could be one of
the mediators of some forms of toxicity associated with
IL-2 injections.

MATERIALS AND METHODS

Blood was obtained from healthy, normal volunteers.
Ficoll-separated PBMC were washed and placed in culture in
RPMI-1640 medium containing 5% fetal calf serum at a density
of 5 X 10^6 cells/ml.   Following stimulation with LPS (Sigma),
rIL-2 (Cetus), rIFN-γ (Schering), or media alone, cells
and supernatants were separated by centrifugation, and
protease inhibitors were added to the supernatants.   Stimulation with rIL-2, IFN-γ, or media alone was done in the
presence of polymyxin B.   Duplicate 0.1 ml aliquots of
supernatant were assayed for the presence of IL-1α, IL-1β,
and TNF-α using specific radioimmunoassays (Lisi et al.,
1987; Van der Meer et al., 1987; Lonnemann et al., 1987).

RESULTS

TABLE 1.   Effect of LPS and rIL-2 on cytokine secretion.

Donor	Cytokine Concentration (ng/ml)								
	IL-1α			IL-1β			TNF-α		
	1	2	3	1	2	3	1	2	3
Media alone	<0.1	<0.1	<0.1	0.8	<0.1	<0.1	0.4	<0.1	–
rIL-2 (1000 U/ml)	0.7	3.9	5.3	6.1	6.8	16.0	6.6	4.8	–
LPS (100 ng/ml)	1.2	0.8	2.7	12.0	5.2	22.0	3.1	3.6	–

PBMC from several donors were stimulated with LPS,
rIL-2, or media alone for 24 hours.   In Table 1, we show
that stimulation with either LPS or rIL-2 leads to the secretion of both IL-1α and IL-1β.   We confirm that TNF-α is

also secreted as shown previously (Nedwin et al., 1985).
For the three donors examined here, the concentration of
IL-1β in the PBMC supernatants at 24 hours following either
LPS or rIL-2 treatment is greater than the corresponding
concentration of IL-1α.

TABLE 2.   Effect of IFN-γ on rIL-2-induced IL-1 secretion.

| | rIL-2 | Cytokine Concentration (ng/ml) | |
IFN-γ	(1000 U/ml)	IL-1α	IL-1β
–	–	<0.1	<0.1
	+	2.3	3.5
10 U/ml	–	<0.1	<0.1
	+	4.8	5.8
100 U/ml	–	<0.1	<0.1
	+	5.0	6.3

IFN-γ has been shown to augment the secretion of TNF-α
(Nedwin et al., 1985) and TNF-β (Svedersky et al., 1985)
in response to IL-2 stimulation.   Therefore, we examined
whether IFN-γ might have a similar enhancing effect on
IL-2-induced IL-1 secretion.   We stimulated PBMC for 24
hours with increasing concentrations of IFN-γ, either alone
or in the presence of rIL-2 (1000 U/ml).   In Table 2, we
show that IFN-γ by itself does not stimulate IL-1 secretion
although it markedly enhances the secretion that occurs in
response to rIL-2 stimulation.   IFN-γ also augments LPS-
induced IL-1 secretion (Gerrard et al., 1987) and the
mechanisms of enhancement may be the same with both inducers.

REFERENCES

Gerrard TL, Siegel JP, Dyer DR, Zoon KC (1987).   Differential
   effects of interferon-α and interferon-γ on interleukin 1
   secretion by monocytes.   J Immunol 138:2535.
Gery I, Gershon RK, Waksman BH (1972).   Potentiation of the
   T-lymphocyte response to mitogens.   I. The responding
   cell.   J Exp Med 136:128.

Handa K, Suzuki R, Matsui H, Shimizu Y, Kumagai K (1983).
  Natural killer (NK) cells as responder to interleukin 2.
  II. IL-2 induced interferon-γ production. J Immunol
  130:988.
Howard M, Matis L, Malek TR, Shevach E, Kell W, Cohen D,
  Paul WE (1983). Interleukin 2 induces antigen-reactive
  T cell lines to secrete BCGF-1. J Exp Med 158:2024.
Kasahara T, Hooks JJ, Dougherty SF, Oppenheim JJ (1983).
  Interleukin 2-mediated immune interferon (IFN-γ) pro-
  duction by human T cells and T cell subsets. J Immunol
  130:1784.
Kaye J, Gillis S, Mizel SB, Shevach EM, Malek TR,
  Dinarello CA, Lachman LB, Janeway CA (1982). Growth of
  a cloned helper T-cell line induced by a monoclonal anti-
  body specific for the antigen receptor: interleukin-1 is
  required for the expression of receptors for interleukin-2.
  J Immunol 133:1339.
Lisi PJ, Chu CW, Koch GA, Endres S, Lonnemann G, Dinarello CA
  (1987). Development and use of a radioimmunoassay for human interleukin-1β. Lymphokine Res 6:229.
Lonnemann G, Endres S, Van der Meer JWM, Ikejima T, Cannon JG,
  Dinarello CA (1987). Development and use of a highly
  sensitive radioimmunoassay for human interleukin-1 alpha:
  comparison of immunoreactive IL-1 alpha and IL-1 beta
  production from stimulated human mononuclear cells.
  Immunobiology 175:81 (abstract).
Nedwin GE, Svedersky LP, Bringman TS, Palladino MA,
  Goeddel DV (1985). Effect of interleukin 2, interferonγ,
  and mitogens on the production of tumor necrosis factors
  α and β. J Immunol 135:2492.
Robb RJ (1984). Interleukin 2: the molecule and its
  function. Im Today 5:203.
Smith K, Gillis S, Baker PE, McKenzie D, Ruscetti FW (1979).
  T-cell growth factor-mediated T cell proliferation.
  Proc Natl Acad Sci USA 332:423.
Svedersky LP, Nedwin GE, Goeddel DV, Palladino MA (1985).
  Interferon-γ enhances induction of lymphotoxin in recom-
  binant interleukin 2-stimulated peripheral blood mono-
  nuclear cells. J Immunol 134:1604.
Van der Meer JWM, Endres S, Lonnemann G, Cannon JG,
  Ikejima T, Okusawa S, Gelfand JA, Dinarello CA (1987).
  Concentrations of immunoreactive human tumor necrosis
  factor alpha produced by human mononuclear cells _in vitro_.
  J Leukocyte Biol in press.

Monokines and Other Non-Lymphocytic Cytokines, pages 141–144

LIPOSOMAL MURAMYL DIPEPTIDE IS MORE POTENT THAN FREE MURAMYL DIPEPTIDE IN INDUCING IL-1 SECRETION FROM MACROPHAGES

Nigel C. Phillips

Montreal General Hospital Research
Institute/McGill University, Montreal,
Quebec H3G 1A4, Canada

INTRODUCTION

N-acetylmuramyl-L-alanyl-D-isoglutamine (MDP) is the minimal structural component of bacterial peptidoglycan possessing immunoadjuvant activity (Ellouz et al, 1974). MDP is capable of inducing Interleukin-1 (IL-1) secretion from macrophages in vitro (Oppenheim et al, 1980). MDP and its lipophilic derivative MDP-glycerol dipalmitate (MDP-GDP) are potent inducers of macrophage tumoricidal activity in vitro, especially when incorporated within liposomes (Phillips et al, 1985, 1987a). In vivo studies have demonstrated significant activation of pulmonary macrophage tumoricidal activity after systemic treatment with liposomal MDP-GDP, and inhibition of experimental pulmonary tumor growth (Phillips et al, 1985,1987a). Potent immunoadjuvant activity is also observed when proteins such as carcinoembryonic antigen are incorporated within liposomes containing MDP-GDP (Phillips et al, 1987b).

IL-1 has been implicated in the adjuvant activity of MDP (Wood et al, 1983), suggesting that the enhanced immunoadjuvant effect of liposomal MDP-GDP may result from efficient IL-1 induction. While a considerable body of data exists on the relative efficacy of free and liposomal muramyl peptides in inducing macrophage tumoricidal activity, no comparable studies have been carried out to determine their ability to induce IL-1 secretion from macrophages.

MATERIALS AND METHODS

Liposomes containing MDP-GDP or the GDP derivative of
an inactive muramyl dipeptide, N-acetylmuramyl-D-alanyl-D-
isoglutamine (MDP(D-D)-GDP) were made as previously
described (Phillips et al, 1987a). Alveolar macrophages
were isolated from male C57BL/6J mice by lung lavage, and
treated with MDP or MDP(D-D), control liposomes or
liposomal MDP-GDP MDP(D-D)-GDP for 24 hr in MEM containing
endotoxin-free fetal calf serum. The adjuvants were then
removed, and IL-1 activity in the supernatant determined
24-96 hrs post stimulation. Alveolar macrophages were
treated <u>in situ</u> by the iv injection of the adjuvants. The
macrophages were isolated 24 hr later, and IL-1 activity in
the supernatants determined at 24-96 hrs. IL-1 activity was
determined by [^{3}H]-thymidine incorporation of C3H/HeJ
thymocytes sub-optimally stimulated with PHA. Activities
were calculated as mUnits, where 1 Unit = 50% maximal [^{3}H]-
thymidine incorporation induced by an LPS-stimulated
macrophage IL-1 preparation.

RESULTS

MDP induced IL-1 production from alveolar macrophages
<u>in vitro</u> in the dose range 5-500 ug/ml. Activity was
observed at 24 and 48 hr post-stimulation: no IL-1 activity
was observed 72 hr post stimulation (Table 1).

TABLE 1. Induction of IL-1 secretion <u>in vitro</u> by MDP and
MDP(D-D)

Treatment			IL-1, mUnits			
		24hr	48hr	72hr	96hr	TOTAL
Control		10	8	12	10	40
MDP	500 ug/ml	750	2600	10	12	4362
	50	740	3000	8	10	3758
	5	600	1000	10	10	1620
MDP(D-D)	500 ug/ml	10	10	10	8	38
	50	10	12	10	10	42
	5	10	10	15	8	43

5 x 10^6 macrophages were incubated in 1.0 ml MEM-FCS.

MDP(D-D) was ineffective in inducing IL-1 secretion from alveolar macrophages in the dose range 5-500 ug/ml (Table 1). Liposomes containing MDP-GDP or MDP(D-D)-GDP in the dose range 0.01-1.0 ug/ml induced levels of IL-1 activity greater than observed for MDP (Table 2). IL-1 activity continued to be secreted for at least 96 hr post stimulation. A major difference between MDP and liposomal MDP-GDP or MDP(D-D)-GDP was the lag-period (24 hr) observed for the liposomal muramyl dipeptides (Table 1, Table 2).

TABLE 2. Induction of IL-1 secretion in vitro by liposomal MDP-GDP and MDP(D-D)-GDP

Liposomal treatment (100 nmols)			24hr	48hr	72hr	96hr	TOTAL
Control			15	10	10	10	35
MDP-GDP	1.0	ug/ml	160	4000	2500	4000	10660
	0.1		100	5000	5000	3600	13700
	0.01		40	4500	4000	3500	12040
MDP(D-D)	1.0	ug/ml	200	8000	6500	3800	18500
-GDP	0.1		450	3200	5500	3650	12800
	0.01		350	3600	4000	4000	11950
Control liposomes			12	15	15	10	52

The systemic treatment of C57BL/6J mice with 100 ug MDP resulted in secretion of IL-1 by alveolar macrophages on subsequent in vitro assay (Table 3). MDP(D-D) was inactive at the same dose (Table 3).

TABLE 3. In situ Induction of IL-I secretion by free and liposomal muramyl dipeptides

Treatment	ug/mouse	IL-1, mUnits				
		24hr	48hr	72hr	96hr	TOTAL
Control		10	10	10	10	40
MDP	100	200	800	80	10	1090
MDP(D-D)	100	10	10	10	15	45
Liposomes (2.5 umols)		10	12	15	15	52
" MDP-GDP	10	50	1600	2000	1800	5450
" MDP(D-D)GDP	10	80	2000	2500	2200	6780

In contrast liposomes containing 10 ug MDP-GDP or MDP(D-D)-GDP induced significant and prolonged secretion of IL-1 activity (Table 3).

DISCUSSION.

Liposomes containing MDP-GDP or MDP(D-D)-GDP are significantly more potent than free MDP in inducing macrophage tumoricidal activity. The relative potencies between free MDP and liposomal MDP-GDP or MDP(D-D)-GDP for tumoricidal activity would appear to be maintained for the induction of IL-secretion from macrophages. The kinetics of IL-1 secretion after liposomal muramyl dipeptide treatment are suggestive of the formation of a long-lived depot capable of inducing prolonged secretion. Such an hypothesis is consistent with the enhanced immunoadjuvant activity of liposomes containing MDP-GDP.

REFERENCES.

Ellouz F, Adam A, Ciorbaru R, Lederer E (1974). Minimal structural requirements for adjuvant activity of bacterial peptidoglycan derivatives. Biochem Biophys Res Commun 59:1317-1325.

Oppenheim JJ, Togawa A, Chedid L, Mizel S (1980). Components of mycobacteria and muramyl dipeptide with adjuvant activity induce lymphocyte activating factor. Cell Immunol 50:71-81.

Phillips NC, Moras ML, Chedid L, Lefrancier P, Bernard JM (1985). Activation of alveolar macrophage tumoricidal activity and eradication of experimental metastases by freeze-dried liposomes containing a new lipophilic muramyl dipeptide derivative. Cancer Res 45:128-134.

Phillips NC, Chedid L, Bernard JM, Level M, Lefrancier P (1987a). Induction of murine macrophage tumoricidal activity and treatment of experimental metastases by liposomes containing lipophilic muramyl dipeptide analogs. J Biol Resp Modif (in press).

Phillips NC, Major PP, Isheda M, Sikorska H (1987b). Liposomal incorporation and immunogenicity of carcinoembryonic antigen. J Biol Resp Modif (in press).

Wood DD, Staruch MJ, Durette PL, Melvin III WV, Graham BK (1983). Role of interleukin-1 in the adjuventicity of muramyl dipeptide in vivo. In Oppenheim JJ (ed): "Interleukins, Lymphokines and Cytokines," New York: Academic Press, pp 691-698.

Monokines and Other Non-Lymphocytic Cytokines, pages 145–151
© 1988 Alan R. Liss, Inc.

CACHECTIN/TNF AND IL-1 SYNTHESIS AND SECRETION ARE INDUCED BY GLUCOSE-MODIFIED PROTEIN BINDING TO HIGH-AFFINITY MACROPHAGE RECEPTOR

Helen Vlassara, Michael Brownlee, Kirk Manogue, Araxi Pasagian, Charles Dinarello and Anthony Cerami

Laboratory of Medical Biochemistry, The Rockefeller University, New York, New York 10021-6399

With the availability of recombinant cachectin/TNF a number of studies have appeared which demonstrate the pluripotential nature of this protein. Included in these diverse bioactivities are the induction of hemorrhagic necrosis (Old, 1985), cachexia and shock (Beutler *et al.*, 1985), as well as the ability to enhance the growth of fibroblasts (Sugarman *et al.*, 1985), release of the degradative enzyme collagenase from several mesenchymal cells (Dayer *et al.*, 1985), and secretion of growth factors including interleukin-1 (IL-1) (Beutler and Cerami, 1987; Dinarello *et al.*, 1986; Nawroth *et al.*, 1986; Le *et al.*, 1987), granulocyte-macrophage colony stimulating factor (GM-CSF) (Munker *et al.*, 1986), and platelet derived growth factor (PDGF) (Nawroth and Stern, 1986; Gajdusek *et al.*, 1986). The dual capacity of a single protein to cause both cell death as well as cell growth suggests that this protein might in fact serve as the mediator of a single important purpose: normal tissue remodelling. What serves as the on and off signal for this coordination has not yet been understood.

Monocyte-derived macrophages have been described as playing an important role in the regulation of extracellular matrix protein and mesenchymal cell turnover which is critical for the maintenance of normal tissue homeostasis in response to time-dependent senescence and local tissue injury (Krane, 1984).

Recently, we have identified a new membrane-associated macrophage receptor that specifically recognizes proteins modified by advanced glycosylation endproducts (AGE) (Vlassara *et al.*, 1985; Vlassara *et al.*, 1986; Radoff *et al.*, *submitted*). This type of irreversible protein modification results from the reversible nonenzymatic addition product of glucose with protein amino

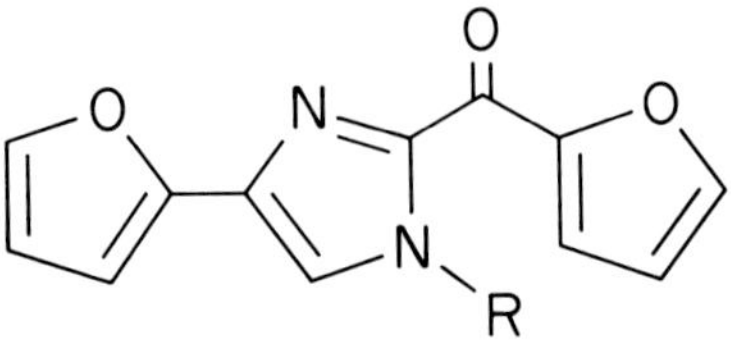

Figure 1. Glucose-derived protein crosslink formed under physiologic conditions. This compound, 2-furoyl-4(5)-(2-furanyl)-1H-imidazole, is a condensation product of two glucose molecules and two lysine-derived amino groups.

groups (the Amadori product) through a series of slowly occurring reactions and rearrangements (Brownlee *et al.*, 1984). One of these adducts has been identified as 2-(2-furoyl)-4(5)-(2-furanyl)-1H-imidazole (FFI) (Pongor *et al.*, 1984) (Fig. 1). AGE, unlike their dissociable precursors, continue to accumulate on proteins with slow turnover rates for the entire life of the molecule. This accumulation results in the progressive formation of glucose-derived protein cross-links (Pongor *et al.*, 1984) and serves as a biologic marker of protein senescence. Proteins with Amadori glycosylation products alone are not recognized by the macrophage AGE-receptor (Vlassara *et al.*, 1986). However, recognition of advanced glycosylation endproducts on proteins such as peripheral nerve myelin by the AGE-receptor increases linearly with age of the individual (Fig. 2).

Since the macrophage AGE-protein receptor would selectively target macrophages to a time-dependent integrator of *in vivo* protein exposure to glucose, we hypothesized that cross-linked and senescent macromolecules could be preferentially removed and replaced by newly synthesized material in a tightly coordinated system mediated by the macrophage receptor binding of AGE-protein, if this binding were coupled to a secretory response involving macrophage polypeptides such as cachectin/TNF.

In order to evaluate this hypothesis, freshly isolated human monocytes were incubated in endotoxin-free media with the interferon-γ and either unmodified bovine serum albumin (BSA), albumin modified with glucose or glucose-6-phosphate (Glu-BSA and G-6-P-BSA), or FFI (FFI-BSA) as described (Vlassara *et al.*, 1984). Immunoreactive human cachectin/TNF was detected using a sensitive ELISA method (Vlassara *et al.*, *submitted*).

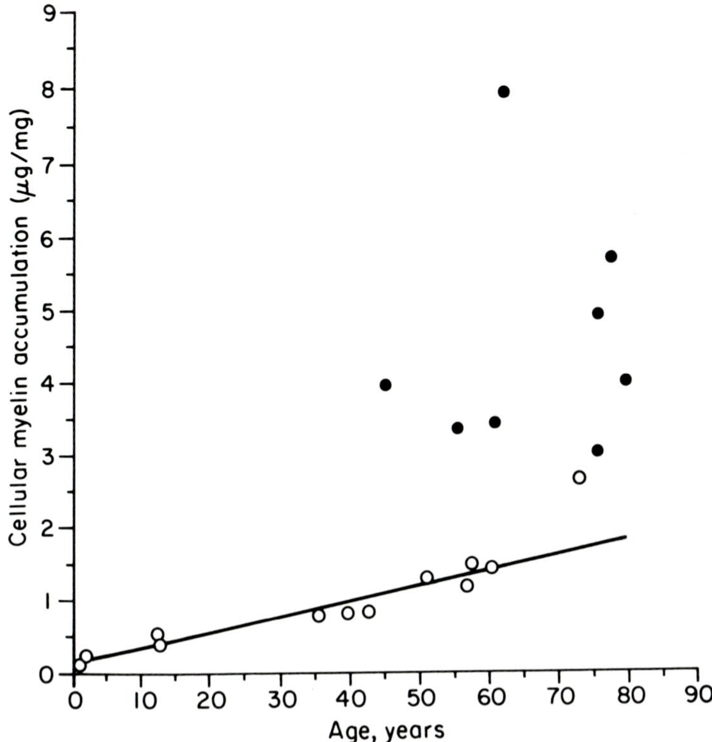

Figure 2.   Intracellular accumulation of iodinated normal (open circles) and diabetic (solid circles) human peripheral nerve myelin by monocyte/macrophages as a function of subject age.

Medium from macrophages incubated with BSA contained minimal levels of cachectin/TNF.   In contrast, medium from macrophages incubated with each of the three AGE-BSA samples contained more than 10 times the amount of cachectin/TNF found in media with unmodified BSA.   Interferon-γ alone elicited no response from monocytes incubated for the same period of time under identical conditions.

In order to determine whether the observed appearance of cachectin/TNF in conditioned media involved induction of new cachectin/TNF mRNA, as opposed to exclusively posttranscriptional events, Northern blot analysis of monocyte cachectin/TNF mRNA was performed.   No cachectin/TNF was detectable in monocyte

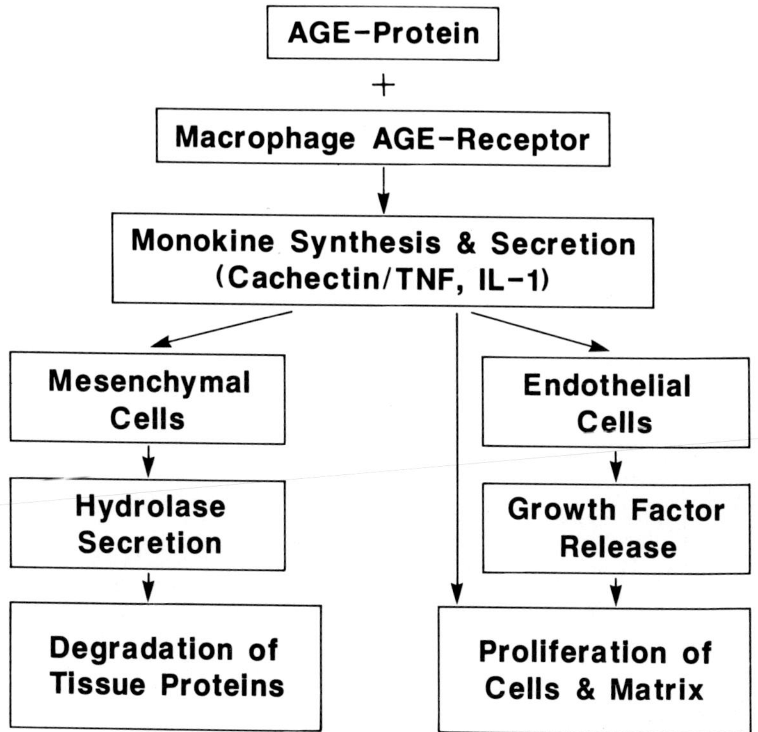

Figure 3.   Schematic representation of potential mechanisms by which advanced glycosylation endproduct-mediated synthesis and secretion of cachectin/TNF and IL-1 might contribute to the regulation of normal tissue remodelling.

preparations incubated with unmodified albumin.   In contrast, cachectin/TNF mRNA was present in monocyte preparations incubated with each of the AGE-modified albumins.   These results indicate that the specific binding of AGE-proteins to their receptor, like the binding of LPS, induce transcription of new cachectin/TNF mRNA.   The relative contribution of transcriptional, translational, and posttranslational events to the cachectin/TNF secretion induced by AGE-protein binding to its receptor remains to be elucidated.

Preliminary data suggest that IL-1 is also produced intracellularly in response to AGE-proteins under similar conditions (Vlassara *et al.*, *manuscript in preparation*). Even though its presence may represent a secondary response via cachectin/TNF, IL-1 shares and quite possibly can amplify several of the activities of cachectin/TNF relating to tissue necrosis and remodelling (Le and Vilcek, 1987).

These data demonstrate that AGE-protein binding to its macrophage receptor stimulates secretion of cachectin/TNF, and possibly IL-1. The mechanisms by which this could affect tissue homeostasis are shown schematically in Figure 3. The degradative enzymes necessary for macrophage removal of AGE-proteins from the tissues, such as vascular wall, do not appear to be secreted by the macrophage itself (*unpublished observations*). Rather, binding of AGE-protein to its macrophage receptor induces the synthesis and secretion of cachectin/TNF, a monokine which then specifically amplifies the original signal by stimulating nearby mesenchymal cells to synthesize and release collagenase and other extracellular proteases (Sugarman *et al.*, 1985; Le *et al.*, 1987). At the same time that this monokine is stimulating protein removal, it can also stimulate the release of growth factors (Le *et al.*, 1987; Munker *et al.*, 1986; Nawroth *et al.*, 1986; Gajdusek *et al.*, 1986).

The *in vivo* modification of matrix proteins by time-dependent formation of glucose-derived AGE's may thus constitute a unique biologic time-clock signalling macrophages to secrete cachectin/TNF, IL-1, and possibly other cytokines that can profoundly alter the degradation and proliferation of tissue components.

REFERENCES

Beutler B, Cerami A (1987). Cachectin: more than a tumor necrosis factor. New Engl J Med 316: 379-385.

Beutler B, Mahoney J, Le Trang N, Pekala P, Cerami A (1985). Purification of cachectin, a lipoprotein lipase-suppressing hormone secreted by endotoxin-induced RAW 264.7 cells. J Exp Med 161: 984-995.

Brownlee M, Vlassara H, Cerami A (1984). Nonenzymatic glycosylation and the pathogenesis of diabetic complications. Ann Intern Med 101: 527-537.

Dayer JM, Beutler B, Cerami A (1985). Cachectin/tumor necrosis factor stimulates collagenase and prostaglandin E_2 production by human synovial cells and dermal fibroblasts. J Exp Med

162: 2163-2168.

Dinarello CA, Cannon JG, Wolff SM, Bernheim HA, Beutler B, Cerami A, Figari IS, Palladino Jr MA, O'Connor JV (1986). Tumor necrosis factor (cachectin) is an endogenous pyrogen and induces production of interleukin 1. J Exp Med 163: 1433-1450.

Gajdusek C, Carbon S, Ross R, Nawroth PP, Stern DM (1986). Activation of coagulation releases endothelial cell mitogens. J Cell Biol 103: 419-428.

Krane SM (1984). Collagen degradation. In Berk PD, Castro-Malaspina H, Wasserman LR (eds): "Myelofibrosis and the Biology of Connective Tissue," New York: Alan R. Liss, vol 54, pp 89-102.

Le J, Vilcek J (1987). Tumor necrosis factor and interleukin 1: cytokines with multiple overlapping biological activities. Lab Invest 56: 234-248.

Le J, Weinstein D, Gubler U, Vilcek J (1987). Induction of membrane-associated interleukin 1 by tumor necrosis factor in human fibroblasts. J Immunol 138: 2137-2142.

Munker R, Gasson J, Ogawa M, Koeffler HP (1986). Recombinant human TNF induces production of granulocyte-monocyte colony-stimulating factor. Nature 323: 79-82.

Nawroth PP, Bank I, Handley D, Cassimeris J, Chess L, Stern D (1986). Tumor necrosis factor/cachectin interacts with endothelial cell receptors to induce release of interleukin 1. J Exp Med 163: 1363-1375.

Nawroth PP, Stern DM (1986). Modulation of endothelial cell hemostatic properties by tumor necrosis factor. J Exp Med 163-740-745.

Old LJ (1985). Tumor necrosis factor (TNF). Science 230: 630-632.

Pongor S, Ulrich PC, Bencsath FA, Cerami A (1984). Aging of proteins: isolation and identification of a fluorescent chromophore from the reaction of polypeptides with glucose. Proc Natl Acad Sci USA 81: 2684-2688.

Radoff S, Vlassara H, Cerami A. Characterization of a solubilized cell surface binding protein on macrophages specific for proteins modified non-enzymatically by advanced glycosylated endproducts. *Submitted*.

Sugarman BJ, Aggarwal BB, Hass PE, Figari IS, Palladino Jr MA, Shepard HM (1985). Recombinant human tumor necrosis factor-α: effects on proliferation of normal and transformed cells *in vitro*. Science 230: 943-945.

Vlassara H, Brownlee M, Cerami A (1984). Accumulation of diabetic rat peripheral nerve myelin by macrophages increases with the presence of advanced glycosylation endproducts. J Exp Med 160: 197-207.

Vlassara H, Brownlee M, Cerami A (1985). High-affinity receptor-mediated uptake and degradation of glucose-modified proteins: a potential mechanism for the removal of senescent macromolecules. Proc Natl Acad Sci USA 82: 5588-5592.

Vlassara H, Brownlee M, Cerami A (1986). Novel macrophage receptor for glucose-modified proteins is distinct from previously described scavenger receptors. J Exp Med 164: 1301-1309.

Vlassara H, Dinarello C, *et al.* *Manuscript in preparation.*

Vlassara H, Manogue KR, Brownlee M, Pasagian A, Cerami A. Cachectin/tumor necrosis factor is induced by proteins modified by advanced glycosylation products: role in normal tissue remodelling. *Submitted.*

Monokines and Other Non-Lymphocytic Cytokines, pages 153–158
© 1988 Alan R. Liss, Inc.

HUMANS TAKING DIETARY OMEGA-3 FATTY ACIDS HAVE DECREASED *IN VITRO* PRODUCTION OF INTERLEUKIN-1

Stefan Endres, Reza Ghorbani,
Joseph G. Cannon, Gerhard Lonnemann,
Jos W. M. van der Meer, Sheldon M. Wolff
and Charles A. Dinarello

Department of Medicine
New England Medical Center Hospitals
and Tufts University School of Medicine
Boston, MA 02111

INTRODUCTION

The aim of this study was to investigate whether dietary supplementation with omega-3 (w-3) fatty acids, contained in fish-oil, affects the synthesis of interleukin-1 (IL-1). The main forms of w-3 fatty acids are eicosapentaenoic acid (EPA) and docosahexaenoic acid. They are scarce in a normal western diet, but are rich in cold water fish.

The rational to study the effect of w-3 fatty acids on the production of IL-1 was based on several lines of evidence (Table 1): 1) there is a low incidence of inflammatory and coronary artery disease in populations with high intake of w-3 fatty acids; 2) some clinical improvement by dietary w-3 fatty acids has been observed in rheumatoid arthritis, where synovial IL-1 have been implicated as a pathogenic link; and 3) arachidonic acid metabolites, which are altered by w-3 fatty acids, are involved in the regulation of IL-1 production (Dinarello et al., 1984; Kunkel et al., 1986).
Alteration of monocyte function by dietary w-3 fatty acid supplementation has previously been shown (Lee et al., 1985; Payan et al., 1987).

TABLE 1. Beneficial Effects of w-3 Fatty Acids
Compared with Evidence for IL-1 Involvement in
Different Disease Models.

	Beneficial Effect of w-3 Fatty Acids	Evidence for IL-1 Involvement
Glomerulo-nephritis	Fish-oil suppresses lupus nephritis in mice (Kelley, 1983)	Mesangial cells produce IL-1 (Lovett, 1986)
Amyloidosis	Fish-oil retards amyloidosis in mice (Cathcart, 1987)	IL-1 induces serum amyloid A (Ramadori, 1985)
Arthritis	Fish-oil results in subjective alleviation in patients with rheumatoid arthritis (Kremer, 1987)	IL-1 in synovial fluid of arthritic joints (Wood, 1985) IL-1 activates synovial cells (Krane, 1985), osteoclasts and induces PGE_2
Diabetes mellitus	Reduced incidence of diabetes mellitus in Eskimo populations (Kromann and Green, 1980)	IL-1 is cytotoxic for pancreatic islet cells (Bendtzen, 1986)
Athero-sclerosis	w-3 fatty acids inhibit athero-sclerosis in hyperlipidemic swine (Weiner, 1986)	IL-1 is expressed by vascular cells (Libby, 1986) and induces smooth muscle proliferation (Libby, 1988)

METHODS

   We designed a longitudinal study with 6 healthy
volunteers. They added 16 g of fish-oil concentrate
(MaxEPA®) per day, containing 2.7 g EPA, to their
normal diet. This supplement, taken as capsules, was

given for a period of six weeks. *In vitro* IL-1 production was assessed during four phases of the study: before beginning the w-3 supplementation, after six weeks of the supplementation; and during the 10th and the 20th week after cessation of the diet. To ascertain reproducibility, the assay was performed on 3 different days within one week for each of the four study phases.

To determine *in vitro* IL-1 production, peripheral blood mononuclear cells were incubated for 24 hours with different stimuli. At the end of the incubation, the cells were lysed by freeze thawing to obtain total, that is cell-associated plus secreted IL-1. IL-1ß was determined by a specific radioimmunoassay (Lisi et al., 1987).

RESULTS

We confirmed compliance of the volunteers by measuring an increase in the plasma concentration of eicosapentaenoic acid.

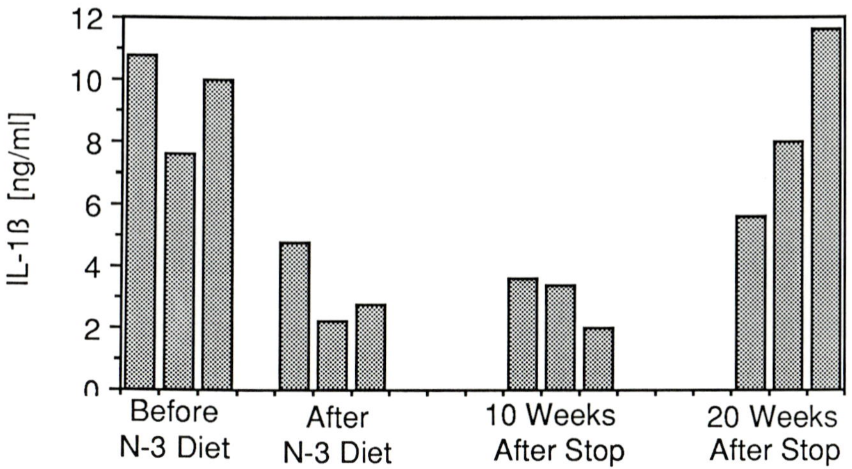

Figure 1. Results for a single subject; *in vitro* IL-1ß production induced by 1 ng/ml endotoxin.

Fig. 1 illustrates the results for a single
subject during the course of the study. Endotoxin
induced production of IL-1ß decreased from 9.5 ng/ml
at base-line to 3 ng/ml after the supplement. Ten
weeks after cessation of the diet IL-1ß production
was still reduced, but had returned to the pre-diet
level by the 20th week after cessation of the diet.
The repeated determinations made on 3 separate days
gave good reproducibility during each phase of the
study. The combined results for all 6 donors showed
the same response as depicted for the individual
donor.

DISCUSSION

The mechanism of decreased IL-1 production
probably involves interference of w-3 fatty acids
with the metabolism of arachidonic acid (Fig. 2).

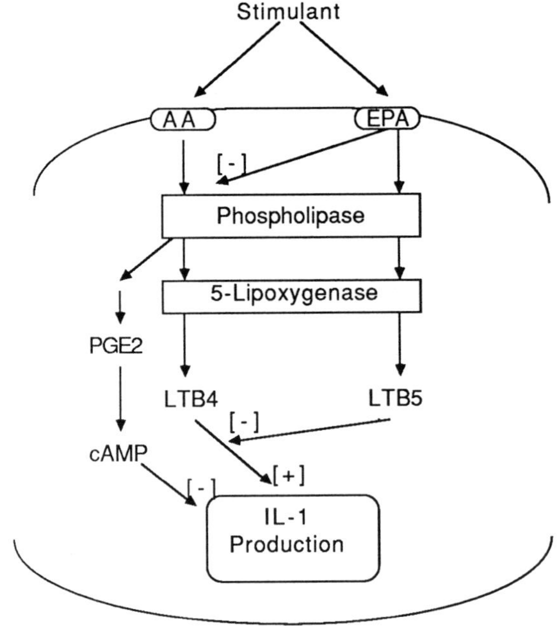

Figure 2. Hypothetical mechanism for effect of w-3
fatty acids on IL-1 production.

In humans taking w-3 fatty acid supplement, EPA is incorporated into the cell membrane. Upon activation of the cell, EPA affects the arachidonic acid metabolism on several levels. In summary, we have shown that: 1) *In vitro* synthesis of IL-1 can be reduced by dietary supplementation; 2) This effect persists as long as 10 weeks after cessation of the diet. At that time production of IL-1 was reduced by 58%; it returned to pre-diet levels after 20 weeks; and 3) The results suggest that the anti-inflammatory effect of n-3 fatty acids may be mediated, in part, by decreased production of IL-1.

REFERENCES

Bendtzen K, Mandrup-Poulsen T, Nerup J, Nielsen JH, Dinarello CA, Svenson M. Cytotoxicity of human pI 7 interleukin-1 for pancreatic islets of Langerhans (1986). Science 232:1545-7.
Cathcart ES, Leslie CA, Meydani SN, Hayes KC. (1987) A fish oil diet retards experimental amyloidosis, modulates lymphocyte function, and decreases macrophage arachidonate metabolism. J Immunol 139:1850-4.
Dinarello CA, Bishai I, Rosenwasser LJ, Coceani F (1984). The influence of lipoxygenase inhibitors on the in vitro production of human leukocytic pyrogen and lymphocyte activating factor (interleukin-1). Int J Immunopharm 6:43-50.
Kelley VE, Ferretti A, Izui A, Strom TB (1985). A fish oil diet rich in eicosapentaenoic acid reduces cyclooxygenase metabolites, and suppresses lupus in mrl-lpr mice. J Immunol 134:1914-9.
Krane SM, Dayer JM, Simon LS, Byrne S (1985). Mononuclear cell conditioned medium containing mononuclear cell factor (MCF), homologous with interleukin-1, stimulates collagen and fibronectin synthesis by adherent rheumatoid synovial cells: effects of prostaglandin E_2 and indomethacin. Collagen Relat Res 5:99-117.
Kremer JM, Jubiz W, Michalek A, et al. (1987). Fish-oil fatty acid supplementation in active rheumatoid arthritis. A double-blinded, controlled, crossover study. Ann Intern Med 106:497-502.

Kromann N, Green A (1980). Epidemiological studies in the Upernavik district, Greenland. Acta Med Scand 208:401-6.

Kunkel SL, Chensue SW, Phan SH (1986). Prostaglandins as endogenous mediators of interleukin 1 production. J Immunol 136:186-92.

Lee TH, Hoover RL, Williams JD, et al. (1985). Effect of dietary enrichment with eicosapentaenoic and docosahexaenoic acids on in vitro neutrophil and monocyte leukotriene generation and neutrophil function. New Engl J Med 312:1217-24.

Libby P, Ordovas JM, Auger KR, Robbins AH, Birinyi LK, Dinarello CA (1986). Endotoxin and tumor necrosis factor induce interleukin-1 gene expression in adult human vascular endothelial cells. Am J Pathol 124:179-186.

Libby P, Warner SJC, Friedman GB (1988). Interleukin-1: a mitogen for human vascular smooth muscle cells that induces the release of growth-inhibitory prostanoids. J Clin Invest in press.

Lisi PJ, Chu CW, Koch GA, Endres S, Lonnemann G, Dinarello CA (1987). Development and use of a radioimmunoassay for human interleukin-1ß. Lymphokine Res 6:229-44.

Lovett DH, Sterzel RB, Ryan JL, Atkins E (1985). Production of an endogenous pyrogen by glomerular mesangial cells. J Immunol 134:670-3.

Payan DG, Wong MYS, Chernov-Rogan T, et al. (1986). Alterations in human leukocyte function induced by ingestion of eicosapentaenoic acid. J Clin Immunol 6:402-10.

Ramadori G, Sipe JD, Dinarello CA, Mizel SB, Colton HR. Pretranslational modulation of acute phase hepatic protein synthesis by murine recombinant interleukin-1 and purified human IL-1 (1985). J Exp Med 162:930-42.

Weiner BH, Ockene IS, Levine PH, et al. (1986). Inhibition of atherosclerosis by cod-liver oil in a hyperlipidemic swine model. N Engl J Med 315:841-6.

Wood DD, Ihrie EJ, Dinarello CA, Cohen PL (1983). Isolation of an interleukin-1-like factor from human joint effusions. Arthritis Rheum 26:975-83.

Monokines and Other Non-Lymphocytic Cytokines, pages 159–163
© 1988 Alan R. Liss, Inc.

REGULATION OF GAMMA INTERFERON PRODUCTION BY EGF: EVIDENCE
FOR A NOVEL INDUCIBLE EGF RECEPTOR ON LYMPHOCYTES

N.A. Abdullah, B.A. Torres, and H.M. Johnson

Department of Comparative and Experimental
Pathology, University of Florida, Gainesville, FL
32610

INTRODUCTION
A major physiological function of individual growth factor families is to modulate cell growth in a tissue specific
manner (Gospodarowicz, 1983). For example, the growth factor interleukin 2 (IL 2) is thought to be restricted to the
lymphoid hematopoietic subpopulation for growth stimulation
(Smith, 1984). Epidermal growth factor (EGF) is capable of
inducing proliferation of many cell types except hematopoietic cells (Carpenter, 1987). However, other functions are
now being attributed to growth factors and their receptors.
The classical growth factors EGF, platelet derived growth
factor (PDGF), and fibroblast growth factor (FGF) have also
been implicated in modulating the immune response. For example, EGF, PDGF, and FGF can replace the IL 2 helper function
for production of murine gamma interferon (IFN$_\gamma$) in vitro
(Johnson and Torres, 1985; Johnson and Torres, 1987). Also,
mononuclear phagocytes, which play a central role in various
immune functions, can produce FGF, PDGF, and EGF-like molecules upon activation (Baird et al, 1985; Martinet et al,
1986; Ross, unpublished data; Shimokado et al, 1985). Thus
these factors are produced by cells that are important for
immune function.
To further study the growth factor replacement of IL 2
for positive regulation of IFN$_\gamma$ production we examine here
the EGF-related factors transforming growth factor α (TGF$_\alpha$;
Marquardt et al, 1984) and vaccinia growth factor (VGF;
Brown et al, 1985) for their ability to provide the helper
signal for IFN$_\gamma$ induction. Both VGF and TGF$_\alpha$ use the same
well-characterized EGF receptor and compete with EGF for
that receptor on mouse 3T3 fibroblasts (Carpenter, 1987;

Eppstein et al, 1985; Massague, 1983).   Functionally, VGF
and TGFα have the same tissue specificity as EGF with regard
to their mitogenic activity (Brown et al, 1985; Carpenter,
1987; Massague, 1983).   A comparison of VGF and TGFα with
EGF for modulating IFNγ production by lymphocytes and for
binding to the EGF receptor on lymphocytes should provide
considerable insight into EGF regulation of immune function
at the level of ligand-receptor interaction.

RESULTS AND DISCUSSION
     Synthetic rat TGFα (Peninsula Labs) and recombinant VGF
(Oncogen, Inc.) were compared with purified mouse submaxil-
lary EGF (Toyobo) for their ability to provide the helper
signal for IFNγ production.   Unlike EGF, neither TGFα nor
VGF could restore competence for IFNγ production by mouse
C57Bl/6 spleen cell cultures that were depleted of helper
cell function (Figure 1).   Both growth factors were as com-

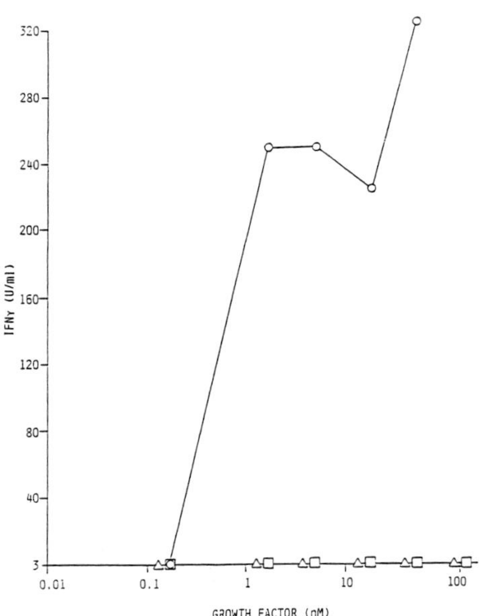

Figure 1. Ability of growth factors to restore competence
for IFNγ production by Lyt 1-, 2+ spleen cells. EGF (O),
TGFα (△), and VGF (□) were incubated with Lyt 1-depleted
spleen cells in the presence of the T-cell mitogen SEA.
IFNγ titers are from day 3 of culture.

petent as EGF in stimulating the proliferation of 3T3 fibroblasts, so their inability to provide the helper signal for
IFNγ production was not due to lack of biological activity
(data not shown). Rather, it is possible that either the
EGF receptor on lymphocytes is different from that on 3T3
cells and thus novel, or that TGFα and VGF can bind to the
EGF lymphocyte receptor but cannot trigger the signal for
IFNγ induction. If the former were true, then TGFα and VGF
should not functionally compete with EGF for the receptor
and thus block its helper signal, whereas if the latter is
true, then they should block the EGF helper signal for IFNγ
production. As shown in Table 1, neither TGFα nor VGF in
molar excess blocked the helper signal of EGF for production
of IFNγ by lymphocytes. Additionally, neither growth factor
blocked IFNγ production by spleen cells that were not depleted of helper cell function (data not shown). Thus, the
functional data suggest that EGF provides its helper signal
for IFNγ production by interaction with a novel receptor on
lymphocytes.

Table 1

Failure of TGFα and VGF to block helper signal
for IFNγ production by mouse spleen cells

SEA-stimulated cultures[a]	IFNγ (U/ml±SD)
Lyt 1[-], 2[+] cells	<7
Lyt 1[-], 2[+] cells + EGF	270±42
Lyt 1[-], 2[+] cells + EGF + TGFα	290±14
Lyt 1[-], 2[+] cells + EGF + VGF	295± 7
Whole spleen cells	215±21

[a]Samples are from day 3 of culture. Concentration of factors: EGF, 30 ng/ml; TGFα, 100 ng/
ml; VGF, 100 ng/ml.

Table 2

Induction of EGF receptor on mouse spleen
lymphocytes[a]

SEA treatment, 0.5 μg/ml	Cold EGF, 3 μM	CPM	p-value
-	-	1115±256	
-	+	1009± 49	N.S.
+	-	1539± 64	
+	+	1158± 54	<0.005

[a]Spleen cells were incubated with SEA for 48 hr,
at which time cultures were depleted of macrophages and red blood cells.

Hematopoietic cells have been reported to lack EGF receptors, thus EGF receptor binding studies were performed on
untreated splenic lymphocytes cultured for 48 hr and splenic
lymphocytes that were stimulated for 48 hr with the T-cell
mitogen staphylococcal enterotoxin A (SEA). As shown in
Table 2, specific binding of ^{125}I-EGF was observed only in
cultures that were stimulated with SEA for 48 hr. Similar
results were observed in at least ten experiments, and specific binding was generally 25 to 50 percent of total binding. The data indicate that the EGF receptor is induced on
lymphocytes and not constitutively expressed as in 3T3

fibroblasts. A saturation binding curve for ^{125}I-EGF on splenic lymphocytes indicated a K_D of 5 to 10 nM.

The functional data presented suggest that EGF exerts its effects on lymphocytes by binding to a novel receptor, since TGFα and VGF could not provide the helper signal for IFNγ production, and could not functionally block the help of EGF. This is supported by the binding competition data where cold EGF blocked ^{125}I-EGF binding to lymphocytes but TGFα at the same concentrations had no effect. It is possible that the binding of mouse ^{125}I-EGF could be due to a contaminant in the EGF preparation, but this is unlikely since purified recombinant human EGF (Scott Labs) inhibited mouse ^{125}I-EGF binding as well as cold mouse EGF.

SUMMARY

We feel that the data presented allow us to draw the following conclusions: a) EGF provides a helper signal for the induction of IFNγ; b) EGF provides its signal by interaction with a novel receptor on lymphocytes based on functional and receptor competition data with TGFα and VGF; c) the novel EGF receptor on lymphocytes is not expressed constitutively but is induced by a T-cell mitogen.

ACKNOWLEDGMENT

This study was supported by NIH Grant CA39048.

REFERENCES

Baird, A, Mormede, P, Bohlen, P (1985). Immunoreactive fibroblast growth factor in cells of peritoneal exudate suggests its identity with macrophage-derived growth factor. Biochem Biophys Res Comm 126:358.

Brown, JB, Twardzik, DR, Marquardt, H, Todaro, GJ (1985). Vaccinia virus encodes a polypeptide homologous to epidermal growth factor and transforming growth factor. Nature 313:491.

Carpenter, G (1987). Receptors for epidermal growth factor and other polypeptide mitogens. Ann Rev Biochem 56:881.

Eppstein, DA, Marsh, YV, Schreiber, AB, Newmann, SR, Todaro, GJ, Nestor, JJ (1985). Epidermal growth factor receptor occupancy inhibits vaccinia virus infection. Nature 318:663.

Gospodarowicz, D (1983). Growth factors and their action in vivo and in vitro. J Pathology 141:201.

Johnson, HM, Torres, BA (1985). Peptide growth factors PDGF, EGF, and FGF regulate interferon-γ production. J Immunol 134:2824.

Johnson, HM, Torres, BA (1987). Lymphokine-like and inter-
    feron regulatory activity of platelet-derived growth
    factor, epidermal growth factor, and fibroblast growth
    factor. Lymphokines 14:253.
Marquardt, H, Hunkapillar, MW, Hood, LE, Todaro, GJ (1984).
    Rat TGF type 1: Structure and relation to EGF. Science
    223:1079.
Martinet, Y, Bitterman, PB, Mornex, J-F, Grotendorst, GR,
    Martin, GR, Crystal, RG (1986). Activated human mono-
    cytes express the c-sis proto-oncogene and release a
    mediator showing PDGF-like activity. Nature 319:158.
Massague, J (1983). Epidermal growth factor-like transform-
    ing growth factor. J Biol Chem 258:13614.
Shimokado, K, Raines, EW, Madtes, DK, Barrett, TB, Benditt,
    EP, Ross, R (1985). A significant part of macrophage-
    derived growth factor consists of at least two forms of
    PDGF. Cell 43:277.
Smith, KA (1984). Interleukin 2. Ann Rev Immunol 2:319.

Section IV. Receptors and Post-Receptor Events

Monokines and Other Non-Lymphocytic Cytokines, pages 167–174
© 1988 Alan R. Liss, Inc.

IMMUNOPRECIPITATION OF INTERLEUKIN-1 RECEPTORS FROM MURINE CELL LINES.

Janet M. D. Plate and Vivek M. Rangnekar

Section of Medical Oncology, Department of Internal Medicine and Department of Immunology, Rush-Presbyterian-St. Luke's Medical Center, Chicago, Illinois

INTRODUCTION

We have successfully immunoprecipitated interleukin-1 (IL-1) receptors solubilized from mouse cell membranes as well as nascent chains of IL-1 receptors with a xenogeneic antiserum. The antiserum was raised in our laboratories against supernates made from draining lymph node cells of skin-graft-primed mice (Plate et al., 1982). These supernates contained mouse skin-graft induced helper factors (SgHF) which led to an antigen specific induction of cytolytic T lymphocytes (Plate et al., 1982) and/or to the induction of IL-2 synthesis (Plate, 1984). The xenogeneic antiserum administered to skin-graft recipients resulted in prolongation of major histocompatibility complex incompatible skin-graft survival and was called rat anti-skin-graft induced helper factor serum (rat anti-SgHF) (McMannis and Plate, 1985a). The rat anti-SgHF inhibited the differentiation of precytolytic effector cells in mixed lymphocyte cultures by blocking the helper T cell pathway (McMannis and Plate, 1985b). Kinetic studies revealed a time dependent modulation of IL-1 function by the antiserum. This modulation appeared to have been the result of antibody mediated internalization of cell surface IL-1 receptor molecules required for helper T cell activation. The strongest evidence had been that the interaction of cells with IL-1, before modulation of the antigenic target by the antiserum was completed, resulted in the reversal of the inhibitory effect of this xenogeneic antiserum on the helper T cell pathway. The present data confirm that the antiserum recognized determinants on IL-1 receptors. The antiserum does not immunoprecipitate free IL-1, but does immunoprecipitate ligand-conjugated IL-1 receptors on mouse thymoma, lymphoma and fibroblast lines.

MATERIALS AND METHODS

<u>Cell Lines</u>: P388D$_1$ monocytes, EL-4 thymoma cells, LBRM-33,1A5 T lymphoma cells and BALB/c 3T3 fibroblast cells were maintained in endotoxin-defined conventional tissue culture medium with 10% fetal calf serum, L-glutamine and antibiotics.

<u>Interleukins</u>: Purified human IL-1-alpha and radiolabeled human IL-1-alpha were generous gifts from Dr. P.L. Kilian and R. Chizzonite, Hoffmann-LaRoche, Nutley NJ (Kilian et al, 1986). Specific activity of radiolabeled IL-1-alpha samples ranged from 1170 to 2049 cpm/femtamole. Purified human IL-1-beta was purchased from Cistron Laboratories, Pinebrook, NJ. Recombinant human IL-2 was a gift from the Cetus Corporation, Emeryville, CA.

<u>Antisera</u>: Antiserum was raised in Fisher F-344 rats against supernates derived from draining lymph node cells of class I MHC disparate mice as described (Plate et al., 1982; McMannis and Plate, 1985a).

<u>^{125}I-IL-1-Alpha Binding</u>: The radiolabeled IL-1-alpha was incubated at 4°C for 16 hr with the IL-1 responsive murine cell lines: LBRM-33,1A5, 3T3 fibroblast, and EL-4 thymoma. In most experiments, 2.5 pM ^{125}I-IL-1-alpha was incubated with 3 x 10^{6} cells. The cells were washed extensively and counted. Specific IL-1-alpha binding was determined by subtracting from the total cpm the number of cpm bound in the presence of unlabeled IL-1 at 25 nM.

<u>Affinity Cross-Linking</u>: The affinity cross-linking reagents dithiobis-succinimidyl propionate (DSP) or disuccinimidyl tartrate (DST) (Pierce Chemical Company, Rockford, IL) were used to covalently bind the radiolabeled IL-1-alpha to their receptors (Dower et al., 1985; Dower et al., 1986).

<u>Immunoprecipitation</u>: Immunoglobulins were conjugated to formalin-fixed protein A bearing <u>Staphylococcus aureus</u> (IgSorb, Monoclonal Antibody Center, Cambridge, MA) by means of an affinity purified goat anti-rat immunoglobulin

(Southern Biotechnology Associates, Birmingham, AL). Rat immunoglobulin conjugated IgSorb was mixed with ^{125}I-ligand labeled and cross-linked cells which had been lysed in phosphate buffered saline containing 1% CHAPS (3-((Cholamidopropyl) dimethyl-ammonio)) 1-propanesulfonate) and 2 mM phenylmethyl-sulphonyl fluoride. Mixtures were incubated for 2 hr at 4°C, then pelleted. The supernates containing all non-immunoprecipitated materials were saved and prepared for SDS-PAGE analyses. Pellets were washed five times with CHAPS lysis buffer and twice with buffer that also contained 0.05% SDS and 0.5 M NaCl before boiling in 50 ul of SDS-sample buffer. The bacterial debris were removed by microfugation and the freed immunoprecipitated materials subjected to SDS-PAGE.

<u>SDS-PAGE, Transblotting, and Autoradiography</u>: Laemmli SDS-PAGE with a 12% acrylamide, N,N'-methylene bis-acrylamide separating gel and a 4% stacking gel were used to separate proteins after cross-linking, lysis, and immunoprecipitation. Prestained protein standards (BRL, Gaithersburg, MD) were used to evaluate separation and determine the molecular weights of the separated proteins. Initial experimental gels were transblotted onto nitrocellulose. The transblots were exposed at -70°C to Kodak X-Omat AR film in the presence of two intensifying screens, then developed for autoradiography.

RESULTS

<u>Cross-linking of IL-1 to Membrane Associated Receptors</u>: LBRM-33,1A5 cells were cross-linked to ^{125}I-IL-1-alpha using the reducible cross-linking reagent, DSP. Lysates of these cells were then subjected to SDS-PAGE analyses. A single radioactive band with an apparent molecular weight of 97 kDa was revealed in non-reduced LBRM-33,1A5 samples (Fig. 1A, Lane 2), whereas under reducing conditions the 97 kDa band disappeared (Fig. 1A, Lane 1). These data demonstrated the effective cross-linking of the IL-1 ligand to cell surface molecules. Specific binding of ^{125}I-IL-1-alpha was demonstrated through the inhibition of the formation of radiolabeled complexes by the addition of excess unlabeled IL-1 into the binding reaction (Fig. 1A, Lane 3; Fig. 1B, Lane 1). Recombinant IL-2, on the other hand, did not inhibit the binding of radiolabeled IL-1 to form a ligand-receptor complex, hence the 97 kDa band was intact (Fig. 1C, Lane 1). These data confirmed that the 17.5 kDa

radiolabeled IL-1 bound specifically to 79.5 kDa cell surface molecules, which apparently were IL-1 receptors.

^{125}I-IL-1-alpha was also cross-linked to the cells
with DST, a non-reducible cross-linker. The receptor IL-1
complex migrated at similar molecular weight position under
both reducing (Fig. 1D, Lane 1) and non-reducing conditions
(Fig. 1D, Lane 2). These data suggested that IL-1 was not
covalently cross-linked to other subunits as part of the
receptor complex.

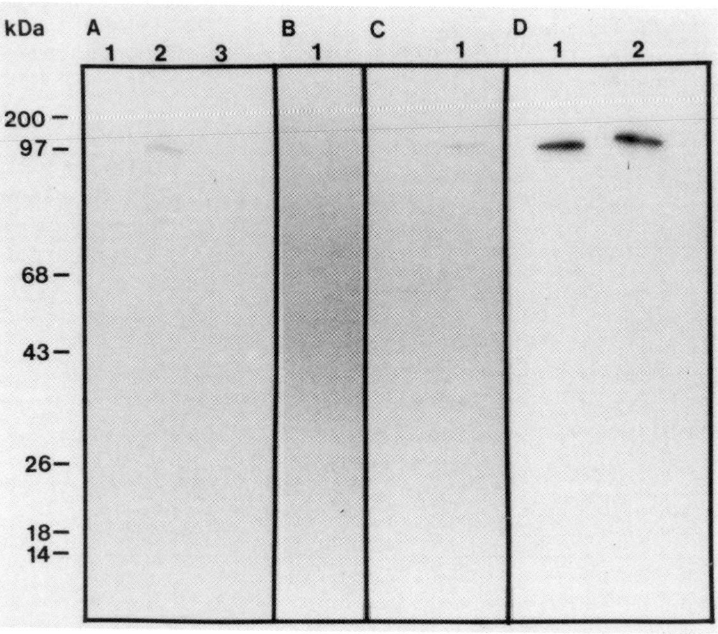

FIGURE 1.   Binding of ^{125}I-IL-1 to LBRM-33,1A5 cell surface
receptors examined by autoradiography of the transblotted
SDS-polyacrylamide gel.   Cells cross-linked to ^{125}I-IL-1
with DSP (Fig. 1A, B, C) or DST (D) were lysed with CHAPS
buffer and electrophoresed under reducing (A, Lane 1; D,
Lane 1) and non-reducing conditions (A, Lanes 2, 3; B, Lane
1; C, Lane 1; D, Lane 2). Specific binding of ^{125}I-IL-1 to
its receptors was inhibited by adding murine P388D$_1$ derived
cold IL-1 (A, Lane 3) and purified human IL-1-alpha (B,
Lane 1).   Addition of cold rIL-2 to the binding reaction
did not inhibit IL-1 binding to the receptors (C, Lane 1).

<u>Immunoprecipitation of IL-1 Receptor Complexes</u>:   SDS-PAGE analyses were performed with radiolabeled immunoprecipitated complexes.   Both the IgSorb pellet (immunoprecipitable complex) and the supernate (non-immunoprecipitable component) from the immunoprecipitation reaction were prepared for electrophoresis.   The rat anti-SgHF immunoprecipitated   a   single sized 97 kDa molecule from   IL-1-alpha radiolabeled lysates of EL-4 (Fig.   2A,   Lane 1), 3T3 (Fig. 2B, Lane 1),   and LBRM-33,1A5 cells (Fig.   2B,   Lane 2). Normal rat immunoglobulins, on the other hand, did not immunoprecipitate the radiolabeled IL-1 receptor complex (Fig. 2C, Lane 2), hence, the supernate from the normal rat immunoglobulin reaction which was comprised of the non-immunoprecipitable material still contained the 97 kDa complex (Fig. 2C, Lane 1). The supernates of the rat anti-SgHF immunoprecipitates contained no detectable radiolabeled material indicating that the majority of the specifically labeled receptors had been immunoprecipitated. The size of the radiolabeled complex immunoprecipitated with rat anti-SgHF was similar to that of the IL-1 receptor complex.   These data further demonstrate that antibodies present in the rat anti-SgHF recognize the IL-1 receptor complex.

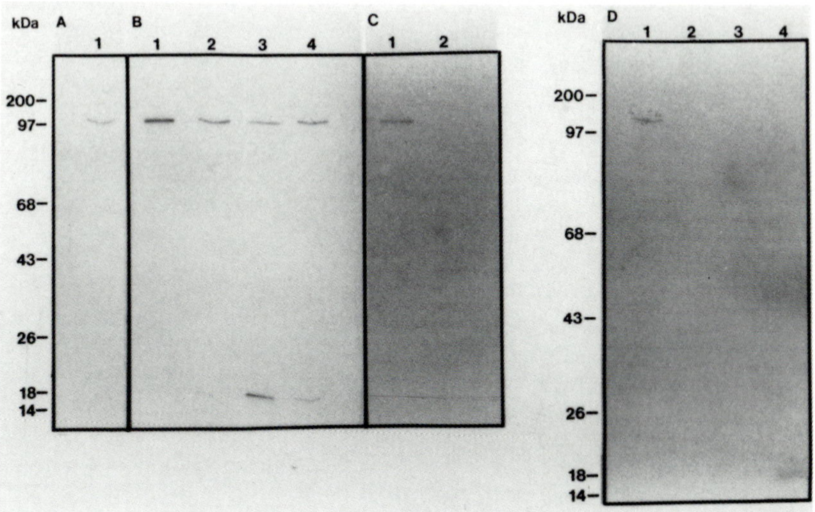

<u>FIGURE 2</u>.   Autoradiographs of immunoprecipitated and SDS-PAGE separated complexes.   Control lysates of radiolabeled

<u>Specificity of the Xenogeneic Antiserum for the IL-1 Recep-</u>
<u>tor Moiety of the Receptor-Ligand Complex</u>:   The immunopre-
cipitated complexes were comprised of both IL-1 and the IL-
1 receptor, hence, the antiserum could have recognized
either IL-1 or receptor molecules.   Experiments were set
up, therefore, to determine 1) whether the antiserum could
directly immunoprecipitate radiolabeled IL-1, or 2) whether
incubation of the IgSorb bound antiserum with unlabeled IL-
1 could inhibit the subsequent immunoprecipitation of the
radiolabeled receptor ligand complex, or 3) whether the
antiserum could immunoprecipitate nonspecifically associated cell bound radiolabeled IL-1.   Free ^{125}I-IL-1-alpha
was not immunoprecipitated by the antiserum (Fig.   2D, Lane
3).   The non-immunoprecipitable component (supernate of the
reaction mixture) still contained the radiolabeled IL-1-
alpha molecules, thus, a band was observed at approximately

IL-1 bound complexes formed after cross-linking ^{125}I-IL-1
to 3T3 and LBRM-33,1A5 are depicted in B, Lanes 3 and 4,
respectively.   Lysates were immunoprecipitated with xenogeneic rat anti-SgHF or normal rat immunoglobulin.   The rat
anti-SgHF immunoprecipitated IL-1 receptor, ^{125}I-IL-1 complex of 97 kDa from EL-4 (A, Lane 1), 3T3 (B, Lane 1), and
LBRM-33,1A5 (B, Lane 2).   Fig. 3C, Lanes 1 and 2, respectively, contained the non-immunoprecipitable (supernate)
and immunoprecipitable (pellet) components of the immunoprecipitation reaction between normal rat immunoglobulin
and lysate from ^{125}I-IL-1 cross-linked EL-4 cells.   The
radiolabeled complex was evident in the supernate (C, Lane
1) demonstrating that the normal rat immunoglobulin did not
immunoprecipitate IL-1 receptor complexes.   Free ^{125}I-IL-1,
without cellular lysates, was used in immunoprecipitation
reactions directly with rat anti-SgHF.   The supernate (D,
Lane 4) and pellet (D, Lane 3) from the immunoprecipitation
reaction were electrophoresed.   The free ^{125}I-IL-1 was not
immunoprecipitated, hence, remained in the supernate (D,
Lane 4).   Also, rat anti-SgHF immunoglobulin was first
mixed with IL-1, then used to immunoprecipitate bound complexes from lysates made after cross-linking ^{125}I-IL-1 to
LBRM-33,1A5 cells.   Fig. 3D, Lanes 1 and 2, respectively,
contained the immunoprecipitable component (pellet) and
supernate (non-immunoprecipitable component) of the reaction.   Preincubation of soluble IL-1 with rat anti-SgHF
immunoglobulin, therefore, did not inhibit the immunoprecipitation of the radiolabeled IL-1 receptor complex (D,
Lane 1).

17.5 kDa (Fig. 2D, Lane 4). Furthermore, incubation of the
IgSorb conjugated rat anti-SgHF immunoglobulins with IL-1,
before immunoprecipitation, did not inhibit immunoprecipitation of the radiolabeled complexes (Fig. 2D, Lane 1).
The supernate of the latter immunoprecipitation reaction
was devoid of radiolabeled receptor complexes, hence, no
reduction of the ability to immunoprecipitate the complexes
was observed (Fig. 2D, Lane 2).

DISCUSSION

We demonstrate that a 97,000 molecular weight receptor
complex that had been affinity cross-linked with the radiolabeled ligand, IL-1, can be immunoprecipitated from mouse
cells with our xenogeneic rat antiserum. Cross-linked
complexes of similar sizes were successfully immunoprecipitated from thymoma, lymphoma, and fibroblast cell lines.
The specificity of interaction between the IL-1 bound receptor complex and the xenogeneic antiserum was demonstrated; 1) unlabeled IL-1 added to the binding reaction
between ^{125}I-IL-1 and murine IL-1 receptors competitively
inhibited radiolabeled IL-1 binding and subsequent immunoprecipitation of a radiolabeled complex; this experiment
also revealed that radiolabeled IL-1 molecules nonspecifically associated with cell membranes were not immunoprecipitated; 2) addition of rIL-2 to the binding reaction did
not affect immunoprecipitation of the radiolabeled complexes; 3) the xenogeneic antiserum neither bound to nor
immunoprecipitated free IL-1 molecules; and finally, we
demonstrated in another manuscript that 4) the xenogeneic
antiserum binds nascent peptide chains which are capable of
specifically binding to the IL-1 ligand. It is apparent,
thus, that antibodies present in the xenogeneic antiserum
can specifically bind to the IL-1 receptor. This antiserum
should now allow us to purify and characterize IL-1 receptor molecules as well as to clone the cDNA encoding the IL-
1 receptor.

ACKNOWLEDGEMENTS

This research was supported in part by NIH Grant No.
CA-25612. The authors gratefully acknowledge Drs. PL
Kilian and R Chizzonite, Hoffmann-LaRoche, Inc., for radiolabeled human IL-1-alpha, and Ms. Donna Dickerson for the
preparation of this manuscript.

REFERENCES

Plate JMD, McDaniel CA, Flaherty L, Stimpfling JH, Melvold RW, Martin NQ (1982). Antigen specific soluble helper activity for murine major histocompatibility complex encoded molecules. I. Kinetics of factor production following skin transplantation and genetic mapping of the H-2 region specificity. J Exp Med, 155:681-697.

Plate JMD (1984). The dissection of helper T cell pathways during T cell responses to class I alloantigens. Proc Am Assoc Cancer Res 25:264.

McMannis JD, Plate JMD (1985). Xenogeneic antisera to soluble products from activated lymph node cells. I. Characterization of reactivity and effects on immune responses. Transplantation 40:405-412.

McMannis JD, Plate JMD (1985). Xenogeneic antiserum to soluble products from activated lymphoid cells inhibits Interleukin-1 mediated fucntions in the helper pathway of cytolytic effector cell differentiation. Proc Natl Acad Sci USA   82:1513-1517.

Kilian PL, Kaffka KL, Stern AS, Woehle D, Benjamin WR, DeChiara TM, Gubler U, Farrar JJ, Mizel SB, Lomedico PT (1986). Interleukin-1-alpha and interleukin-1-beta bind to the same receptor on T cells. J Immunol, 136:4509-4514.

Dower SK, Kronheim SR, March CJ, Conlon PJ, Hopp TP, Gillis S, Urdal DL (1985). Detection and characterization of high affinity plasma membrane receptors for human interleukin-1. J Exp Med, 162:501-515.

Dower SK, Call SM, Gillis S, Urdal DL (1986). Similarity between the interleukin-1 receptors on a murine T lymphoma cell line and on a murine fibroblast cell line. Proc Natl Acad Sci USA, 83:1060-1064.

Monokines and Other Non-Lymphocytic Cytokines, pages 175–178
© 1988 Alan R. Liss, Inc.

STRUCTURE AND PROPERTIES OF THE RECEPTOR FOR INTERLEUKIN 1

Michael Martin, Roswitha Kroggel, Marta Szamel
and Klaus Resch

Institute of Molecular Pharmacology, Medical
School Hannover, D-3000 Hannover 61, FRG

INTRODUCTION

Similar to the polypeptide hormones the biological activity of the cytokine IL-1 is mediated by high affinity
binding to plasma membrane receptors (Oppenheim et al.,
1986; Dower and Urdal, 1987; Martin and Resch, 1988). As
this receptor is not abundant on cells, its properties have
not been fully established. IL-1 binding proteins have been
described in different cells with molecular masses ranging
from about 60 to 100 kDa (Dower et al., 1986; Matsushima
et al., 1986; Bird and Saklatvala, 1987; Bron and MacDonald,
1987). Part of this heterogeneity can be explained by a
variable degree of glycosylation (Bron and MacDonald,1987).
Very little is known about the intracellular signals generated by the IL-1 receptor. Recently, phosphorylation of a
cytoplasmic protein was shown in response to IL-1, suggesting activation of protein kinases as part of the signal
transduction (Matsushima et al., 1987).

RESULTS AND DISCUSSION

We have shown earlier that purified murine IL-1 inhibited the growth of several tumor cell lines, including
the human myelogenous leukemia cell line K 562, and the
murine T-lymphoma EL-4 (Lovett et al., 1986). Similar results were obtained with recombinant human IL-1 alpha or
IL-1 beta. In all instances, concentrations of 1-10 U/ml
were effective.

In isolated plasma membranes of these cells, natural

and recombinant IL-1 selectively induced at 4° C the phosphorylation of a single protein of M_r of 41 (K 562) or 43 (EL-4) kDa (Martin et al., 1986; Resch et al., 1988). The stimulation of this protein phosphorylation by IL-1 was time and concentration dependent, and independent of cAMP, cGMP, or Ca^{2+}. Analysis of the phosphoaminoacids of this protein revealed that after induction with IL-1 radioactiv label was exclusively present in tyrosine phosphate. Experiments with the radioactive affinity labelling ATP analogue fluorosulfonylbenzoyl-adenosine (FSBA) led to a labelling of the 41 to 43 kDa protein suggesting that it possessed an ATP binding and cleaving capacity (M. Martin, D. Lovett, M. Szamel and K. Resch, submitted to Eur. J. Biochem). This is consistant with the notion that this protein contains the tyrosine kinase activity, and that phosphorylation is the result of an autophosphorylation. Protein-tyrosine kinases with ligand induced capacity of autophosphorylation are characteristic for many growth regulating receptors .

IL-1 binding proteins so far have been reported in the range of 60 to 100 kDa. In experiments, in which ^{125}I-labelled rh IL-1alpha was crosslinked for 60 min at room temperature with disuccinimidyl suberate (DSS), the usual crosslinking conditions, to EL-4 cells, two labelled products of M_r of about 97 and 140 kDa were found. When the crosslinked IL-1 is substracted, this corresponds to putative receptor (glyco)proteins of about 80, or 143 kDa. As the larger binding site could be the complex of the 80 kDa and a 43 kDa protein, crosslinking was performed also at conditions minimizing the formation of larger protein aggregates. The Fig. shows that indeed at short crosslinking times at 4° C (5 min) a distinct band at 60 kDa became apparent, which became weaker after longer time periods of crosslinking. After substraction of IL-1 this band corresponds to a 43 kDa IL-1 binding protein (Kroggel et al., 1988).

From these experiments a model for the IL-1 receptor can be deduced. The receptor for IL-1 may consist of two noncovalently linked chains, the alpha chain with a M_r of about 80 kDa and the beta chain with a M_r of 41 to 43 kDa. Both chains contribute to IL-1 binding, and as a dimer may represent the high affinity receptor, as described in EL-4 cells (Lowenthal and MacDonald, 1986). The beta chain

contains a cytoplasmic portion, which carrries a tyrosine
protein kinase with autophosphorylating properties. This
two chain model has similarities to the recently revealed
structure of the receptor for IL-2 (Smith, 1986). It also
reveales the general structure of receptors for growth regulating hormones, such as the insulin receptor .

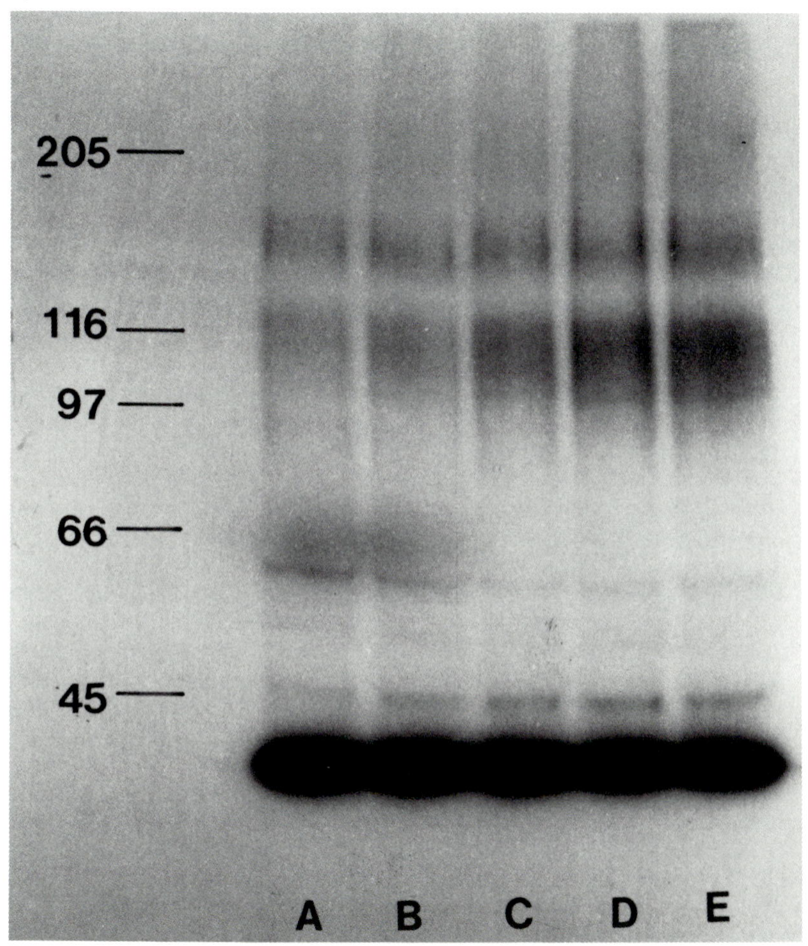

10^7 EL-4 cells were incubated with 0.1 µCi of human recombinant ^{125}I IL-1 alpha at 4° C for 1 hour, washed twice
and crosslinked with 0.5 mM DSS at 25° C for 5,15,30,60,
or 120 minutes (lane A to E). The cells were washed twice
and lysed with 1% Triton in PBS, pH 7.4. The membrane proteins were denaturated and separated by SDS-PAGE as in
(9, 12).

Bird TA and Saklatvala J (1987). Studies on the fate of receptor-bound ^{125}I-interleukin 1beta in porcine synovial fibroblasts. J Immunol 139:92-97.

Bron C and MacDonald HR (1987). Identification of the plasma membrane receptor for interleukin 1 on mouse thymoma cells. FEBS Lett 219:365-368.

Dower SK, Call SM, Gillis S, and Urdal DL (1986). Similaryty between the interleukin receptors on a murine T lymphoma cell line and on a fibroblast cell line. Proc Natl Acad Sci 83:1060-1063.

Dower SK and Urdal DL (1987). The interleukin-1 receptor. Immunol Today 8:46-51.

Kroggel R, Martin M, Pingoud V, Dayer JM, and Resch K (1988). Two chain structure of the interleukin 1 receptor. FEBS Lett; accepted for publication.

Lovett D, Kozan B, Hadam M, Resch K, and Gemsa D (1986). Macrophage cytotoxicity: Interleukin 1 as a mediator of tumor cytostasis. J Immunol 136:340-347.

Lowenthal JW and MacDonald HR (1986). Binding and internalization of interleukin 1 by T cells: Direct evidence for high and low affinity classes of interleukin 1 receptor. J Exp Med 164:1060-1074.

Martin M, Lovett D, and Resch K (1986). Interleukin 1 induces specific phosphorylation of a 41 kDa plasma membrane protein from the human tumor cell line K 562. Immunobiol 171:165-169.

Martin M and Resch K (1988). Interleukin 1: More than a mediator between leukocytes. Trends Pharmacol Sci, in press

Matsushima K, Akahoshi T, Yamada M, Furutani Y, and Oppenheim JJ (1986). Properties of a specific interleukin 1 (IL-1) receptor on human Epstein Barr-virus transformed B-lymphocytes: Identity of the receptor for IL-1alpha and IL-1beta. J Immunol 136:4496-4502.

Matsushima K, Kobayashi Y, Copeland TD, Akahoshi T, and Oppenheim JJ (1987). Phosphorylation of a cytosolic 65-kDa protein induced by interleukin 1 in glucocorticoid pretreated normal human peripheral blood mononuclear leukocytes. J Immunol 139:3367-3374.

Oppenheim JJ, Kowacs EJ, Matsushima K, and Durum SK (1986). There is more than one interleukin 1. Immunol Today 7:45-56.

Resch K, Kroggel R, Kyas U, and Martin M (1988). Biological and molecular properties of the receptor for interleukin 1 on tumor cells. In Bonavida B et al. (eds): "Proc. of the Int.Conf.on TNF and rel.cytotoxins. Basel: Karger, in press.

Smith KA (1986). The two-chain structure of high affinity IL-2 receptors. Immunol Today 8:11-13.

Monokines and Other Non-Lymphocytic Cytokines, pages 179–184

EVIDENCE FOR DIFFERENCES IN THE MOLECULAR PROPERTIES OF
INTERLEUKIN-1 RECEPTORS

Richard Horuk, James J. Huang, Maryanne Covington,
and Robert C. Newton
Medical Products Division; E.I. Du Pont De Nemours &
Co., Glenolden Laboratory, Glenolden, PA 19036

INTRODUCTION

Interleukin 1 (IL-1) is a macrophage-derived
polypeptide hormone of molecular weight 17,500 (Oppenheim
et al., 1986). Numerous reports, (Dower and Urdal, 1987)
have demonstrated that IL-1 interacts with cellular
receptors to elicit its biologic effects. Despite
mediating a wide range of biologic activities in a
diverse number of cell types, (Oppenheim and Gery, 1982,
Dinarello, 1984, Durum et al., 1985, Whicher and
Chambers, 1984) the IL-1 receptor binding region is
thought to be tightly conserved (see evidence cited by
Dower and Urdal, 1987). It is not clear, however,
whether all cells share a common IL-1 receptor or whether
receptors in different target tissues have undergone
evolutionary change and thus acquired new roles. In this
report we demonstrate fundamental differences in the
molecular properties of the IL-1 receptor in two cell
lines, Raji (human B-lymphoma) and EL4 (murine
T-lymphoma) cells.

RESULTS AND DISCUSSION

Several studies have recently shown that IL-1
receptors internalize at 37°C (Lowenthal and MacDonald,
1986, Matsushima et al., 1986, Bird and Saklatvala,
1986). To determine the extent of internalization of
IL-1 receptors at 37°C, Raji and EL4 cells were incubated
with [^{125}I]-IL-1 in the presence or absence of sodium

azide and subjected to the acid stripping procedure
described by Haigler et al., 1980. With this approach,
non acid-extractable material is taken as a measure of
internalized radioactivity and extractable material is
considered to be surface bound $[^{125}I]$-IL-1. At 37°C EL4
cells internalized 59% of the radiolabeled IL-1 after
only 2 h. In contrast, IL-1 binding to Raji cells at
37°C was almost exclusively cell surface, 91%, even after
6 h.

Endocytosis is known to be an energy-dependent
process inhibitable by agents such as cyanide or azide.
Thus, we examined the ability of sodium azide to inhibit
the of IL-1 receptors at 37°C. The addition of sodium
azide to EL4 cells at 37°C dramatically altered the
distribution of radioligand in these cells such that 93%
of binding was to cell surface receptors compared to only
41% in the absence of azide. In contrast sodium azide
had no effect on IL-1 binding in Raji cells. Incubation
with sodium azide did not appear to have any deleterious
effects on the cells as judged by trypan blue exclusion.

Scatchard analysis (Scatchard, 1949) of equilibrium
binding data for $[^{125}I]$-IL-1 at 37°C to EL4 and Raji
cells is shown in Figure 1. The linear plots are
indicative of a single class of IL-1 receptor binding
sites in both cell types. For EL4 cells the calculated
apparent K_D was 0.4 ± 0.088 nM with 241 ± 85 binding
sites per cell (average from four separate experiments),
and for Raji cells the calculated apparent KD was 2.1 ±
0.12 nM with 7709 ± 950 binding sites per cell. The
parameters of IL-1 binding in these two cell types thus
differ both in terms of cell number and in the receptor
binding affinity.

The specificity of IL-1 receptors in EL4 and Raji
cells was further investigated with the aid of IL-1
analogs generated by site specific mutagenesis, Figure 2
(Huang et al., 1987). The analogs were able to inhibit
the binding of $[^{125}]$-I labeled IL-1 in Raji and EL4
cells, Figure 2. The relative binding affinities of
clone 18 and Glu 4, calculated from competition curves,
was 200 and 0.2% respectively in EL4 cells. In Raji
cells the relative binding affinities of clone 18 and

Glu 4 were 90 and 25% respectively. The marked
differences in the relative binding affinities of these
analogs in EL4 and Raji cells suggests that there are
structural differences in the way IL-1 is seen by
receptors on these two cell lines.

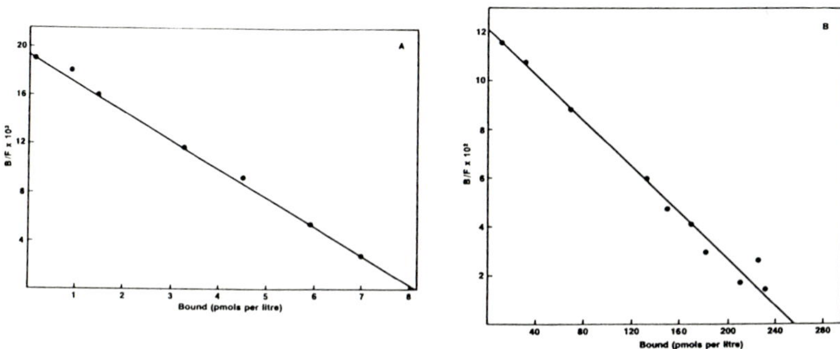

Figure 1. Scatchard analysis of [^{125}I]-IL-1 binding to
(A) EL4 and (B) Raji cells at 37°C. Cells (2 x 10^7) were
incubated with varying concentrations of radiolabeled
IL-1 for 3 h. Data were analyzed as described by
McPherson, 1983.
Binding represents specific binding.

Residue #	115	116	117	118	119	120	121	Relative Receptor Binding Affinity (%)	
								EL4	Raji
nβ-IL1			ALA	PRO	VAL	ARG	SER	100	100
rβ-IL1	THR	ASN	ALA	PRO	VAL	ARG	SER	100	100
Clone 18			THR	MET	VAL	ARG	SER	189–210	90–110
Glu-4			THR	MET	VAL	GLU	SER	0.2–0.3	20–30

Figure 2. Comparison of the N-terminal amino acid
sequences of human IL-1-β with human recombinant IL-1-β
and analogs. Relative receptor binding affinities of the
analogs were calculated as the ratio between the
concentration of unlabeled IL-1 giving half maximal
inhibition of radiolabeled IL-1 receptor binding, and the
concentration of analog giving half maximal inhibition x
100. Data represent the range from 3 separate
experiments.

The IL-1 receptor on these two cell types was further characterized by chemical crosslinking with ^{125}I-labeled IL-1 in the presence or absence of an excess of unlabeled IL-1, Figure 3. Both cell lines showed covalent incorporation of radiolabeled IL-1 into one protein band. In Raji cells a protein of molecular weight 85 KDa was labeled while in EL4 cells the molecular size of the labeled band was 98 KDa. In both cases labeling was specific since it could be inhibited by the addition of excess IL-1.

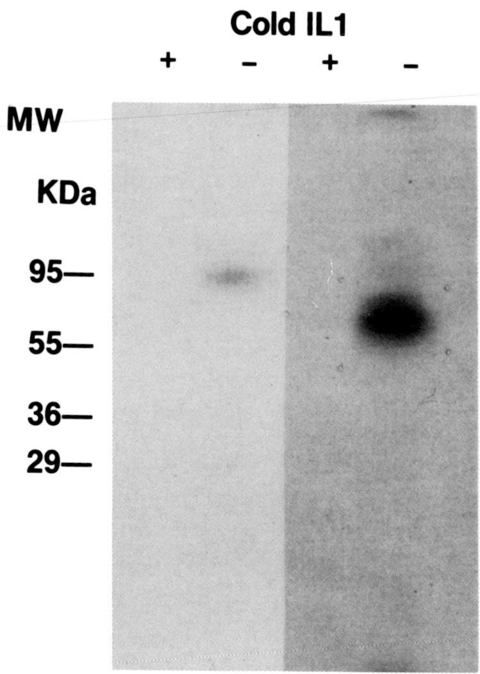

Figure 3. SDS-PAGE analysis of IL-1 receptors in EL4 and Raji cells covalently crosslinked with [^{125}I]-IL-1. Cells were covalently labeled with radiolabeled IL-1 in the presence or absence of unlabeled IL-1 (as indicated) and subjected to SDS-PAGE as previously described (Horuk, et al., 1986). The molecular weights indicated in the left margin were estimated from standards.

Raji cells are B-lymphocytes infected with Epstein
Barr Virus (EBV) derived from a patient with Burkitt's
lymphoma (Minowada et al., 1982). Given the observation
that Burkitt's lymphoma is characterized by the presence
of large numbers of undifferentiated B-cells (Carbone,
1983) and that IL-1 is known to promote the
differentiation of pre B- to mature B-cells (Giri et al.,
1984) it seems reasonable to speculate that the changes
observed in the Raji IL-1 receptor could be contributory
factors to the cancerous nature of these cells.

Comparison of the Raji IL-1 receptor cDNA sequence
with those from other cells will be useful in determining
whether the strikingly different biochemical properties
of the IL-1 receptor observed here i.e., failure to
internalize, altered receptor binding affinities with
IL-1 analogs, decrease in molecular size, could be due to
the deletion of an integral polypeptide domain in the
protein. Such studies with the Raji IL-1 receptor might
provide a clearer understanding of receptor function,
intracellular trafficking and receptor mediated signaling
processes and should help to unravel the complex sequence
of biochemical events that accompany IL-1 action in the
cell.

REFERENCES

Bird TA, Saklatvala J (1986). Nature 324:263-266.

Carbone PA (1983). In: Cecils Textbook of Medicine,
  Wyngaarden JB, Smith LH (eds) W. B. Saunders,
  Philadelphia: p953.

Dinarello CA (1984). Rev Infect Dis 6:51-95

Dower SK, Urdal DL (1987). Immunology Today 8:46-51.

Durum SK, Schmidt JA, Oppenheim JJ (1985). Ann Rev
  Immunol 3:263-287.

Giri JG, Kincade PW, Mizel SB (1984). J Immunol
  132:223-228.

Haigler HT, Maxfield FR, Willingham MC, Pastan
  I (1980). J Biol Chem 255:1239-1241.

Horuk R, Matthaei S, Olefsky JM, Baly DL, Cushman SW,
  Simpson IA (1986). J Biol Chem 261:1823-1828.

Huang JJ, Newton RC, Pezzella K, Covington M,
   Tamblyn T, Rutledge SJ, Kelley M, Lin Y (1987).
   Mol Biol and Med 4:169–181.

Lowenthal JW, MacDonald HR (1986). J Exp Med
   164:1090–1074.

Matsushima K, Yodoi J, Tagaya Y, Oppenheim JJ
   (1986). J Immunol 137:3183–3188.

McPherson GA (1983). Comp Prog in Biomed 17:107–114.

Minowada J, Sagawa K, Trowbridge IS, Kung PD, Goldstein G
   (1982). In Rosenberg SA, Kaplan HS (eds): Malignant
   Melanomas, New York: Academic Press, p 53.

Oppenheim JI, Gery T (1982). Immunology Today 3:113–119.

Oppenheim JI, Kovacs EJ, Matsushima K, Durum SK (1986).
   Immunology Today 7:45–56.

Scatchard G (1949). Ann NY Acad Sci 52:660–672.

Whicher J, Chambers R (1984). Immunology Today 5:3–4.

Monokines and Other Non-Lymphocytic Cytokines, pages 185–190

EVIDENCE FOR AN ESSENTIAL DISULFIDE BOND REQUIRED FOR BINDING ACTIVITY OF THE INTERLEUKIN-1 RECEPTOR

Kathryn Paganelli Parker and Patricia L. Kilian

Department of Immunopharmacology, Hoffmann-La Roche Inc., Nutley, New Jersey 07110

SUMMARY

Treatment of membrane-bound or detergent solubilized interleukin-1 (IL-1) receptors with the disulfide reducing agents dithiothreitol (DTT) or 2-mercaptoethanol (2-ME) results in the inhibition of ^{125}I-IL-1 binding to its receptor. The observed decrease in binding is primarily due to a reduction in the number of IL-1 receptor sites. When the receptor is preincubated with IL-1 prior to addition of dithiothreitol, no loss in binding is seen. These experiments suggest that the interleukin-1 receptor requires the presence of an intact disulfide bond for binding activity. The disulfide bond may be located in the IL-1 receptor protein itself or in another protein intimately associated with it.

INTRODUCTION

High affinity receptors for IL-1 have been identified on the murine EL-4 thymoma cell line as well as other cell types (Dower et al. 1985, Kilian et al. 1986, Lomedico et al. 1986, Matsushima et al. 1986, Mizel et al. 1987). In addition, methods for assaying binding of radioiodinated recombinant IL-1-alpha to EL-4 membranes and detergent solubilized receptor have been described (Paganelli et al., 1987). Very little characerization of the IL-1 receptor has been reported to date. Sulfhydryl groups are known to be important for the activity of a number of receptors. The objective of this report is to examine the effect of sulfhydryl reagents on the binding activity of the IL-1 receptor.

RESULTS AND DISCUSSION

Recombinant human and murine IL-1 alpha were radioiodinated as previously described (Kilian et al. 1986, Paganelli et al. 1987). Membranes were prepared from murine EL-4 thymoma cells and assayed for binding of ^{125}I-IL-1 alpha as described (Paganelli et al. 1987).

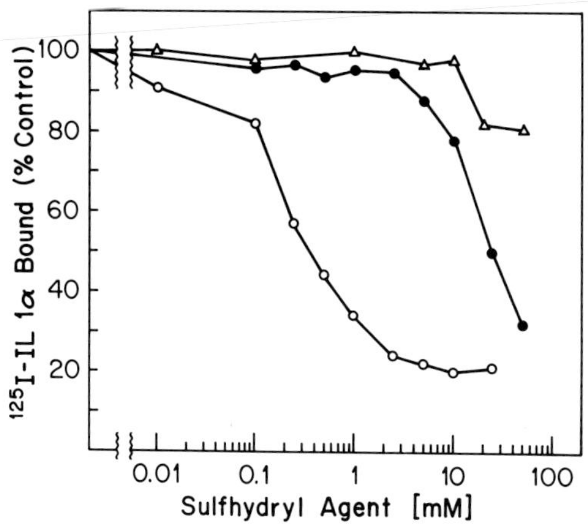

Figure 1.   Effect of DTT, 2-ME and NEM on binding of ^{125}I-human IL-1-alpha to EL-4 membranes.   EL-4 membranes were incubated with the indicated concentrations of DTT (O), 2-ME ( ), or NEM ( ) and 4 x 10^{-11} M ^{125}I-IL-1 for 60 min at 37°C. Values are expressed as percent of total ^{125}I-IL-1 binding in the absence of sulfhydryl reagents.

The effect of sulfhydryl reagents on binding of ^{125}I-human IL-1-alpha to EL-4 membranes was examined. The ^{125}I-IL-1 binding is reduced in a dose-dependent manner upon addition of the disulfide reducing agents DTT or 2-ME to the assay (Figure 1).

Complete inhibition of binding (to the level of nonspecific binding) occurs at DTT concentrations greater than 1 mM, with 50% inhibition of binding observed at 0.25-0.5 mM DTT. Much higher concentrations of 2-ME are required, with maximal inhibition achieved only at 2-ME concentrations of >50 mM (Figure 1). In contrast, the sulfhydryl alkylating agent N-ethylmaleimide (NEM) has little effect on IL-1 binding (Figure 1).

Binding of ^{125}I-human IL-1-alpha to DTT-treated and untreated EL-4 membranes was determined as a function of radioligand concentration (Table 1). There is a marked reduction in receptor number (B_{max}) in the DTT-treated as compared to untreated preparations.

TABLE 1.   IL-1 receptor number decreases upon treatment of EL-4 membranes with DTT

| SH-reagent | ^{125}I-IL-1-alpha Binding | | |
	K_d (pM)	B_{max} fmol/mg protein	r
None (control)	77	106 (100%)	0.97
DTT, 0.5 mM	114	48 (45%)	0.90

EL-4 membranes were incubated with ^{125}I-human IL-1-alpha concentrations ranging from 2.5-50 x 10^{-11}M in the presence or absence of 0.5 mM DTT. Data was analyzed by Scatchard plot analysis and linear regression.

To demonstrate that reduced IL-1 binding results from alteration of the receptor itself and not the IL-1 protein, membranes were treated with DTT and NEM and then washed to remove the sulfhydryl reagents (Table 2). In comparison to control (group 1), IL-1 binding was reduced only in membranes treated with DTT and NEM (group 2), and not in NEM-treated membranes (group 3). Since sulfhydryl reagents were removed prior to the

binding assay, we conclude that the decreased binding
is due to alteration of the receptor protein. To
confirm this, the effect of DTT on binding of murine
IL-1 alpha to membranes was tested and found to have
identical effects. As murine IL-1 has no cysteine
residues, this rules out an effect of DTT on the
single cysteine present in human IL-1.

The effect of sulfhydryl reagents was also evaluated
on the detergent solubilized IL-1 receptor. EL-4
membranes were solubilized with CHAPS, as described
(Paganelli et al. 1987).   DTT and NEM have the same
effects on the solubilized IL-1 receptor as on the
membrane receptor (Table 3).

TABLE 2.   Effect of removal of sulfhydryl reagents on
subsequent binding of ^{125}I-human IL-1-alpha to EL-4
membranes

| Group | Pre-Treatment | | ^{125}I-IL-1-alpha bound |
	T_{60}	T_{30}	fmol/mg
1	PBS[a]	PBS	31.2
2	DTT	NEM	00.8
3	PBS	NEM	42.4

EL-4 membranes were pre-treated at $37^{O}C$ with 1) PBS
(control) for 60 min, 2) 5 mM DTT (30 min) followed by
10 mM NEM (30 min), 3) PBS (30 min) followed by 10 mM
NEM (30 min).   Membranes were washed 3 x with PBS by
centrifugation at 18,000 rpm for 20 min.   The
membranes were assayed for binding with 6.5×10^{-11}
M ^{125}I-human IL-1-alpha. Values represent specific
binding.

[a]PBS, phosphate buffered saline

TABLE 3.   Effect of DTT and NEM on binding of
[125]I-murine   IL-1-alpha   to   EL-4   membranes and
CHAPS-solubilized IL-1 receptor

[125]I-Murine IL-1-alpha, cpm/assay

	Membranes	Detergent Extract
Control	3586	4950
DTT	27	403
NEM	3206	4422

EL-4 membranes or detergent extracts were incubated in
the absence of sulfhydryl agents (control) or in the
presence of 10 mM DTT or 10 mM NEM, and assayed for
binding of 1.2 x 10^{-10}M ^{125}I-murine IL-1.

Occupation   of   the   receptor   by   IL-1   affords
protection of the receptor from the effect of DTT.
Binding   of   ^{125}I-IL-1-alpha to   its   receptor   is
essentially   irreversible, as demonstrated by measuring
the dissociation of the labeled IL-1 at various time
points (Kilian et al. 1986, Paganelli et al. 1987).
This   irreversible   association   is   unaffected by
addition of DTT following binding of IL-1 (data not
shown).   To rule out an effect of DTT on IL-1 binding
by chelation of metal ions, 10 mM EDTA was added to
the membrane binding assay.   There was no effect of
EDTA on IL-1 binding (data not shown).

In   conclusion,   these results indicate that intact
disulfide   bonds   are   critical   for maintaining the
binding   activity   of   the   IL-1 receptor protein.
Occupation of the receptor with IL-1 blocks the effect
of   the   sulfhydryl   reagents,   suggesting that the
disulfide may be located at the binding site of the
receptor.   Alternatively, binding of IL-1 to the
receptor protein may induce a conformational change,

making a disulfide bond distal to the binding site inaccessible to chemical reduction. Results of experiments with the detergent solubilized receptor clearly suggest that the essential disulfide is present in the receptor protein itself or a protein very intimately associated with the receptor. While the exact locus cannot be defined at this time, more detailed characterization of the receptor protein will help resolve these issues.

REFERENCES

Dower SK, Kronheim SR, March CJ, Conlon PJ, Hopp TP, Gillis S, Urdal DL (1985). Detection and characterization of high affinity plasma membrane receptors for human interleukin-1. J. Exp Med 162:501–515.

Kilian PL, Kaffka KL, Stern AS, Woehle D, Benjamin WR, DeChiara TM, Gubler U, Farrar JJ, Mizel SB, Lomedico PT (1986). Interleukin-1-alpha and interleukin-1-beta bind to the same receptor on T cells. J. Immunol 136:4509–4514.

Lomedico PT, Kilian PL, Gubler U, Stern AS, Chizzonite R (1986). Molecular biology of interleukin-1. Cold Spring Harbor Symposium in Quantitative Biology 51:631–639.

Matsushima K, Akahoshi T, Yamada M, Furutani Y, Oppenheim JJ (1986). Properties of a specific interleukin-1 (IL-1) receptor on human Epstein-Barr virus-transformed B lymphocytes:identity of the receptor for IL-1-alpha and IL-1-beta. J. Immunol 136:4496–4469.

Mizel SB, Kilian PL, Lewis JC, Paganelli KA, Chizzonite RA (1987). The interleukin 1 receptor. Dynamics of interleukin 1 binding and internalization in T cells and fibroblasts. J. Immunol 138:2906–2912.

Paganelli KA, Stern AS, Kilian PL (1987) Detergent solubilization of the interleukin-1 receptor. J. Immunol 138:2249–2253.

Monokines and Other Non-Lymphocytic Cytokines, pages 191–196
© 1988 Alan R. Liss, Inc.

MAPPING THE RECEPTOR BINDING SITE OF HUMAN INTERLEUKIN-1β

JAMES J. HUANG, ROBERT C. NEWTON, RICHARD
HORUK, AND YUAN LIN
From the Medical Products Department,
E. I. du Pont de Nemours & Company,
Glenolden Laboraory, Glenolden, Pennsylvania
19036.

1. INTRODUCTION

Human interleukin-1 (IL-1) is a nonglycosylated
polypeptide hormone, primarily released by activated
monocytes and macrophages, which mediates a diverse array
of biological functions (Oppenheim et al 1986; Dinarello,
1982). These activities include induction of various
immunological and inflammation responses and possible
involvement in tumoricidal and hematopoietic activities
(Mizel, 1984; Durum et al 1985).

At present, there are at least two different forms of
IL-1, designated α and β, based on isoelectric point
hetergeneity (Matushima et al 1986; March et al 1985).
Complementary DNA encoding IL-1α and -β have been cloned,
sequenced, and expressed in Escherichia coli (Auron et al
1984; March et al 1985). The amino acid sequence analyses
revealed that the homology between the two IL-1 species is
only 23% (March et al 1985). It is striking that two
distinct and distantly related molecules compete for the
same receptor (Dower et al 1986). It is therefore of
interest to define specific residues which are involved in
receptor binding and are important for biological
activities.

Through the use of an expression system in E. coli
large amounts of fully active recombinant IL-1 (r-IL-1)
are now available for structural and functional

characterization (Kronheim et al 1987; Wingfield et al
1986). However there is a sparsity of information on the
structure/function relationship of IL-1. We report a
high-level expresion system for the production of r-IL-1
in E. coli (Huang et al 1987b). The r-IL-1 was soluble
and was prepared by a simplified procedure to a greater
than 99% purity. The purified r-IL-1 possess specific
activity comparable to that of monocyte-derived IL-1. In
the same communication, we also showed that the deletion
of residues at the amino-terminus led to a total loss of
biological activity of IL-1. This suggests that this
region of the molecules is essential for structure and/or
function. These studies have prompted us to construct a
series of N-terminal analogs of IL-1 with which to further
define the role of this region of the molecule.

2.   MATERIALS AND METHODS
     E. coli strain JM101, complementary DNA encoding IL-1β
and the parental plasmid (pDP506Δ) used in this study were
previously described (Auron et al 1984; Huang et al
1987b). Plasmid pDP506Δ was digested with EcoRI and Hind
III and replaced with oligomer (A A T T C C A T A G A G G
G T A T T A C A T A T G G C A C C T G T A A G A T C T C T
G A A C T G C A C G C T C C G G G A C T C A C A G C A A A
A A) to generate mature form IL-1β. The oligomer (73
mer), flanked by EcoRI and Hind III restriction site,
includes a Shine Dalgarno (S/D) sequence (dotted line),
translational initiation codon ATG (underlined) and a
silent change at Arg_4-Ser_5 coding sequence to generate a
new restriction site Bgl II. A series of 35 mers (from
EcoRI to Bgl II) with proper coding sequence mutated, was
made and used to generate various amino-terminal mutants.

     Purification and bioassay of mutein IL-1, circular
dichroism (CD) spectroscopy, receptor binding assay,
analytic electrophoresis, DNA sequencing were described
elsewhere (Huang et al 1987a,b).

3.   RESULTS AND DISCUSSIONS

     Table 1 shows the biologic activity of the analogs
determined by the thymocyte proliferation assay. The
biological activity of r-IL-1(DP506) is about 10% that of
native form IL-1 (THP-1). Note that DP506 contains 15
exogenous amino acid residues (Huang et al 1987b) that

were contributed by the expression vector and the pro-IL-1
sequence. By deleting most of the exogenous residues
(DP516), the r-IL-1 bioactivity improves dramatically.
DP516 possesses a specific activity (as measured by both
the Gingival Fibroblast PGE_2 induction and the thymocyte
proliferatin assays) equivalent to that of the native form
IL-1 (THP-1).

Table 1 Bioactivity of recombinant interleukin-1 used in
this study.

Clone Designation	Sequence at Amino-Terminus	Specific[a] Activity (%)	Receptor[b] Binding (%)
DP506	Fusion-IL-1 (166)[d]	10	ND[c]
DP516	TNAPVR-IL-1 (155)	100	100
C-12	des 7-IL-1 (146)	<0.1	1
THP-1	APVR-IL-1 (153)	100	100
C-22a	TPVR-IL-1 (153)	380	ND
C-18	TMVR-IL-1 (153)	700	200
Glu-4	TMVD-IL-1 (153)	0.14	0.2

A)The specific activity and receptor binding affinity were
   normalized against that of DP516. The specific activity
   of DP516, as measured by LAF and PGE_2 assays, was
   $1 \sim 2 \times 10^7$ unit/mg.
B)Relative receptor-binding affinity was determined by
   free competition binding to EL4/9 murine T-lymphoma
   cells. DP516 and native IL-1 exhibits super-imposable
   binding curves with an apparent $K_D \sim 200$ pM.
C)ND not determined.
D)Numbers are amino acid residue of IL-1 analogs.
   One-letter codes for amino acid are given.

   Recombinant protein C-12 which has seven N-terminal
residues deleted, showed no bioactivity, indicating that
integrity of the IL-1 molecule is important for its
function. Clone 22a, which has the substitution alanine
to threonine at the amino-terminus of IL-1, shows a 4-fold
increase in bioactivity (Huang et al 1987a). Another
mutant (clone 18), which has the first two amino acids
replaced, demonstrated 7-fold enhanced activity. It has
been shown that the flexibility and accessibility of the
amino terminus of a protein modulate its stability and
function (Thornton et al 1983). It is possible that the
improved activity of these analogs is due to structural

rearrangements that result in enhanced receptor bindings.
    The three dimensional structure of a polypeptide chain
is determined by the total number of interatomic
interactions and hence by the amino acid sequence.
Examining the amino-end of the IL-1 sequence revealed that
a protonated arginine (position 4 of IL-1β) might be
involved in salt-bridge formation or hydrogen bonding
which plays a role in stablizing the protein structure.
Substitution of arginine by glutamic acid (Glu-4),
resulted in a total loss of bioactivity. This suggested
that the positively charged arginine residue is important
in the structure and/or biological activity of IL-1.

All the recombinant clones described in this
communication are produced in a similar fashion. The
expression system and purification procedure of each clone
are identical. Thus, it is possible that the variation in
bioactivity is a result of the protein's secondary and
tertiary structure. It is surprising that analyses of
circular dichroism spectra reveal no detectable
difference in the secondary structure between DP516, C-18,
and Glu4 (Huang et al 1987a). From a CD scan of heat
inactivated IL-1 a rearrangement in secondary structure
indicative of increased beta sheet formation was observed.
We concluded that the differences in activity of these
recombinant proteins are not due to denaturation of the
protein but rather are attributed by changes in folding of
the polypeptides.

The receptor binding affinity of these muteins to
murine EL4/9 cells correlated well with the bioactivity
(Table 1). The munteins which showed enhanced activity,
also demonstrate a higher receptor binding affinity. On
the contrary, analogs which exhibited a dramatic loss of
activity showed a low receptor binding affinity. In the
receptor completion assay, the individual competetion
curves were paralleled suggesting receptors are of a
single class (Horuk et al 1987). Thus, the altered
bioactivity of these analogs appear to result from changes
in receptor binding rather than to post-receptor mediated
events.

In summary, we utilized site specific mutagenesis to
engineer a series of recombinant IL-1s which have various
degrees of bioactivity. Manipulation of the

amino-terminal sequence of IL-1 generated recombinant proteins that showed increased or decreased bioactivity as compared to native IL-1. Generally speaking, the terminal regions of proteins are less likely to be involved in the active center (Thornton et al 1983); nevertheless, we have shown that the arginine at the amino-end of the IL-1 molecule is one of the key residues in the function of IL-1. The side chain of Arg_4 might be directly involved in receptor binding or critical in maintaining the tertiary structure of the receptor binding site.

Auron PE, Webb AC, Rosenwasser LJ, Mucci SF, Rich A, Wolff SM, Dinarello CA (1984). Nucleotide sequence of human monocyte interleukin 1 precursor cDNA. Proc. Natl. Acad. Sci. USA. 81,790-791.

Dower SK, Kronheim SR, March CJ, Conlon PJ, Hopp TP, Gillis S, Uradl DL (1985). Detection and characterization of high affinity plasma membrane receptors for humane interleukin 1. J. Exp. Med. 162-501-511.

Durum SK, Schmidt JA, Oppenhein JJ. (1985). Interleukin-1: an immunological perspective. Annu. Rev. Immunol. 3:263-287.

Huang JJ, Newton RC, Horuk R, Matthew JB, Covington M, Pezzella K, Lin Y (1987a). Muteins of human interleukin-1 that show enhanced bioactivities. FEBS LETTERS (In Press).

Huang JJ, Newton RC, Pezzella K, Covington M, Tamblyn T, Rutledge SJ, Kelley M, Lin Y (1987b). High-level expression in Escherichia coli of a soluble and fully active recombinant interleukin-1β. Mol Biol Med 4:169-181.

Horuk R, Huang JJ, Covington M, Newton RC (1987). A biochemical and kinetic analysis of the interleukin-1 receptor. J Biol Chem 262:22553-22557.

Kronheim SR, Cantrell MA, Deeley MC, March CJ, Glackin PJ, Anderson DM, Hemenway T, Merriam JE, Cosman D, Hopp TP (1986). Purification and characterization of humane interleukin-1 expressed in Escherichia coli. Bio/Technology. 4:1078-1081.

Matsushima K, Copeland TD, Onozaki K, Oppenheim JJ (1986b). Purification and biochemical characteristics of two human interleukins 1 from the Myelomonocytic THP1 cell line. Biochem. 25:3424-3429.

March CJ, Mosley B, Larsen A, Cerretti DC, Braedt G, Price V, Gillis S, Henney CS, Kronheim SR, Grabstein K, Conlon PJ, Hopp TP, Cosman D (1985). Cloning, sequence and expression of two distinct human interleukin-1 complementary DNAs. Nature 31:641–647.

Mizel JB (1982). Interleukin 1 and T cell activation. Immunol Rev 63:51–72.

Oppenheim JJ, Kovacs EJ, Matsushima K, Durum SK (1986). There is more than one interleukin 1. Immunology Today 7:45–56.

Thornton JM, Sibanda BL (1983). Amino and carboxyl-terminal regions in globular proteins. J Mol Biol 167:443–460.

Wingfield P, Payton M, Tavernier J, Barnes M, Shaw A, Rose K, Simona MG, DeMczuk S, Williamson K, Dayer J-M (1986). Purification and characterization of human interleukin-1β expressed in recombinant Escherichia coli. Eur J Biochem 160:491–497.

Monokines and Other Non-Lymphocytic Cytokines, pages 197–202
© 1988 Alan R. Liss, Inc.

MONOCLONAL ANTIBODIES TO HUMAN INTERLEUKIN 1ß FOR ANALYSIS
OF THE STRUCTURE-FUNCTION RELATIONSHIP

Diana Boraschi, Gianfranco Volpini, Stefano
Censini, Paola Bossù, Paolo Ghiara, Giuseppe
Scapigliati, Annalisa Massone, Cosima Baldari,
John L. Telford and Aldo Tagliabue

Sclavo Research Center, 53100 Siena, Italy

INTRODUCTION

Interleukin 1 (IL-1) is a family of related proteins
(IL-1α and IL-1ß) with immunostimulatory and inflammatory
activities both <u>in vitro</u> and <u>in vivo</u> (Dinarello, 1984;
Oppenheim et al., 1986). For IL-1ß, the biological
activities are exerted by the 17.5 kD fragment 117-269,
derived from a 31 kD precursor. Attempts have been made to
define functional domains within the mature protein, both by
the use of synthetic peptides and of N-terminal or
C-terminal truncated recombinant polypeptides (Antoni et
al., 1986; Nencioni et al., 1987; Palaszynski, 1987; Mosley
et al., 1987). However, removal of a few amino acids from
either termini always resulted in a drastic decrease of the
receptor-binding capacity of hu IL-1ß, thus of its
biological activity (Mosley et al., 1987), possibly due to
the inability of truncated proteins to fold correctly into
an active structure (Baldari et al., 1987a).

The question of the structure-function relationship in
the hu IL-1ß protein has been thus approached by the use of
monoclonal antibodies (mAbs) which recognize different sites
of the protein. The relevance of the recognized regions for
the biological activities of hu IL-1ß has been

assessed by the capacity of these mAbs to inhibit IL-1ß in three different <u>in vitro</u> assays.

RESULTS AND DISCUSSION

MAbs were raised against either the recombinant hu IL-1ß fragment 121-269 (Baldari et al., 1987b) or against the synthetic nonapeptide 163-171 (Antoni et al., 1986). Mapping of the epitopes recognized by mAbs was performed by immunoblotting of a series of overlapping hu IL-1ß peptides, obtained by expression of truncated cDNAs in <u>E. coli</u> or yeast (Baldari et al., 1987a). Table 1 summarizes the immunoblotting reactivities of the recombinant peptides with the different mAbs obtained. Four families of mAbs were defined by reactivity with the recombinant fragments. Seven mAbs (MhC) recognize epitopes within the region 133-147, two (MhD) bind to the stretch 148-192, four (MhG) to the region 218-243, and one (MhI) to the fragment 251-269.

TABLE 1. Specificity of Monoclonal Antibodies to hu IL-1ß

IL-1ß	Immunoblotting reactivity with			
peptides	MhC	MhD	MhG	MhI
121-269	+	+	+	+
121-197	+	+	−	−
198-269	−	−	+	+
121-192	+	+	−	−
133-269	+	+	+	+
148-269	−	+	+	+
121-217	+	+	−	−
121-243	+	+	+	−
121-250	+	+	+	−
Specificity	133-147	148-192	218-243	251-269

Six of these mAbs and a mAb raised against the synthetic peptide 163-171 were further characterized (Table 2) and then assayed for the ability to inhibit the biological activity of IL-1ß. None of the mAbs could inhibit

TABLE 2. Characteristics of Monoclonal Antibodies to hu IL 1ß.

mAb	Epitope recognized	K^* (1/moles)	Ig class
MhC1	133-147	1.3×10^9	IgG_1
MhC2	133-147	1.7×10^9	IgG_1
MhD1	148-192	5.5×10^8	IgG_1
MhG1	218-243	1.3×10^8	IgG_1
MhG2	218-243	6.1×10^8	IgG_1
MhI	251-269	1.3×10^9	IgG_1
Vhp20	163-171	4.6×10^8	IgG_{2a}

$*$ Affinity constant for hu r IL-1ß measured in solid-phase RIA.

hu IL-1α in any of the _in vitro_ assays used, i.e. murine thymocyte co-stimulation assay, D10.G4.1 proliferation, and PGE_2 induction from human fibroblasts (not shown). On the other hand, mAbs could inhibit hu IL-1ß activity by different degrees in all three assays (Table 3). Both mAbs MhC (recognizing the fragment 133-148) and MhI (C-terminal region 251-269) were highly efficient in blocking the biological activity of IL-1ß, whereas only partial inhibition could be attained by mAbs MhG. In contrast, mAbs MhD1 and Vhp20 were completely unable to inhibit IL-1ß activities.

These data thus allow the identification of distinct

TABLE 3. Inhibition of hu IL-1ß Activities by Monoclonal
         Antibodies

	Percent inhibition of hu IL-1ß[+] on		
mAb[*]	Thymocytes	D10.G4.1	Fibroblasts
MhC1	93.1	59.3	67.7
MhC2	78.9	n.t.	41.0
MhD1	4.3	6.8	0.0
MhG1	60.7	n.t.	24.6
MhG2	53.9	n.t.	19.1
MhI	99.3	n.t.	78.2
Vhp20	5.2	0.0	0.0

[*] 250 μg/ml on thymocytes and fibroblasts; 100 μg/ml on
D10.G4.1.

[+] 5U/ml in the thymocyte and fibroblast assays; 0.2 U/ml in
the D10.G4.1 test.

regions of hu IL-1ß critical for the optimal expression of
its biological activity. Both the N-terminal and the
C-terminal moieties of the protein, recognized by mAbs MhC
and MhI, appear to play a major role for the IL-1ß activity
on different target cells. This is in agreement with
previous reports, which suggested the importance of these
regions for binding of hu IL-1ß to its receptor (Mac Donald
et al., 1986; Mosley et al., 1987; Palaszynski, 1987).
On the other hand, mAbs directed to epitopes within the
internal IL-1ß region 148-192 (MhD and Vhp20) did not affect
the biological activity of IL-1ß, possibly because the
recognized epitopes are not involved in receptor-binding. In
this respect, it is interesting to note that the 163-171

fragment possibly represents one of the active immunostimulatory sites of IL-1ß (Antoni et al., 1986; Nencioni et
al., 1987), although unable to bind efficiently to the IL-1
receptor (unpublished). This observation, together with
previous data on the lack of biological activity of a
receptor-binding synthetic peptide of hu IL-1ß (Palaszynski,
1987), suggests the hypothesis of the dissociation of active
sites from receptor-binding moieties of IL-1ß.

REFERENCES

Antoni G, Presentini R, Perin F, Tagliabue A, Ghiara P,
    Censini S, Volpini G, Villa L, Boraschi D (1986). A short
    synthetic peptide fragment of human interleukin 1 with
    immunostimulatory but not inflammatory activity. J Immunol
    137: 3201-3204.
Baldari C, Massone A, Macchia G, Telford JL (1987a).
    Differential stability of human interleukin 1 beta
    fragments expressed in yeast. Prot Engineer in press.
Baldari C, Murray JAH, Ghiara P, Cesareni G, Galeotti CL,
    (1987b). A novel leader peptide which allows efficient
    secretion of a fragment of human interleukin 1ß in
    Saccharomyces cerevisiae. EMBO J 6: 229-234.
Dinarello CA (1984). Interleukin-1. Rev Infect Dis 6: 51-95.
Mac Donald HR, Wingfield P, Schmeissner U, Shaw A, Clore GM,
    Gronenborn AM (1986). Point mutations of human inter-
    leukin-1 with decreased receptor binding affinity. FEBS
    Lett 209: 295-298.
Mosley B, Dower SK, Gillis S, Cosman D (1987). Determination
    of the minimum polypeptide lenghts of the functionally
    active sites of human interleukins 1 and 1ß. Proc Natl
    Acad Sci USA 84: 4572-4576.
Nencioni L, Villa L, Tagliabue A, Antoni G, Presentini R,
    Perin F, Silvestri S, Boraschi D (1987). In vivo
    immunostimulating activity of the 163-171 peptide of human
    IL-1ß. J Immunol 139: 800-804.
Oppenheim JJ, Kovacs EJ, Matsushima K, Durum SK (1986).

There is more than one interleukin 1.   Immunol Today 7: 45-56.
Palaszynski EW (1987).   Synthetic C-terminal peptide of IL-1 functions as a binding domain as well as an antagonist for the IL-1 receptor.   Biochem Biophys Res Commun 147:   204-211.

Monokines and Other Non-Lymphocytic Cytokines, pages 203–208
© 1988 Alan R. Liss, Inc.

EFFECT OF TRANS-RETINOIC ACID ON INTERLEUKIN-1 RECEPTOR ACTIVITY

Patricia L. Kilian

Department of Immunopharmacology, Hoffmann-La Roche Inc., Nutley, New Jersey 07110

INTRODUCTION

Retinoids, a family of synthetic and naturally occurring molecules structurally related to Vitamin A (retinol), have a wide range of biological acivities (Jetten, 1984; Lotan, 1980; Pawson et al., 1982; Sporn and Roberts, 1983) including the ability to modulate immune function. Retinoids have been shown to regulate both humoral and cell-mediated immunity and specific effects of retinoids on T and B lymphocytes, natural killer cells, and macrophages have been reported (see, e.g., Abb and Deinhardt, 1980; Dennert, 1986; Katz et al., 1987, Rhodes and Oliver, 1980, Shapiro and Edelson, 1984; Sidell et al. 1984, Valone and Payan, 1985). Much remains to be elucidated, however, concerning the precise mechanisms by which retinoids elicit these effects.

The objective of this study was to examine the effect of retinoids on Interleukin-1 (IL-1) receptor expression. Two major types of IL-1 proteins, designated IL-1-alpha and IL-1-beta have been described (Auron et al., 1984; Gubler et al., 1986; Lomedico et al, 1984; March et al., 1985). Both IL-1 proteins are produced in varying ratios by activated macrophages as well as other cell types but differ significantly in their amino acid sequences (e.g., there is less than

30% homology between human IL-1-alpha and IL-1-beta).
Despite this difference, however, both IL-1-alpha and
IL-1-beta have similar biological activities. These
activities are quite diverse and include effects of
IL-1 on immune function (for refs. see Dinarello,
1986; Lomedico et al., 1986; Oppenheim et al., 1986).
Receptors for IL-1 which recognize both IL-1-alpha and
IL-1-beta have previously been identified on the
murine EL-4 thymoma cell line (Kilian et al., 1986).
These cells show increased Interleukin-2 production in
response to Il-1. The EL-4 cells provide a model
system for evaluating the effect of retinoids on IL-1
receptor activity.

RESULTS AND DISCUSSION

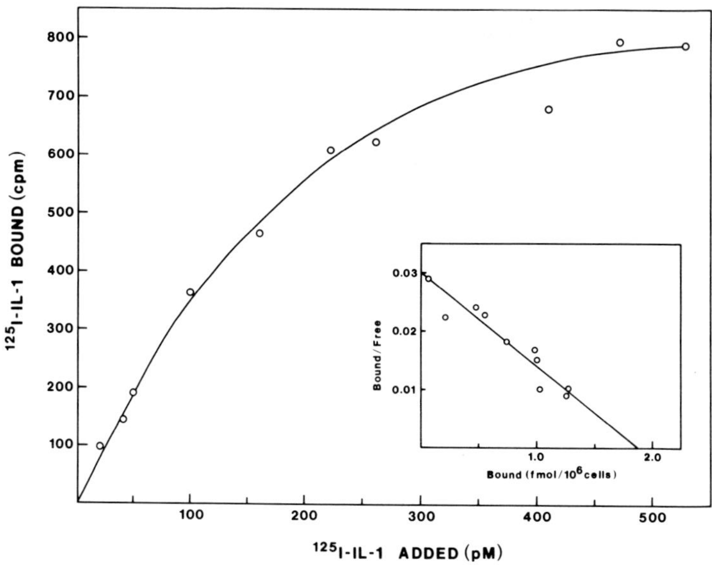

Figure 1. Specific binding of murine ^{125}I-IL-1 as a
function of its concentration to EL-4 cells.
(Reprinted, with permission, Kilian et al, 1986).

Pure E. coli-derived recombinant murine IL-1-alpha was labeled with ^{125}I to high specific activity and with retention of biological activity (Kilian et al., 1986). The ^{125}I-IL-1 binds to the murine EL-4 thymoma cells in a specific and saturable manner (Fig. 1). Scatchard plot analysis (Fig. 1, Inset) reveals a single type of high affinity binding site with an apparent dissociation constant (Kd) of approximately 2 x 10^{-10}M and the presence of approximately 1200 binding sites per cell.

The effect of trans-retinoic acid on IL-1 receptors was examined. The EL-4 cells were maintained in culture in the presence or absence of 2 x 10^{-6}M trans-retinoic acid for three days. The cells were subsequently evaluated for ^{125}I-IL-1 binding. As shown in Table 1, binding to the trans-retinoic acid treated cells is approximately 1.6-fold higher compared with untreated cells at all concentrations of ^{125}I-IL-1 tested.

TABLE 1.   Effect of Trans-Retinoic Acid on ^{125}I-murine IL-1-alpha Binding to EL-4 Cells

^{125}I-IL-1 Added x 10^{-10}M	^{125}I-IL-1 Bound Control (A)	RA*-Treated (B) cpm/4 x 10^6 cells	(B/A)
4.9	240	386	1.6
9.5	527	783	1.5
42.0	1400	2366	1.7

* RA = trans-retinoic acid

In addition, we also find that trans-retinoic acid increases Interleukin-2 production in response to IL-1 (Kilian et al., in preparation).

These results show that trans-retinoic acid increases expression of IL-1 receptors on EL-4 cells and thereby modulates the responsiveness of these cells to IL-1. Whether retinoids mediate this effect via a transcriptional, translational or post-translational mechanism remains to be determined. Further characterization of the receptors for both IL-1 (see Paganelli et al., 1986) and the retinoids (see Shubeita et al., 1987) will help clarify this issue. Whether the observed effect of retinoids on IL-1 receptor activity underlies known in vivo effects of retinoids on immune function also warrants additional study.

REFERENCES

Abb J and Deinhardt F. (1980). Effects of retinoic-acid on the human lymphocyte responses to mitogens. Expl Cell Biol 48:169-179.

Auron PE, Webb AC, Rosenwasser LF, Mucci SF, Rich A, Wolff SM, Dinarello CA (1984). Nucleotide sequence of human monocyte interleukin 1 precursor cDNA. Proc Natl Acad Sci USA 71:7907-7911.

Dennert G (1985). Immunostimulation by retinoic acid. In Nugent J., Clark S (eds): "Retinoids, Differentiation and Disease," London:Pitman Publishing, pp 117-131.

Dinarello CA (1986). Multiple biological properties of recombinant human interleukin 1 (beta). Immunobiol 172:301-315.

Gubler UA, Chua AO, Stern, AS, Hellmann CP, Vitek MP, DeChiara TM, Benjamin WR, Collier KG, Dukovich M, Familletti PC, Fiedler-Nagy C, Jenson J, Kaffka K, Kilian P, Stremlo D, Weittreich BH, Woehle D, Mizel SB, Lomedico PT (1986). Recombinant human interleukin 1:purification and biological character-ization. J. Immunol 136:2492-2497.

Jetten AM (1984). Modulation of cell growth by retinoic and and their possible mechanism of action. Fed Proc 43:134-139.

Katz DR, Drzymala M, Turton JA, Hicks RM, Hunt R, Palmer L, Malkovsky M (1987). Regulation of accessory cell function by retinoids in murine immune responses. Br J Exp Path 68:343-350.

Kilian PL, Kaffka KL, Stern AS, Woehle D, Benjamin WR, DeChiara TM, Gubler U, Farrar JJ, Mizel SB, Lomedico PT (1986). Interleukin 1-alpha and Interleukin 1-beta bind to the same receptor on T cells. J Immunol 136:4509-4514.

Lomedico PT, Gubler U, Hellmann CP, Dukovich M, Giri JG, Pan Y-CE, Collier K, Semionow R, Chua AO, Mizel SB (1984). Cloning and expression of murine interleukin-1 cDNA in Escherichia coli. Nature 312:458-462.

Lomedico PT, Kilian PL, Gubler U, Stern AS, Chizzonite R (1986). Molecular biology of interleukin 1. Cold Spring Harbor Symp Quan Biol 51:631-639.

Lotan R (1980). Effects of Vitamin A and its analogs (retinoids) on normal and neoplastic cells. Biochim Biophys Acta 605:33-91.

March CJ, Mosley B, Larsen A, Cerretti DP, Braedt G, Price V, Gillis S, Henney CS, Kronheim SR, Gradbstein K, Conlon PF, Hopp TP, Cosman D (1985). Cloning, sequence, and expression of two distinct human interleukin-1 complementary DNAs. Nature 315:641-648.

Oppenheim JJ, Kovacs EJ, Matsushima K, Durum SK (1986) Immunology Today 7:45-56.

Paganelli KA, Stern AS, Kilian PL (1987). Detergent solubilization of the interleukin 1 receptor. J. Immunol 138:2249-2253.

Pawson BA, Ehmann CW, Itri LM, Sherman MI (1982). Retinoids at their threshold: Their biological significance and therapeutic potential. J Med Chem 25:1269-1277.

Rhodes J and Oliver S (1980) Retinoids as regulators of macrophage function. Immunology 40:467-472.

Shubeita HE, Sambrook, JF, McCormick AM (1987). Molecular cloning and analysis of functional cDNA and genomic clones encoding bovine cellular retinoic acid-binding protein. Proc Natl Acad Sci USA 84:5645-5649.

Shapiro PE, Edelson RL (1984). Effect of retinoids on the immune system. In Saurat JH (ed): "Retinoids: New Trends in Research and Therapy," Basle: Karger, pp 225-235.

Sidell N, Rieber P, Golub SH (1984). Immunological aspects of retinoids in humans. Cell Immunol 87: 118-125.

Sporn MB and Roberts AB (1983). Role of retinoids in differentiation and carcinogenesis. Cancer Res 43: 3034-3040.

Valone FH, Payan DG (1985). Potentiation of mitogen-induced human T-lymphocyte activation by retinoic acid. Cancer Res 45:4128-4131.

Monokines and Other Non-Lymphocytic Cytokines, pages 209–212

COVALENT DISULFIDE BINDING OF IL-1 TO α_2-MACROGLOBULIN

Marius Teodorescu, John L. Skosey, Carol
Schlesinger, and Jeanette Wallman

Departments of Microbiology/Immunology (M.T.,C.S.,
J.W.) and Medicine (J.L.S.), University of Illinois
College of Medicine, Chicago, IL 60612

INTRODUCTION

Cytokines, IL-1 in particular, are likely to play significant roles in the chronic inflammation of rheumatoid arthritis (RA). IL-1α and β have free SH groups of unpaired cys-
teines and, therefore, could bind covalently to serum proteins
with free SH groups. Three such proteins, C3, C4 and α_2-
macroglobulin (α_2M) have labile internal thioester bonds which
are capable of generating free SH groups "spontaneously" or,
much faster, as the result of reaction with primary amines.
α_2M also develops free SH groups when it binds proteinases
(see Harpel and Brower, 1983).

We hypothesize that some cytokines form disulfide bonds
to α_2M, which results with an extension of their half life and
hence of their effects in chronic inflammation. Thus, drugs
used in the therapy of RA, such as gold compounds and peni-
cillamine (D-pen), or cell products which prevent the formation of these bonds may exert an anti-inflammatory effect.
To test this hypothesis we determined whether: (a) IL-1 bound
to α_2M treated with methylamine; (b) the binding was prevented
by D-pen or by a protein with free SH groups produced in abun-
dance by activated lymphocytes (SH-LyP) and (c) α_2M-bound IL-1
remained biologically active.

MATERIALS AND METHODS

Treatment of serum or α_2M with IL-1. Aliquots of normal
human serum (NHS) or partially purified human α_2M (Sigma) were
treated with 0.2 M methylamine. Human rIL-1β, non-labeled
(Cistron) or ^{125}I-labeled (New England Nuclear), was added and

the mixtures incubated at 37°C for 2h and 4°C overnight.

Polyacrylamide gel electrophoresis(PAGE). Two PAGE systems were used: native, in a tris/EDTA/borate buffer (Hall and Roberts, 1978) and denaturing, in SDS in a phosphate buffer. The gels were stained and autoradiographed.

Preparation of lymphocyte-produced proteins with free SH (SH-LyP). Rabbit lymphocytes activated by Concanavalin A and Streptococcal mitogen were incubated for two days at 39°C in medium with 5% normal rabbit serum and for 18h without serum. The supernatant was collected and dialyzed.

RESULTS AND DISCUSSION

Binding of IL-1 to methylamine-treated α_2M (MA-α_2M). Normal human serum was treated with methylamine (MA/NHS) or with diluent buffer and was incubated with ^{125}I-rIL-1β. To block free SH groups 10^{-3} M D-pen (Merck, Sharp and Dohme) was added to some aliquots of MA/NHS. Substantial radioactivity was associated with α_2M in MA/NHS. This association was completely inhibited by D-pen at 10^{-3} M (Fig. 1, lanes 1-3) and by about 50% at 10^{-4} M (therapeutic concentration).

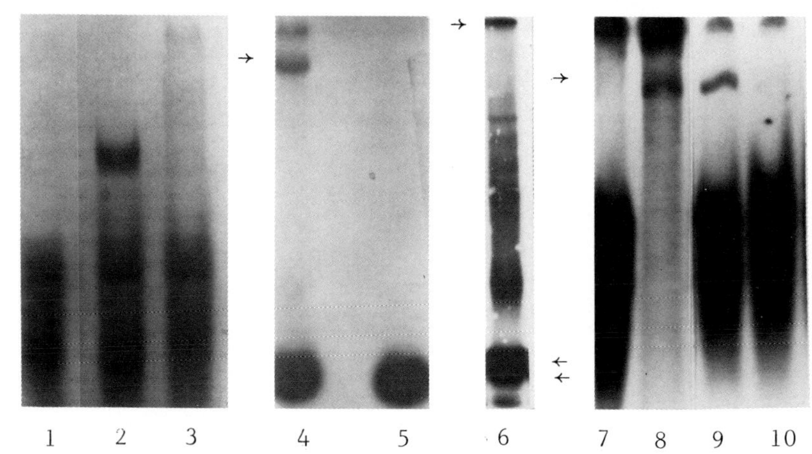

Figure 1. Composite of autoradiographs which show the binding of ^{125}I-rIL-1 and of ^{125}I-SH-LyP to α_2M. Lanes 1-3 and 7-10: native PAGE (tris buffer); lanes 4 and 5: SDS-PAGE (phosphate buffer). Single arrow: position of α_2M. Contents of lanes: 1: IL-1; 2: IL-1+MA/NHS; 3: IL-1+D-pen+MA/NHS; 4: IL-1+α_2M (nonreduced); 5: IL-1+α_2M (reduced); 6: Laemmli gel of ^{125}I-supernatant containing SH-LyP (double arrow); 7: IL-1; 8: ^{125}I-SH-LyP+α_2M; 9: IL-1+α_2M; 10: ^{125}I-IL-1+SH-LyP+α_2M.

Much less radiolabel was observed in the α_2M bands when human serum was not pretreated with MA (not shown). Thus, IL-1 bound most likely to the SH groups resulting from the cleavage of the internal thioester bonds of α_2M.

Aliquots of IL-1+MA/α_2M mixtures prepared as shown above were boiled in SDS in the presence or absence of 2-mercapto-ethanol (2-ME). ^{125}I-IL-1 remained in the α_2M band in the absence of 2-ME but was absent from it when it was reduced by 2-ME (Fig. 1, lanes 4 and 5). Thus, a covalent disulfide bond had been formed between IL-1β and α_2M.

<u>Proteins with free SH groups produced by lymphocytes (SH-LyP)</u>. We have recently described a protein produced by activated rabbit B cells (or human B cell line RPMI-1788) in quantities about 10 times higher than Ig (Schlesinger et al.,1987; submitted). It is a noncovalent dimer of 12+13 Kd chains (Fig. 1,lane 6), has free SH groups and binds covalently to MA/α_2M. In the presence of serum it is rapidly degraded but remains apparently unaltered when it is bound to α_2M. The biologic function of SH-LyP is still unknown. However, its production in large quantity suggested that it may play a regulatory role in preventing other cytokines from binding to α_2M. Indeed, like D-pen, supernatants containing SH-LyP inhibited the binding of ^{125}I-rIL-1 to MA-α_2M (Fig. 1, lanes 7-10).

Based on either biologic activity or binding studies several cytokines have been found associated with α_2M: a macrophage activating factor (McDaniel et al.,1976), lymphotoxin (Papermaster et al.,1979), a polyclonal B cell activator (see Teodorescu,1983), nerve cell growth factor (Ronne et al., 1979) and platelet derived growth factor (PDGF) (Huang et al.,1984). PDGF, which does not have free SH groups, appears to bind as a result of a disulfide bond interchange, suggesting that a noncovalent binding as the first stage.

<u>Two stages of binding and the biologic effects of α_2M-bound Il-1</u>. In the serum-containing native PAGE no other radiolabeled protein band was detected other than those caused by ^{125}I-rIL-1 (Fig. 1). Thus, IL-1 probably bound only to the SH of α_2M and not to those of C3 and C4. The same was true for SH-LyP. This observation suggested that the presence of free SH groups was not sufficient for a protein to bind IL-1.

Human α_2M treated with ^{125}I-rIL-1 or ^{125}I-SH-LyP in the presence or absence of D-pen was precipitated and washed with 12% polyethylene glycol. The control contained no α_2M. The precipitates were analyzed by SDS-PAGE under reducing and non-reducing conditions. We found that: (a) ^{125}I was detected only in the samples containing α_2M; (b) in the nonreduced samples ^{125}I was present both in α_2M band and in the Il-1 band;

(c) in the presence of D-pen ^{125}I was present only in the IL-1 band; (d) in the reduced samples ^{125}I was present only in the Il-1 band. Thus, IL-1 was bound both non-covalently and covalently to α_2M. Similar results were obtained with SH-LyP from ^{125}I-labeled supernatant. Whether these were two stages of the same process and whether other unrelated proteins with similar m.w. also bind to α_2M remains to be determined.

An experiment similar to that described above was performed with non-radiolabeled rIL-1β in bovine serum albumin. The redissolved precipitate was tested for biologic activity in the mouse thymocyte assay. The sample treated without α_2M had no detectable biologic activity. Both samples containing α_2M, with or without D-pen, were biologically active (contained about 10% of the added IL-1). Thus, non-covalently bound IL-1 α_2M was biologically active. Whether the covalently bound IL-1 was also biologically active could not be determined in this experiment.

To obtain further support in favor of our hypothesis, it remains to be shown that IL-1 or other cytokines maintain biologic activity when they are covalently bound to α_2M. In addition, it remains to be shown that α_2M carrying cytokines has a reduced clearance rate in the inflammatory milieu.

REFERENCES

Hall PK, Roberts RC (1978). Physical and chemical properties of human α_2-macroglobulins. Biochem J 173:27-37.

Harpel PC, Brower MS (1983). α_2-Macroglobulin: an introduction. Ann NY Acad Sci 421:1-9.

Huang JS, Huang SS, Deuel TF (1984). Specific covalent binding of platelet-derived growth factor to human plasma α_2-macroglobulin. Proc Natl Acad Sci USA 81:342-346.

McDaniel MC, Laudico R, Papermaster BW (1976). Association of macrophage-activating factor from a human cultured lymphoid cell line in crowded lymphoid cell cultures. Clin Immunol Immunopathol 5:91-104.

Papermaster BW, Gilliland CD, Smith M, Buchok S, McEntire JE, Butler RC, Spector S, Friedman H (1979). Tumor regression induced in mice by partially purified lymphokine fractions. Ann NY Acad Sci 332:451-459.

Ronne H, Anundi H, Rask L, Peterson PA (1979). Nerve cell growth factor binds to serum α_2-macroglobulin. Biochem Biophys Res Commun 87:330-336.

Teodorescu M (1983). B cell activating lymphokine and its natural inhibitor in the serum of patients with autoimmune diseases. Lymphokines 8:81-141.

Monokines and Other Non-Lymphocytic Cytokines, pages 213–216

KINETICS OF GROWTH INHIBITION AND RECEPTOR BINDING BY INTERLEUKIN-1.

Edwin Gaffney, Shiow Tsai, George Koch, Richard Malovarca
Department of Molecular and Cell Biology, The Pennsylvania State University, University Park, PA 16802 (E.G., S.T.) and Cistron Biotechnology, Pine Brook, NJ 07058 (G.K., R.M.)

INTRODUCTION

IL-1 influences tumor cell growth by promoting monocyte-mediated tumoricidal activity (Onozaki et al., 1985a) and by inducing cytotoxic T-cell responses. IL-1 also exerts direct antiproliferative effects when tested with cells established from malignant breast tissues (Tsai and Gaffney, 1986). Inhibition was not mediated by prostaglandin production. Highly purified IL-1 was reported by others (Onozaki et al., 1985b) to be cytocidal or cytostatic for some tumor lines. Subsequent studies showed that direct inhibitory activity was common to both native and recombinant human IL-1 from a variety of sources (Gaffney and Tsai, 1986) and that IL-1 stimulated growth with certain cells (Tsai and Gaffney, 1987). The current study begins to eluciate the kinetics of IL-1 mediated growth inhibition.

RESULTS

The effect of human rIL-1 on the induction of growth inhibition was measured by [^{3}H]-TdR incorporation. MDA-MB-415 cells were seeded at 10^4 in 200 µl medium in wells of 96-well microtiter plates. rIL-1α or β was added 24 hours later at 1ng/well. A reduction in incorporation was observed at 3 hours and reached a maximum by 24 hours. DNA synthesis was decreased 80-90% by day 1 (Fig. 1). Although RNA synthesis decreased slightly by day 1, an increase to 60% above control was observed by day 3. Protein synthesis increased 20% above control 2 days after IL-1 addition and declined to control levels thereafter.

The reversibility of inhibition was shown by
incubating 24 hour cultures with 1ng of rIL-1β. Each day,
sets of control and treated cultures were washed 3 times
and refed with fresh medium. Cultures were incubated with
[³H]-TdR on subsequent days. Following exposure to 1ng of
rIL-1, DNA synthesis resumed within 1 day regardless of the
length of exposure. However, the level of incorporation
did not return to control levels (Fig. 2).

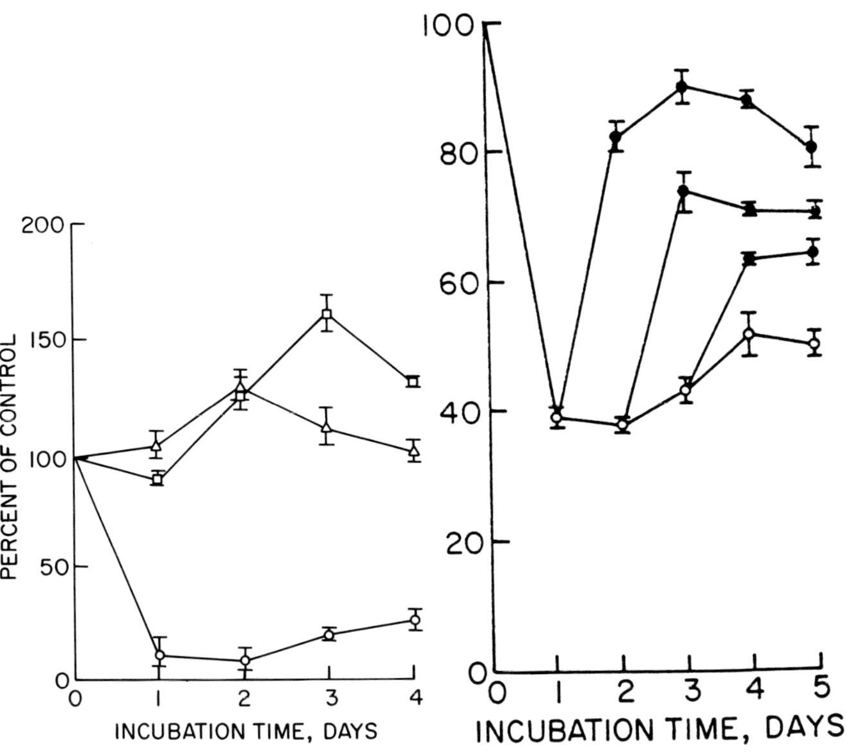

Figure 1. Macromolecular
synthesis. Triplicate
control and treated (1ng
(IL-1β) cultures incubated
3h in 1µCi [³H]-TdR (O) or
6h in 1µCi [³H]-leucine (Δ)
or 0.5 µCi [³H]-Urd (□).
Average cpm/cell was used to
calculate % control ± S.D.

Figure 2. Reversibility of
arrest. Control and treated
cultures fluid changed to
fresh medium each day (●) or
maintained (O). Cultures
from each set incubated in
0.5 µCi [³H]-TdR for 4h/day.
Average ± S.D.

The relation between incubation time and receptor
binding was studied using ^{125}I-rIL-1ß. Purity of the
^{125}I-IL-1 was confirmed by electrophoresis and biological
activity was retained when measured in a thymocyte assay.
Confluent 35mm cell cultures were incubated at 4°C in 1 µCi
^{125}I-IL-1 contained in 0.8 ml buffer consisting of DMEM, 2%
FBS and 20mM Hepes. Cells were hydrolyzed in 2N NaOH.
Specific binding was observed with a maximum at 2 hours of
incubation (Fig. 3). Binding of ^{125}I-IL-1ß was also dose
dependent (Fig. 4). Specific binding was again demonstrated by incubating cells in the presence or absence of a
100-fold excess of unlabeled rIL-1ß.

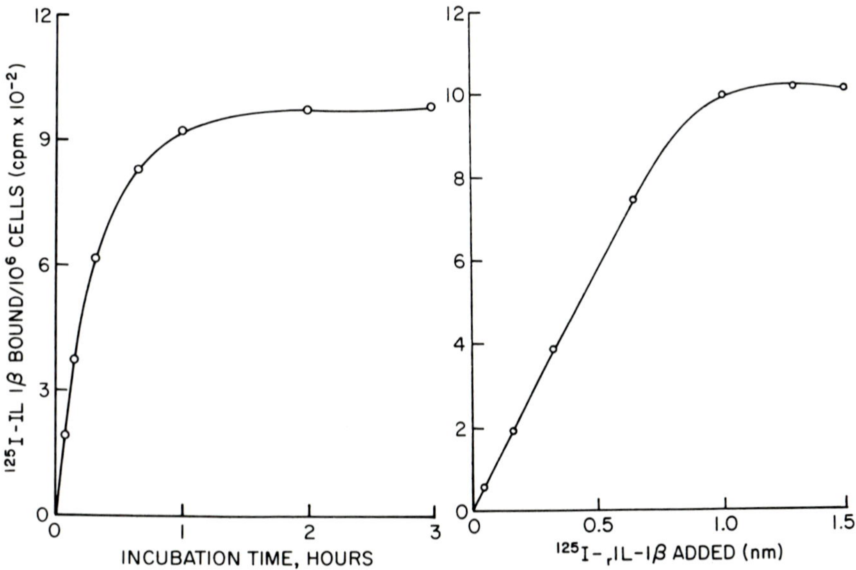

Figure 3. Time dependent
specific binding of ^{125}-I-
rIL-1ß to MDA-MB-415 cells

Figure 4. Binding of ^{125}-I-
IL-1ß as a function of
ligand concentration. Data
represent specific binding.

DISCUSSION

IL-1 is growth inhibitory or cytocidal when tested
with the melanoma line, A375, the mouse fibroblast, L929,
and the myleoid leukemia line, K562 (Onozaki et al., 1985b;
Lovett et al., 1986). The mouse cell line, M1, is also
inhibited by IL-1 but inhibition appears to correlate with
the induction of differentiation. We previously reported

that IL-1 stimulates, inhibits or has no significant effect
on the replication of a variety of target cells. Lines
established from malignant mammary tissue were among the
growth inhibited cells.

This study initiates an effort to analyze the kinetics
and mechanism by which IL-1 inhibits the replication of the
mammary cell line, MDA-MB-415. The response of MDA-MB-415
is dose dependent and at a concentration of 1ng IL-1 was
observed to significantly inhibit [^{3}H]-TdR incorporation by
cells maintained in microtiter well cultures. Inhibition
was maximum by 24 hours and was maintained in the presence
of IL-1 over a 5 day period. Inhibition was rapidly reversible following removal of the monokine, but DNA synthesis
did not completely return to control levels.

The biological response induced by IL-1 has been correlated with the presence of a low number of surface receptors in T-cells. Both IL-1α and IL-1β appear to bind the
same receptors with equal affinities, although some evidence disputes this. Our preliminary findings show that
MDA-MB-415 cells also bind ^{125}I-IL-1β in a saturable
manner. Thus, growth inhibition may be related to receptor
occupancy.

REFERENCES

Gaffney EV, Tsai S-C (1986). Lymphocyte-activating and
     growth-inhibitory activities for several sources of
     native and recombinant interleukin 1. Can Res
     46:3834-3837.
Lovett D, Kozan B, Hadam M, Resch K, Gemsa D (1986).
     Macrophage cytotoxicity: Interleukin 1 is a mediator
     of tumor cytostasis. J Immunol 136:340-347.
Onozaki K, Matsushima K, Klimerman EB, Saito T,
     Oppenheim JJ (1985a). Role of interleukin-1 in
     promoting human monocyte-mediated tumor cytotoxicity.
     J Immunol 135:314-320.
Onozaki K, Matsushima K, Aggarwal BB, Oppenheim JJ
     (1985b). Human interleukin 1 is a cytocidal factor
     for several tumor cell lines. J Immunol
     135:3962-1968.
Tsai S-C, Gaffney EV (1987). Modulation of cell
     proliferation by human recombinant interleukin-1 and
     immune interferon. J Natl Cancer Inst 79:77-81.

Monokines and Other Non-Lymphocytic Cytokines, pages 217–222
© 1988 Alan R. Liss, Inc.

SIGNAL REQUIREMENT FOR INTERLEUKIN 1-DEPENDENT IL2 PRODUC-
TION AND IL2 RECEPTOR INDUCTION BY HUMAN LEUKEMIA-DERIVED
HSB.2 SUBCLONES

Tadashi Kasahara, Naofumi Mukaida, Hitoshi Yagisawa,
Tadashi Kawai and Kohei Shioiri-Nakano

Departments of Medical Biology and Parasitology, and
Clinical Pathology, Jichi Medical School,
Minamikawachi-machi, Tochigi-ken, 329-04, Japan

INTRODUCTION

Interleukin 1(IL1) is produced by a variety of cell
types and has multiple biologic function including enhanced
IL2 production, induction of IL2 receptor (IL2R) on T and
natural killer cells, prostaglandin and collagenase production on fibroblasts or synovial cells, as well as production
of acute phase proteins by hepatocytes (Oppenheim et al,
1986). Recent success of molecular cloning of murine and
human IL1 revealed the presence of two distinct IL1 species
and their common receptors. Direct or indirect effects of
IL1 are being analysed in such systems as the activation of
various lymphokine genes in T cell lymphoma LBRM33 subclones
(Hagiwara et al, 1987), interferon (IFN)-β2/BSF-2 induction
from fibrolasts (Van Damme et al, 1987) or class III major
MHC gene expression in hepatoma cells (Perlmutter et al,
1986). The mechanism of IL1 action on various cells and the
post-receptor system are, however, not yet fully understood.
Activation of various receptor-mediated cellular responses
has been shown to be Ca^{2+}-dependent and mediated by breakdown of membrane phosphatidylinositols (PI).
We have previously established subclones from a human
leukemic cell line, HSB.2, that produce high levels of IL2
and IFN-γ in an IL1-dependent manner (Kasahara et al, 1985;
Mukaida et al, 1987). Using these subclones, we investigated
the role of IL1 in the lymphokine gene activation particularly in view of the involvement of protein kinase C (PKC)
activation, intracellular $Ca^{2+}([Ca^{2+}]i)$ level, PI metabolism
and cyclic nucleotides.

MATERIALS AND METHODS

<u>IL2</u> <u>and</u> <u>IFN-γ</u> <u>Production</u>: HSB.2 subclones (1×10^6 cells/ml) were incubated with 20μg/ml of phytohemagglutinin (PHA, DIFCO) in the presence or absence of rIL1α (Dainippon Pharmaceutical Co., Osaka) or rIL1β (Otsuka Pharmaceutical Co., Tokushima) for 24hr. IL2 and IFN-γ activity was determined as described elsewhere (Kasahara et al, 1985).
<u>Measurement</u> <u>of</u> <u>Cytosol</u> <u>PKC</u> <u>Activity,</u> <u>Intracelluar</u> <u>Ca^{2+}</u> <u>Level</u> <u>and</u> <u>Inositol</u> <u>Phosphates</u> <u>(InsPs)</u>: PKC activity in the cytosol fraction was determined using histon type IIIS as a substrate in the presence of $CaCl_2$, phosphatidylserine and 1,3-diolein. For the measurement of cytosolic free Ca^{2+}, cells were loaded with quin-2 AM and fluorescence was measured by Hitachi 650 spectrophotometer using excitation of 339 nm and emission of 492 nm. To determine InsPs, cells were labeled with [^{3}H]myo-inositol for 12hr in Medium-199 supplemented with 10% dialysed FCS. Total and individual InsPs were eluted stepwise from a Dowex 1-X8 anion exchange column. Detail methods on these procedures were described elsewhere (Mukaida et al, 1987).
<u>IL2R</u> <u>Induction</u>: After cells were incubated with rIL1β or phorbol-myristate-acetate (PMA) for 16hr, they were labeled with monoclonal anti-Tac antibody (1:1,000 dilution; donated by Dr.T.Uchiyama) and FITC-conjugated anti-mouse IgG (1:10 dilution, TAGO). Immunofluorescence was measured by a Coulter Epics C flow cytometry.
<u>RNA</u> <u>Blot</u> <u>Analysis</u> <u>for</u> <u>IL2</u> <u>and</u> <u>IL2R</u>: Total cellular RNA from stimulated and unstimulated cells were separated by guanidine thiocyanate and subsequent ultracentrifugation on a CsCl density gradient. Northern blot analysis was done using nick-translated ^{32}P-labeled cDNA probes for human IL2 (p3-16, provided by Dr.T.Taniguchi), IL2R (pKCR Tac-2, provided by Dr.J.Yodoi) or IFN-γ (provided by Dr.W.Drohan).

RESULTS AND DISCUSSION

IL1 signal is essential for the optimal IL2 and IFN-γ production: We have already established several subclones from HSB.2-C5B2 cells, which produced high levels of IL2 in an IL1-dependent manner. One of the subclones, C5B2#28, which produced low levels of IL2 (5.8 ± 2.2 u/ml) and IFN-γ (280 ± 110 u/ml) when stimulated with PHA (20 μg/ml), produced higher levels of IL2 (95 ± 18 u/ml) and IFN-γ ($3,050 \pm 620$ u/ml) when stimulated with PHA plus rIL1β (20 u/ml). In this

system, PHA signal could be substituted with PMA (20nM) plus
ionomycin (200nM), whereas IL1 signal was still indispen-
sable for maximal IL2 and IFN-γ production, indicating that
PKC activation and increase of Ca^{2+} are needed but not
sufficient. The involvement of PKC activation was clearly
demonstrated by a PKC inhibitor, H-7 (Mukaida et al, 1987).

IL1 is essnential for the IL2 and IFN-γ mRNA expression:
Above observation obtained based on the biological activity
of IL2 and IFN-γ was confirmed as well as on the level of
transcription of these lymphokine genes. Northern blot
analysis indicated that rIL1α or rIL1β markedly augmented
mRNA expression of IL2 induced by PHA or PMA+ionomycin (Fig.
1A). IFN-γ mRNA expression was similarly enhanced by the
presence of rIL1. These data suggested that IL1 regulates
these lymphokine genes at a pretranslational level.

IL1 has a direct effect on Tac antigen expression: Although
IL1 acted as a costimulator with PHA or PMA+ionomycin in the
lymphokine production, IL1 as well as PMA by itself could
induce Tac antigen expression on C5B2 subclones to a marked
degree. This observation was evidenced by an immunofluorescence staining and subsequent analysis on a flow cyto-
metry (Table 1). As expected, PMA-induced but not IL1-in-
duced Tac antigen expression was mostly abrogated by H-7.
The augmented Tac antigen expression was confirmed by the
northern blot analysis shown in Fig.1B.

Effect of IL1 on PKC activation, intracellular $[Ca^{2+}]i$ level,
and PI turnover: It is of great interest to examine what

Table 1. Induction of Tac antigen on a HSB.2-C5B2 subclone

	no drug		H-7 25 µM	
stimulants	% positive cells	MFI	% positive cells	MFI
medium	17.9	200.0	n.t.	n.t.
rIL1β 20 u/ml	47.8	345.4	41.8	319.9
PMA 20 nM	73.7	507.7	39.6	298.0

HSB.2-C5B2 cells were incubated with stimulants for 16 hr.
Tac antigen was stained by anti-Tac and FITC-goat anti-mouse
IgG. Mean Fluorescence intensity was measured on an Epics-C.

signals are involved in these IL1-transmitted lymphokine genes activation.   First, PKC activity was measured in the cells treated briefly with stimulants.   Marked reduction of PKC activity in the cytosol fraction of PHA or PMA-treated cells was observed (18% in PHA treated cells and 0.2% in PMA treated cells compared with med control). Neither did IL1 induce PKC activity reduction (94% of med control), nor did IL1 augment further the PHA-induced PKC activity reduction.
    Next, we looked at whether these stimulants increased the $[Ca^{2+}]i$ level. PHA or ionomycin induced more than 100 nM of

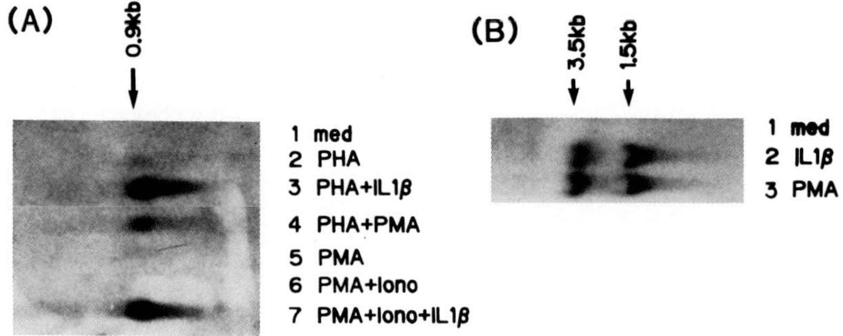

Figure 1. Expression of IL2 (A) and IL2R (B) mRNA in a HSB.2-C5B2 subclone incubated with various stimulants.

Table 2. Measurement of $[Ca^{2+}]i$ level in the PHA and rIL1β-treated HSB.2-C5B2 subclone

stimulants	$[Ca^{2+}]i$ (nM)	(No of Exp)	net increment of $[Ca^{2+}]i$ (nM)
medium	122 ± 9	(29)	0
PHA 20 µg/ml	223 ± 13	(11)	101
rIL1β 20 u/ml	126 ± 8	(5)	4
PMA 20 nM	131 ± 8	(4)	9
PMA+rIL1β	127 ± 9	(2)	5
PHA+rIL1β	253 ± 11	(6)	131
PHA+ PMA	260 ± 11	(3)	140
Ionomycin 200nM	339 ± 12	(3)	217

$[Ca^{2+}]i$ was determined during 10 min after stimulation, using a quin 2-AM probe in the presence of 1 mM $CaCl_2$.

net [Ca2+]i elevation, whereas rIL1β or PMA treatment alone
had no such effect with a mild augmentation of $[Ca^{2+}]i$ level
induced by PHA (Table 2).

The accumulation of InsPs during 60 min of stimulation
was observed markedly by PHA but not by rIL1β at all. Nor
did rIL1β augment the PHA-induced InsPs accumulation. It may
be noteworthy that the combination of PMA, ionomycin plus
rIL1β, which did not accompany accumulation of InsPs, stimulated significant levels of IL2 production and IL2 mRNA
expression (Fig.1), suggesting that pathyways utilized by
this combination are essentially different from that by PHA.

Finally, participation of cyclic nucleotides in these
IL1-mediated activation was studied. PHA but not rIL1β induced significant level of cAMP production within 15 min and
moreover, rIL1β did not augment the level induced by PHA.
However, reagents increasing cAMP levels such as forskolin,
dibutyryl cAMP or 8-bromo-cAMP failed to substitute IL1
action with only modest elevation of IL2 production.

Our observation on the role of cAMP sharply contrasts
with that observed by Mary et al. (1987) that such drugs
increasing cAMP levels remarkably inhibited IL2 production
by PHA+PMA-induced Jurkat cells. On the contrary, it was
found by Narumiya et al. (1987) that forskolin is able to
induce Tac antigen and IL2R level on a human NK-like cell
line, YTC3 cells, although the same drug did not induce Tac
antigen on our HSB.2-C5B2 cells at all. Taken collectively,
it seems that cAMP affects differently on IL2 production and
IL2R induction. In contrast, cGMP level was significantly
dropped off by not only PHA- but also by rIL1β-stimulation
in C5B2 cells. The cGMP level decreased less than 50 %
within 10 min after incubation with these stimulants. Although we don't know exactly the reason and the consequence
of the decrease of cGMP at present, this phenomenon should
be noteworthy in that IL1 directly modulates its level on
the otherwise refractory HSB.2-C5B2 cells.

CONCLUSION

The role of IL1 during IL2 production and Tac antigen
(IL2R) expression has been studied on human leukemic HSB.2-
C5B2 subclones. On these cell lines, IL1 is prerequisite
for maximal IL2 and IFN-γ production regardless of the
stimulation with PHA, or with a combination of PMA plus
ionomycin. Although PHA by itself induced PKC activation,
$[Ca^{2+}]i$ level and InsPs accumulation markedly, IL1 neither

affected these parameters at all, nor augmented the levels induced by PHA stimulation. While PHA induced high level of InsPs accumulation during a brief incubation, it was considered that this accumulation was not always necessary, since a combination of PMA, ionomycin plus rIL1 induced significant level of IL2 production and IL2 mRNA activation without accumulation of InsPs. In contrast, IL1 as well as PMA directly induced Tac antigen by itself without accompanying any increase of these parameters. It should be of note that Tac antigen expression was induced not only by PMA which activated PKC greatly, but also by IL1 which did not activate PKC at all.

REFERENCES

Hagiwara H,Huang HJS, Arai N, Herzenberg LA, Arai KI, Zlotnik A (1987). Interleukin 1 modulates messenger RNA levels of lymphokines and of other molecules associated with T cell activation in the T cell lymphoma LBRM33-1A5. J Immunol 138: 2514-2519.
Kasahara T, Mukaida N, Hatake K, Motoyoshi K, Kawai T, Shioiri-Nakano K (1985). Interleukin 1(IL1)-dependent lymphokine production by human leukemic T cell line, HSB.2 subclones. J Immunol 134: 1682-1689.
Mary D, Aussel C, Ferrua B, Fehlmann M (1987). Regulation of interleukin 2 synthesis by cAMP in human T cells. J Immunol 139: 1179-1184.
Mukaida N, Kasahara T, Yagisawa H, Shioiri-Nakano K, Kawai T (1987). Signal requirement for interleukin 1 (IL1)-dependent IL2 production by a human leukemia-derived HSB.2 subclone. J Immunol 139: in press.
Narumiya S, Hirata M, Nanba T, Nikaido T, Taniguchi Y, Tagaya Y, Okada M, Mitsuya H, Yodoi J (1987). Activation of interleukin 2 receptor gene by forskolin and cyclic AMP analogues. Biochem Biophys Res Commun 143:753-760.
Oppenheim JJ, Kovacs EJ, Matsushima K, Durum SK (1986). There is more than one interleukin 1.Immunol Today 7:45-56.
Perlmutter DH, Goldberger G, Dinarello CA, Mizel SA, Colten HR (1986). Regulation of class III major histocompatibility complex gene products by interleukin 1. Science 232:850-852.
Van Damme J, Opdenakker G, Simpson RJ, Rubira MR, Cayphas S, Vink A, Van Snick J (1987). Identification of the human 26-kd protein, interferon β2, as a B cell hybridoma/ plasmacytoma growth factor induced by interleukin 1 and tumor necrosis factor. J Exp Med 165: 914-919.

Monokines and Other Non-Lymphocytic Cytokines, pages 223–228
© 1988 Alan R. Liss, Inc.

INTERLEUKIN-1-STIMULATED EL-4 CELLS RELEASE LINOLEIC ACID,
WHICH AUGMENTS TRANSLOCATION OF PROTEIN KINASE C AND
PRODUCTION OF INTERLEUKIN-2

Philip L. Simon, Mike A. Clark, Linda S.
Henderson and Shouki Kassis

Depts. of Immunology (P.L.S., S.K.), Molecular
Pharmacology (M.A.C.), and Pharmacology (L.S.H.),
Smith Kline & French Laboratories, King of
Prussia, PA 19406

INTRODUCTION

Interleukin-1 (IL-1) acts as a helper factor for the
production of interleukin-2 (IL-2) by EL-4 cells when the
cells are co-stimulated with calcium ionophores, phorbol
myristate acetate (PMA), or a combination of the two
agents (Simon 1984; Simon et al., 1985; Truneh et al.,
1987). The mechanism of action of calcium ionophore is to
raise the intracellular level of calcium, while that of
PMA is to activate protein kinase C (PKC). Although IL-1
induces a small increase in intracellular calcium levels
in EL-4 cells (Truneh et al., 1987), its ability to act in
a synergistic fashion with calcium ionophores such as
A23187 or ionomycin makes it unlikely that this is the
mechanism of action of IL-1 on EL-4 cells. Similarly,
IL-1 has not been shown to directly activate PKC, and the
fact that it acts in concert with PMA to induce IL-2
production makes it unlikely that IL-1 and PMA act in
exactly the same fashion. However, IL-1 has been
previously shown to activate phospholipase A2 (PLA2)
activity in chondrocytes (Chang et al., 1986). In the
series of experiments described in this paper, we investigated the activation of phospholipases in EL-4 cells by
IL-1, and in addition studied the potential role of unsaturated fatty acids that might be released by the action
of PLA2 on the subsequent activation of PKC and IL-2
production. We found that IL-1 caused an early, transient
rise in EL-4 PLA2 activity, which was followed by the
release of linoleic acid from the cells. Linoleic acid

was capable of acting in concert with PMA to induce both
PKC translocation and IL-2 production.

MATERIALS AND METHODS

Recombinant human IL-1 beta was cloned, expressed, and
purified as described previously (Meyers et al., 1987).
Radiolabeled phospholipids and fatty acids, and radioactive P-32 were obtained from Dupont NEN (Boston, MA).
Unlabeled fatty acids were obtained from Nuchek Prep
(Elysian, MN). PMA and calcium ionophore A23187 were
obtained from Sigma Chemical Co. (St. Louis, MO). Culture
of EL-4 cells, assays for IL-1 and IL-2, and calculation
of data were performed as described previously (Simon et
al., 1985). Phospholipase assays were done on the cell-
free sonicates of EL-4 cells as described previously
(Clark et al., 1987). PKC was assayed as previously
described (Patel and Kassis, 1987).

RESULTS AND DISCUSSION

EL-4 cells were cultured for varying periods of time
in the presence or absence of 5 units/ml of recombinant
human IL-1 beta, and then sonicated and centrifuged at
high speed. The cell-free sonicates were then assayed for
phospholipase activity by incubation with labeled phospho-
lipid substrates, and subsequent analysis of the reaction
mixtures by thin layer chromatography. As shown in
Table 1, IL-1 caused a transient rise in phosphatidyl-
choline-specific PLA2 activity, which reached a maximum
within 2 to 3 min, and returned to baseline levels within
10 min after stimulation. No change in PLA2 activity was
observed when phosphatidylethanolamine was used as a substrate nor was there an effect on phospholipase C activity
(data not shown).

We next looked for the more commonly associated consequence of PLA2 activation, the release of arachidonic acid
from cellular phospholipids. However, in several experiments, we were unable to detect the release of radioactivity when the cells were labeled with tritiated
arachidonic acid and then stimulated with IL-1 (data not
shown). This was not due to either a failure of the cells
to take up the labeled fatty acid or to incorporate it

TABLE 1. Stimulation of PC-Specific Phospholipase A2
Activity in EL-4 Cells by IL-1

Time (min)	PLA2 activity[*] (μmol/min/mg protein)
0	3.0 +/- 1.3
1	5.5 +/- 4.0
2	11.7 +/- 7.6
3	17.0 +/- 5.6
4	5.0 +/- 4.4
5	1.9 +/- 1.6
6	1.8 +/- 1.1

---

[*] 1×10^5 EL-4 cells were treated with 5 units/ml of
IL-1 for the indicated time periods before being
sonicated. The sonicates were assayed for PLA2
activity by incubation with ^{3}H-phosphatidylcholine
for 1 hr, followed by separation by TLC. The results
shown are the means +/- S.D. of 3 separate experiments, each of which was assayed in triplicate.

into cellular phospholipids (data not shown). As an
alternative method of labeling the various lipid pools in
the cells, we used tritiated linoleic acid, which is an
established precursor of arachidonic acid. As shown in
Table 2, this procedure enabled us to detect the release
of radiolabeled metabolites from IL-1-stimulated EL-4
cells. The maximum increase in the rate of release was
seen between three and five min after stimulation with
IL-1, and fell back to baseline levels within 10 min. In
the same experiment, no effect on the release of radioactivity was seen when labeled arachidonic acid was used
instead of labeled linoleic acid. Subsequent HPLC
analysis of the released radioactivity demonstrated that
the linoleic acid had not been converted into arachidonic
acid, but instead was a mixture of linoleic acid and other
unidentified metabolites (data not shown).

Several investigators have demonstrated that certain
unsaturated fatty acids can directly activate PKC in cell-

TABLE 2. Release of radioactivity from EL-4 cells labeled
with either linoleic acid or arachidonic acid and
stimulated with IL-1

Time (min)	Linoleic	Arachidonic
0	40	20
1	90	20
2	51	35
3	755	63
4	1015	94
5	1050	85
6	731	10
7	81	11
8	63	19
10	21	10

* EL-4 cells were grown in the presence of tritiated
linoleic or arachidonic acid (10 µCi/ml) for 14 hr.
The cells were then washed 3 times before stimulation
with IL-1 (5 units/ml) or control for the indicated
periods of time. The results shown are the cpm of
radioactivity released by 1 x 10^5 cells stimulated
with IL-1 less the counts released by unstimulated
cells, and are derived from 3 separate experiments
each assayed in duplicate. The standard deviation was
less than 10% of the mean for all values.

free assays of PKC activity (McPhail et al., 1984; Hansson
et al., 1986). We investigated the possibility that
increased extracellular levels of linoleic acid might
effect the translocation of PKC in EL-4 cells, and
subsequent activation of IL-2 production. As shown in
Table 3, stimulation of EL-4 cells with 1 ng/ml PMA
produced neither translocation of PKC from the cytosol to
the membrane (at 1 hr), nor increased production of IL-2
(at 24 hr). Linoleic acid and IL-1 each had a slight
effect on PKC translocation, but no effect on IL-2
production. However, when linoleic acid or IL-1 was added
to PMA at 1 ng/ml, PKC activity was increased. The
relatively high concentration of linoleic acid that was

necessary to achieve these results may be the result of
the fact that the fatty acid partitioned into the serum in
the medium, reducing its effective concentration.

TABLE 3. Augmentation of PMA-induced PKC translocation and
IL-2 production in EL-4 cells by linoleic acid and IL-1

Treatment	PKC activity		IL-2 (U/ml)	
	Exp. 1	Exp. 2	Exp. 1	Exp. 2
Control	8.6	9.5	<2.0	<2.0
PMA (1 ng/ml)	15.4	9.2	2.5	<2.0
Linoleic Acid (200 µM)	22.8	6.8	<2.0	<2.0
IL-1 (5 units/ml)	20.7	9.1	<2.0	<2.0
PMA + Linol.	36.9	34.7	14.6	21.6
PMA + IL-1	30.1	16.3	51.6	41.3
PMA (10 ng/ml)	50.3	47.9	127.5	210.5

*   EL-4 cells at 2×10^5 cells/ml were stimulated with
the indicated agents for 1 hr. One ml aliquots of
each culture were saved and cultured an additional
23 hr for measurement of IL-2 production. The remain-
ing cells were washed with ice cold saline, processed
into cytosol and membrane fractions, which were then
assayed for PKC activity. The results for PKC activity are expressed as the percent of the total activity
detected in the membrane fraction.

The preceding experiments led us to construct a working hypothesis on the role of IL-1 in the augmentation of
IL-2 production by EL-4 cells. Following the binding of
IL-1 to its cell surface receptor, activation of a PC-
specific PLA2 ensues, with the result that the levels of
intracellular and extracellular free unsaturated fatty
acids are increased. PKC activity, which has been sub-
optimally stimulated by PMA, calcium ionophore, T-cell
lectins, or other agents, is then boosted by the increased
level of fatty acid. Once a minimum threshold of PKC
activity is achieved, IL-2 production is initiated.
Experiments using normal T-cells or other T-cell lines

will hopefully let us determine if this hypothesis can be
expanded beyond IL-1-stimulated EL-4 cells.

REFERENCES

Chang J, Gilman SC, Lewis AJ (1986). Interleukin 1
  activates phospholipase A2 in rabbit chondrocytes: a
  possible signal for IL 1 action. J Immunol
  136(4):1283-1287.
Clark MA, Conway TM, Shorr RGL, Crooke ST (1987).
  Identification and isolation of a mammalian protein
  which is antigenically and functionally related to the
  phospholipase A2 stimulatory peptide melittin. J Biol
  Chem 262(9):4402-4406.
Hansson A, Serhan CN, Haeggstrom J, Ingleman-Sundberg M,
  Samuelson B (1986). Activation of protein kinase C by
  lipoxin A and other eicosanoids. Intracellular action
  of oxygenation products of arachidonic acid. Biochem
  Biophys Res Comm 134(3):1215-1222.
McPhail LC, Clayton CC, Snyderman R (1984). A potential
  second messenger role for unsaturated fatty acids:
  activation of Ca2+-dependent protein kinase. Science
  224:662-665.
Meyers CA, Johanson KO, Miles LM, McDevitt PJ, Simon PL,
  Webb RL, Chen M-J, Holskin BP, Lillquist JS, Young PR
  (1987). Purification and characterization of human
  recombinant interleukin-1 beta. J Biol Chem
  262:11176-11181.
Patel J, Kassis S. (1987). Concanavalin A prevents
  phorbol esters-mediated redistribution of protein kinase
  C and ß-adrenergic receptors in rat glioma C6 cells.
  Biochem Biophys Res Comm 144:1265-1272.
Simon PL (1984). Calcium mediates one of the signals
  required for interleukin 1 and 2 production by murine
  cell lines. Cell Immunol 87:720-726.
Simon PL, Laydon JT, Lee JC (1985). A modified assay for
  interleukin-1 (IL-1). J Immunol Meth 84:85-94.
Truneh A, Simon PL, Schmidt-Verhulst A-M (1986).
  Interleukin 1 and protein kinase C activator are
  dissimilar in their effects on IL-2 receptor expression
  and IL-2 secretion by T lymphocytes. Cell Immunol
  103:365-374.

Monokines and Other Non-Lymphocytic Cytokines, pages 229–234
© 1988 Alan R. Liss, Inc.

DETECTION OF PROTEIN PHOSPHORYLATION IN HUMAN PERIPHERAL
BLOOD MONONUCLEAR CELLS IN RESPONSE TO INTERLEUKIN 1 (IL 1)

Kouji Matsushima, Masahiro Shiroo, Wook Lew,
Yoshiro Kobayashi, Tohru Akahoshi and Joost J.
Oppenheim

Laboratory of Molecular Immunoregulation,
Biological Response Modifiers Program, Division
of Cancer Treatment, National Cancer Institute,
Frederick, MD 21701-1013

INTRODUCTION

Although IL 1 has been reported to have diverse
biological activities on a variety of cells (Oppenheim et
al., 1986), little is known about the intracellular
molecular events that occur after binding of IL 1 to its
receptor. Since it has been believed that selective
phosphorylation of cell-associated proteins is essential in
regulating the differentiation and growth of many cell types
after treatment with hormones, growth factors, and cytokines
(Greengard and Robinson, 1984), we have studied the effect
of IL 1 on protein phosphorylation. We chose to study
glucocorticoid treated normal human peripheral blood
mononuclear cells (PBMC) because glucocorticoids
dramatically up-regulate the expression of IL 1 receptors on
PBMC (Akahoshi et al., in press) and the background levels
of protein phosphorylation in PBMC is very low in contrast
with that observed in tumor cell lines. We could identify a
cytosolic 65 kDa protein which is selectively phosphorylated
at serine residues in response to IL 1 stimulation. This 65
kDa protein has been purified and a partial amino acid
sequence has been obtained.

MATERIALS, METHODS AND RESULTS

Induction of Protein Phosphorylation in Human PBMC by IL 1.

Normal human PBMC were isolated from buffy coats by

Ficoll-Hypaque density method and cultured for 5 hrs in RPMI
1640, and 10% fetal calf serum in the presence of different
doses of prednisolone. Cells were washed 3 times with
phosphate-free RPMI 1640 medium and cultured in the presence
of 100 μCi/ml ^{32}P-orthophosphate for an additional 2 hrs.
Cells were further stimulated with carrier-free purified
recombinant human IL 1α (generously provided by Dainippon
Pharmaceutical Company, Osaka, Japan). As shown in Fig. 1,
IL 1 selectively and dramatically induced protein
phosphorylation of a 65 kDa protein (pp65) within one minute
and the phosphorylation reached a maximal level at 10 to 15
min. The induction of protein phosphorylation by IL 1
correlated well with the increase in the number of IL 1
receptors by prednisolone (Akahoshi et al., in press).
Using two dimensional gel electrophoresis, the pp65 was
identified at about pI 5 to 5.5. As little as 1 ng/ml IL 1
was sufficient to induce significant levels of
phosphorylation of this protein. The same degree of
phosphorylation of p65 was observed by using recombinant
human IL 1β (generous gift from Otsuka Pharmaceutical
Company, Tokushima, Japan). Phosphoamino acid analysis of
the pp65 by thin layer chromatography showed that only
serine residues were phosphorylated after IL 1 stimulation.
We did not observe any increase in the phosphorylation of
plasma membrane associated proteins after stimulation of
PBMC with IL 1. Fractionation of cell extracts by
ultracentrifugation revealed that pp65 is located
exclusively in the cytosol, suggesting that pp65 is not an
auto-phosphorylated form of the IL 1 receptor (Matsushima et
al; 1987).

Time Course of the IL 1-Induced P65 Phosphorylation

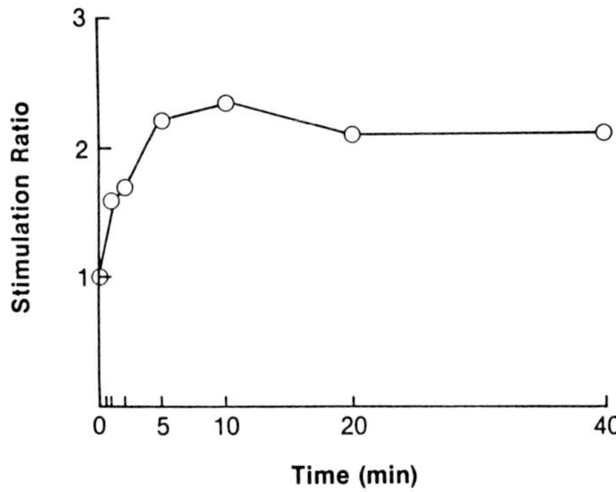

Figure 1.

Purification of pp65 to Homogeneity.

In order to identify the pp65, we purified the pp65 to homogeneity. Prednisolone pretreated PBMC were first labeled with ^{32}P-orthophosphate and stimulated with 1 ug/ml recombinant IL 1α. The cytosol fraction, which was obtained by sonicating PBMC in a buffer consisting of 25 mM HEPES, 2 mM EDTA, 5 mM EGTA, 1 mM PMSF, 4 mM 2-ME, 1 ug/ml leupeptin, 50 mM sodium fluoride, and 1 mM sodium vanadate, followed by ultracentrifugation at 100,000 g for 60 min, was fractionated by sequential chromatography on Sephacryl S-200, HPLC anion exchange (AX 300), and HPLC hydroxyapatite. ^{32}P-labeled pp65 was detected by SDS-PAGE followed by autoradiography. The purified pp65 yielded a single band on SDS-PAGE. The unphosphorylated form of 65 kDa protein (p65), which was adjacent to pp65, was also purified to homogeneity by HPLC anion exchange. About 80 ug of p65 and pp65 was obtained from the cytosolic fraction of 1 x 10^9 PBMC (24 mg protein). 30 to 60% of pp65 was obtained in the phosphorylated form. Both p65 and pp65 yielded identical amino acid composition after hydrolysis. Analysis of hydrolysates on thin layer chromatography revealed that pp65 was phosphorylated only at serine residues. Although the amino terminal of pp65 was blocked, one of the fragments of CNBr digested pp65 was successfully sequenced by the Edman degradation method as shown in Fig. 2. A computer assisted sequence homology comparison of pp65 with other known protein sequences revealed that this protein has an unique protein sequence. Therefore, we initiated cDNA cloning of pp65 using oligonucleotide probes which were constructed based on the partial amino acid sequence. A 2.5 kb cDNA has been obtained and analysis of the nucleotide sequence is in progress.

```
 1    2    3    4    5    6    7    8    9   10   11

Ala-Arg-Lys-Ile-Gly-Ala-Arg-Val-Tyr-Ala-Leu

12   13   14   15   16   17   18   19   20   21   22

Pro-Glu-Asp-Leu-Val-Glu-Val-Asn-Pro-Lys-(Thr)
```

Figure 2. Amino acid sequence of a CNBr fragment from pp65.

Antibody Preparation and Western Blotting Analysis of
p(p)65.

Polyclonal antibody was prepared by immunizing a rabbit
with purified pp65. Using the antibody, Western blotting
analysis of various types of human cell extracts was
performed to detect the presence of p(p)65. Western
blotting analysis revealed a specific 65 kDa band in many
types of leucocytes including monocytes, B lymphocytes,
large granular lymphocytes, T lymphocytes and myeloid cells,
but no p(p)65 was detected in human dermal fibroblasts,
melanoma cells, or Hela cells. A similar results was also
obtained by Northern blotting analysis of mRNA (2.7 kb)
expression by various type of human cells using pp65 cDNA.
These data suggest some selectivity of expression of pp65 in
human cells. The physiological functions of this protein
remain to be established.

Identification of Protein-Kinase(s) Involved in
Phosphorylation of p65.

To identify the protein kinase(s) which is involved in
phosphorylating p65 after stimulation of PBMC with IL 1,
protein kinase inhibitors, HA-1004, H-7 and W-7 were added
to the culture before addition of IL 1. H-7, which is
relatively specific in blocking protein kinase C, did not
block the induction of phosphorylation of p65, whereas H-A
1004, which is a cyclic nucleotide dependent protein kinase
inhibitor, and W-7, which is an inhibitor of calmodulin
kinase both significantly inhibited the induction of
phosphorylation of p65 by IL 1 (Matsushima et al., 1987).
This suggests that protein kinase C is not involved in
phosphorylation of p65 by IL 1. Direct in vitro
phosphorylation of unphosphorylated p65 by cAMP dependent
protein kinase, protein kinase C, and calmodulin kinase was
performed and showed that p65 was a substrate only for cAMP
dependent protein kinase. On the other hand, we could not
observe the induction of cAMP in response to IL 1 in PBMC
before and after treatment with prednisolone, which suggests
that cAMP dependent protein kinase is not physiologically
involved in phosphorylating p65 only after stimulation with
IL 1. Therefore, we are in the process of identifying
protein kinases present in cell extracts of human PBMC. At
least three different protein kinases, which differ in
molecular weight have been detected in IL 1 stimulated human

PBMC cytosol that can phosphorylate p65 in vitro. The
purification and further characterization of these protein
kinases is in progress.

DISCUSSION

     The induction of phosphorylation at serine residues of
a cytosolic 65 kDa protein in normal human PBMC in response
to IL 1 has been identified. Although no specific protein
kinase has been reported to be requisite for the action of
IL 1, our data indicate that unidentified serine protein
kinase(s), which can phosphorylate a 65 novel kDa protein,
may be functionally connected with the IL 1 receptor.

     We believe that IL 1 is necessary for the polyclonal B
lymphocyte activation by glucocorticoids, because
glucocorticoid-treated PBMC responded to IL 1 with an
increase in the number of immunoglobulin producing cells.
Conversely, polyclonal B lymphocyte activation could be
blocked by mouse monoclonal anti-human IL 1β (Tosato et al.,
unpublished data). Furthermore, since the most
glucocorticoid responsive subset of PBMC that shows the
greatest increase in the number of IL 1 receptors is
enriched in B lymphocytes, the induction of p65
phosphorylation may be involved in this IL 1 induced B
lymphocyte activation to produce immunoglobulins.

     Interestingly, several other laboratories have
described phosphorylation of a 65 kDa protein in different
cell types after stimulation with phorbol esters (Ishii et
al., 1987), lipopolysaccharides (Prpie et al., 1987),
lectins (phytohemagglutinin, concanavalin A, and pokeweed
mitogen, Chaplin et al; 1980), interleukin 2 (Ishii et al;
1987), and interleukin 3 (Evans et al., 1986), suggesting
that p65 may be a common substrate for these cytokine and
mitogen induced protein kinases. We have recently also
purified a 65 kDa cytosolic protein in PBMC whose
phosphorylation is augmented by PMA and have established
that this 65 kDa phosphoprotein is identical to the pp65
whose phosphorylation is augmented in response to IL 1. The
identification of the phosphorylation sites of these two
preparations is in progress.

     In conclusion, the identification and purification of a
cytosolic 65 kDa protein whose phosphorylation is augmented

by IL 1 stimulation should lead to a greater understanding
of the intracellular molecular events following IL 1
receptor signal transduction.

REFERENCES

Akahoshi T, Oppenheim JJ, Matsushima K. Induction of
   high affinity interleukin 1 receptor on human peripheral
   blood lymphocytes by glucocorticoid hormones. J Exp Med
   (in press).
Chaplin DO, Wedner HJ, Parker CW (1980). Protein
   phosphorylation in human peripheral blood lymphocytes:
   Mitogen-induced increases in protein phosphorylation in
   intact lymphocytes. J Immunol 124:2390-2398.
Evans SW, Rennick D, Farrar WL (1986). Multilineage
   hematopoietic growth factor interleukin 3 and direct
   activators of protein kinase C stimulated phosphorylation
   of common substrates. Blood 68:906-913.
Greengard P, Robinson GA (1984). Phosphorylation Research
   vol. 18. New York: Raven Press.
Ishii T, Kohno M, Nakamura M, Hinuma Y, Sugamura, K (1987).
   Characterization of interleukin 2 - stimulated
   phosphorylation of 67 and 63 kDa proteins in human T
   cells. Biochem J 242:211-219.
Matsushima K, Kobayashi Y, Copeland TD, Akahoshi T,
   Oppenheim JJ (1987). Phosphorylation of a cytosolic 65
   kDa protein induced by interleukin 1 in glucocorticoid-
   pretreated normal human peripheral blood mononuclear
   leukocytes. J Immunol 139:3367-3374.
Oppenheim JJ, Kovacs EJ, Matsushima K, Durum SK (1986).
   There is more than one interleukin 1. Immunol Today 7:45-
   66.
Prpie V, Weiel JE, Somers SD, DiGuiseppi J, Gonias SL,
   Pizzo SV, Hamilton TA, Herman B, Adams DO (1987). Effects
   of bacterial lipopolysaccharide on the hydrolysis of
   phosphatidylinositol-4,5-bisphosphate in murine peritoneal
   macrophages. J Immunol 139:526-533.

Monokines and Other Non-Lymphocytic Cytokines, pages 235–242
© 1988 Alan R. Liss, Inc.

RECOMBINANT HUMAN GRANULOCYTE-MACROPHAGE COLONY-
STIMULATING FACTOR (rh GM-CSF) INDUCES DIFFERENT
INTRACELLULAR SIGNALS IN MATURE AND IMMATURE MYELOID
CELLS.

Lopez, A.F.*, Hardy, S.J.[§], Eglinton, J.*, Gamble,
J.*, To, L.B.[+], Dyson, P.[+], Wong, G.[+], Clark, S.[+],
Murray, A.W.[§] and Vadas, M.A.*.
From the *Department of Human Immunology and [+]Hema-
tology, the Institute of Medical and Veterinary
Science, Frome Road, Adelaide; [§]The School of Bio-
logical Sciences, Flinders University, Bedford Park,
South Australia, and +Genetics Institute, Cambridge,
MA, USA.

INTRODUCTION

Human GM-CSF is a glycoprotein of 19,000MW produced
by lymphocytes and other cells after stimulation (1).
Originally, this molecule was shown to have growth factor
activity for hemopoietic progenitor cells stimulating
their survival, proliferation and differentiation into
post-mitotic cells of the neutrophil, macrophage and
eosinophil lineages (2). Recently however, it has become
clear that GM-CSF can also affect these differentiated
and post-mitotic cells by stimulating their function (3-
5). This dual role of GM-CSF takes place in a lineage-
specific fashion presumably by interacting with receptors
which neutrophils, macrophages and eosinophils conserve
throughout differentiation. Indeed, specific binding of
GM-CSF has been shown on bone marrow progenitor cells,
hemopoietic cell lines and differentiated granulocytes
(6). It is not known however, what intracellular signals
are triggered following the binding of GM-CSF that lead
to such diverse phenomena as proliferation/differentia-
tion, and functional activation. We show here that rh
GM-CSF induces different intracellular signals in immature and mature myeloid cells suggesting that there may
be differences in their GM-CSF receptors or that these
receptors are coupled to different transducing mechanisms
on myeloid cells at different stages of differentiation.

MATERIALS AND METHODS

Preparation of Myeloid Cells

Mature human neutrophils were obtained from the peripheral blood of normal volunteers after density-gradient centrifugation on Lymphoprep (Nycomed, Oslo, Norway) and hypotonic lysis of erythrocytes. The human promyelocytic cell line HL-60 was used as a model of immature myeloid cells.

rh GM-CSF and other stimuli

rh GM-CSF, a gift from Genetics Institute (Cambridge, MA), was 97.2% pure and had an activity of 4.7 x 10^6 U/mg protein. The tumour-promoter phorbol ester 12-0-tetradecanoyl phorbol-13-acetate (TPA) was obtained from P-L Biochemicals Inc., Milwaukee, Wis. and the bacterial tripeptide formyl-methionyl-leucyl-phenylalanine (FMLP) was purchased from SIGMA.

Protein Kinase-C assay

Neutrophils or HL-60 cells (2ml containing 1.5 x 10^7 cells/ml) were incubated at 37°C for different times with rh GM-CSF and other stimuli. After incubation, the cells were disrupted by sonication as described (7), centrifuged at 100,000g for 30 minutes at 4°C and the pellets resuspended by sonication in 2mls of 20mM Tris-HCl, 2mM EDTA, 5mM EGTA, 0.25M sucrose, 0.01% (w/v) leupeptin, 2mM PMSF, 0.2% (w/v) Triton X-100 and 50mM 2-mercaptoethanol, pH 7.5 at 4°C. After incubation at 2°C for 30 minutes centrifugation was performed as above and the supernatant collected and assayed for protein kinase activity essentially as described (8).

Inositol phosphates assay

Neutrophils or HL-60 cells at 2 x 10^7/ml were incubated overnight in the presence of 10-15uCi/ml myo[^{3}H]-inositol (Amersham, U.K.). After the incubation, the cells were washed 4 times and resuspended to 3 x 10^7/ml in medium containing 10mM Li_2CO_3, pH 7.4 before incubation with stimuli for different times. The reaction was stopped by the addition of ice-cold trichloroacetic acid

(15% w/v) containing 2mM Na_2 EDTA. Samples were stood on
ice for 20 minutes and the precipitated proteins and
lipids were separated by centrifugation. The separation
of water-soluble inositol polyphosphates by anion
exchange chromatography and the extraction of the phosphoinositides were carried out as described (9,10).

Biological assays.

Neutrophils were assayed for their capacity to produce superoxide anion as described (5), and HL-60 cells
for their loss of clonogenicity in response to rh GM-CSF
as described (11).

RESULTS AND DISCUSSION

In the first instance rh GM-CSF was examined for its
capacity to stimulate protein kinase activity in the
membrane fraction of human neutrophils. It is shown in
Table 1 that FMLP and TPA but not rh GM-CSF induced
accumulation of protein kinase activity in the neutrophil
membrane after 30 seconds. No stimulation was observed
over a 30 min period with concentrations of rh GM-CSF
ranging from 1-100ng/ml (data not shown). In parallel
experiments rh GM-CSF did not significantly stimulate the
production of O_2^- by neutrophils directly, however it
enhanced the O_2^- produced after stimulation with 10^{-7}M
FMLP from 15.1 to 27.0 nmoles $O_2^-/10^6$ cells while 10^{-7} M
TPA stimulated O_2^- production to 53.5 nmoles $O_2^-/10^6$
cells.

In contrast to its effect on neutrophils, rh GM-CSF
directly induced the accumulation of protein kinase in
the membrane of the human promyelocytic cell line HL-60
(Table 2). This activity increased rapidly (15-30 sec)
and returned to basal levels after 5 minutes, but was not
as strong and sustained as that induced by TPA. This is
probably due to TPA being less readily broken down than
diacylglycerol. In parallel experiments rh GM-CSF was
also shown to act biologically on HL-60 as it inhibited
their clonogenicity from 28.3 to 16.2 colonies per 10^2
seeded cells after 14 days of incubation.

Table 1 - rh GM-CSF does not Induce Accumulation of Protein Kinase Activity in the Membrane Fraction of Human Neutrophils

Treatment	Phosphate incorporation (pmoles $PO_4^=$/min)	
	$+Ca^{++}$/PS	+EGTA
none	0.072*	0.046
rh GM-CSF (100ng/ml)	0.098	0.050
FMLP (10^{-7} M)	0.146	0.069
TPA (10^{-7} M)	0.291	0.082

* Mean protein kinase specific activity in the presence of Ca^{++} and phosphatidylserine (PS), or EGTA. The incubation time was 30 sec. Values obtained with FMLP and TPA but not rh GM-CSF were significantly ($p < 0.05$) different from "none" control.

From Table 2 and other data it appeared that a Ca/PS dependent protein kinase, probably PK-C, was being stimulated on HL-60 cells by GM-CSF. Thus it was important to examine inositol metabolism, as activation of PK-C by a variety of hormones is preceded by increased metabolism of phosphoinositides, particularly hydrolysis of phosphatidylinositol 4,5-bisphosphate (PIP_2) to yield diacylglycerol and inositol trisphosphate (IP_3).

Table 2 - rh GM-CSF Induces Accumulation of Protein Kinase Activity in the Membrane Fraction of the Human Promyelocytic Cell Line HL-60

Treatment	Phosphate incorporation (pmoles $PO_4^=$/min)	
	$+Ca^{++}$/PS	+EGTA
none	0.451*	0.459
rh GM-CSF (100ng/ml)	0.582	0.518
TPA (10^{-7} M)	1.011	0.642

* Mean protein kinase specific activity. The incubation time was 30 sec. Values obtained with rh GM-CSF and TPA were significantly ($p < 0.05$) different from "none".

Stimulation of human neutrophils with rh GM-CSF did not increase formation of inositol phosphates, however, these could be generated following stimulation with FMLP (Table 3). Incubation of neutrophils with various concentrations of rh GM-CSF over a 30 min period did not increase generation of inositol phosphates. In contrast, rh GM-CSF stimulated inositol phosphate generation in HL-60 cells (Table 4) as did 2% ethanol used as a positive control. In this experiment HL-60 cells responded to rh GM-CSF which inhibited their clonogenicity from 13.1 to 6.2 clones/10^2 seeded cells.

Table 3 - Inositol Phosphate Generation in Neutrophils

Treatment	Lipid	Inositol Phosphates $(dpm/3 \times 10^7$ cells)		
		IP	IP_2	IP_3
none	182,512	5,625	2,317	445
rh GM-CSF (100ng/ml)	170,412	5,038	2,040	357
FMLP (10^{-7} M)	172,879	4,973	5,904	2,252

Incubation was for 30 sec at 37°C. The IP_2 and IP_3 values obtained with FMLP but not with rh GM-CSF were significantly different ($p < 0.01$) from "none" control.

Table 4 - Inositol Phosphate Generation in HL-60 Cells

Treatment	Lipid	Inositol Phosphates $(dpm/3 \times 10^7$ cells)		
		IP	IP_2	IP_3
none	667,977	2,489	4,163	1,235
rh GM-CSF (10ng/ml)	629,376	7,573	5,111	2,261
ethanol (2%)	635,518	7,817	5,903	2,540

Incubation with rh GM-CSF and ethanol was for 30 sec at 37°C. Values obtained with rh GM and ethanol were significantly different ($p < 0.02$) from "none" control.

The inability of rh GM-CSF to stimulate the generation of inositol phosphates and protein kinase on neutrophils is consistent with the lack of direct stimulation of O_2^- production. The production of O_2^- takes place when surface receptors such as for FMLP stimulate certain G proteins, phospholipases, phosphoinositide metabolism, changes in intracellular Ca^{2+} concentrations and protein kinase activity (12). Neutrophils, however, responded to rh GM-CSF by showing enhanced response to FMLP as shown previously (4,5). The exact mechanism of this activation or "priming" by GM-CSF is still unknown although it may involve modulation of surface receptors. For example, GM-CSF has been shown to increase the expression of the C3bi receptor (5), to downregulate the G-CSF receptor (13) and to alter the affinity, but not the number, of the FMLP receptor itself (14).

By contrast, rh GM-CSF stimulated inositol phosphate generation and membrane-associated protein kinase activity in HL-60 cells. These cells have been shown to respond to rh GM-CSF by proliferation followed by differentiation and reduced clonogenicity (11). Stimulation of growth accompanied by activation of these pathways has been shown with other growth factors such as platelet derived growth factor (15); however they may not be a mandatory requirement as the hemopoietic growth factors interleukin-3 and CSF-1 have been shown to stimulate mouse macrophage proliferation without causing inositol phosphate generation (16).

While the results shown here point to different biochemical responses between mature and immature cells a few points of caution should be raised. Firstly, it is possible that some accumulation of protein kinase activity occurs on the neutrophil membrane after rh GM-CSF stimulation which may be small and localised and which cannot be detected in our system. Secondly, in our hands, HL-60 cells have shown substantial variabilty in their response to rh GM-CSF and may not be the ideal model to study immature cell responses. Similar variations have been observed by previous workers in the colony assay (11). Ideally, normal immature myeloid cells purified at different stages of differentiation should be used; however their utilisation is hindered by the relatively large number of cells required for the present methods of assessment.

The difference in intracellular signals generated by GM-CSF on proliferating and non-proliferating cells suggest heterogeneity in the coupling of the receptor, or of the GM-CSF receptor itself. Heterogeneity at the level of receptor coupling has been shown for the M2 muscarinic receptor subtype where agonist stimulation leads to inhibition of adenylyl cyclase and activation of phosphoinositide hydrolysis (17).   Alternatively,the differential response may be due to differences in the GM-CSF receptor itself. In structural studies, specific binding has been demonstrated on immature and mature myeloid cells (6) and there is no evidence so far for GM-CSF receptor subtypes. In addition, the same small region in the aminoterminus of the GM-CSF molecule seems to be necessary for proliferation/differentiation, and activation of myeloid cells (18).

On the other hand, although GM-CSF has been shown to bind to high affinity binding sites on HL-60 cells and neutrophils (6) it appears that there is also a low affinity binding site on HL-60 cells but not on neutrophils (N. Nicola, personal communication). This is consistent with our observation (unpublished) that maximal levels of colony formation are attained with higher concentrations of GM-CSF (100ng/ml) than required for maximal stimulation of neutrophil function (10ng/ml). It could be speculated, therefore, that the binding of GM-CSF to low and high affinity receptors may be triggering different intracellular signals with the low affinity receptor being coupled to inositol metabolism and leading to cell proliferation, and the high affinity receptor coupled to an as yet unidentified signalling mechanism.

While the intracellular mechanisms of GM-CSF stimulation of immature and mature myeloid cells awaits elucidation, this differential signalling may represent an example of a more generalised mode of action of growth factors acting on one cell lineage at different stages of differentiation.

REFERENCES

1. Clarke, S.C. and Kamen, R.   (1987)   Science 236:1229-1237.
2. Metcalf, D.   (1984) Elsevier North/Holland, Amsterdam, The Netherlands.
3. Lopez, A.F., Nicola, N.A., Burgess, A.B., Metcalf, D., Battye, F.L., Sewell, W.A. and Vadas, M.A.   (1983)   J. Immunol. 13:1983-1988.
4. Weisbart, R.H., Golde, D.W., Clark, S.C., Wong, G.G., Gasson, J.C.   (1985)   Nature (Lond) 314:361-363.
5. Lopez, A.F., Williamson, D.J., Gamble, J.R., Begley, C.G., Harlan, J.M., Klebanoff, S.J., Waltersdorph, A., Wong, G., Clark, S.C. and Vadas, M.A.   (1986)   J. Clin. Invest. 78:1220-1228.
6. Gasson, J.C., Kaufman, S.E., Weisbart, R.H., Tamonaga, M. and Golde, D.W.   (1986)   Proc. Natl. Acad. Sci. USA 83:669-673.
7. Tapley, P.M. and Murray, A.W.   (1985)   Eur. J. Biochem. 151:419-423.
8. Roskoski, R. Jr.   (1983)   Method. in Enzym. 99:3-6.
9. Creba, J.A., Downes, C.P., Hawkins, P.T., Brewster, G., Mitchell, R.H. and Kirk, C.J.   (1983)   Biochem. J. 212:733-747.
10. Berridge, M.J., Dawson, R.M.C., Downes, C.P., Heslop, J.P. and Irvine, R.F.   (1983)   Biochem. J. 212:473-482.
11. Begley, C.G., Metcalf, D., Nicola, N. (1987)   Int. J. Cancer 39:99-105.
12. Babior, B.M. (1987) TIBS 12:241-243.
13. Nicola, N.A., Vadas, M.A. and Lopez, A.F.   (1986)   J. Cell. Physiol. 128:501-510.
14. Atkinson, Y., Lopez, A.F., Marasco, W., Lucas, C., Burns, G., Wong, G., Vadas, M.   Submitted for publication.
15. Berridge, M., Heslop, J.P., Irvine, R.F. and Brown, K.D. (1984) Biochem. J. 222:195-201.
16. Whetton, A.D., Monk, P.N., Consalvey, S.D., Downes, C.P.   (1986)   EMBO J 5:3281-3286.
17. Ashkenazi, A., Winslow, J.W., Peralta, E.G., Peterson, G.L., Schimerlik, M.I., Capron, D.J., Ramachandran, J.   (1987)   Science 238:672-675.
18. Clark-Lewis, I., Lopez, A.F., Vadas, M., Schrader, J.W., Kent, S.B.H.   (1987)   Proc. 5th Intern. Lymph. Work. Pierce, C.W. (ed) Human Press, Clifton N.J. (in press).

Monokines and Other Non-Lymphocytic Cytokines, pages 243–248
© 1988 Alan R. Liss, Inc.

STUDIES ON THE NIH 3T3 CELLS SENSITIZED TO TUMOR NECROSIS
FACTOR BY THE EXPRESSION OF ADENOVIRUS E1A ONCOGENE

M.-J. Chen[1], C. Q. Earl[1], B. Holskin[1], M.
Anzano[1], D. Shalloway[2], and J. L. Cook[3]
[1]SmithKline & French Laboratories, King of
Prussia, PA 19406-0939, [2]The Pennsylvania State
University, University Park, PA 16802,
[3]National Jewish Center for Immunology and
Respiratory Medicine, Denver, Colorado 80206

INTRODUCTION

The ability of tumor necrosis factor (TNF) to kill
selectively some tumor cells (Sugarman, 1985) prompted us
to search for a possible correlation between the
expression of specific oncogene(s) and cellular
sensitivity to TNF. Using purified recombinant human TNF-α
and a modified in vitro cytotoxicity assay with NIH 3T3 or
BRK derived cells expressing exogenous oncogenes as the
targets, we found that the expression of adenovirus E1A
oncogene induces cellular cytolytic susceptibility to TNF
(Chen et al. 1987). Several other oncogenes examined were
not effective, including myc and polyoma large T antigen
which share functional similarity with E1A. These E1A
expressing NIH 3T3 cells were also susceptible to
activated macrophage cell-mediated killing. Their degree
of sensitivity to activated macrophages correlated closely
with their degree of sensitivity to TNF. These results
strongly suggest that TNF is a major cytolytic factor of
activated macrophages responsible for the killing of E1A
expressing cells. We also obtained preliminary data
suggesting that TNF susceptible phenotype is associated
with the conversion of a class of higher affinity TNF
receptors on the parental cell into one with lower
affinity on E1A expressing cells. Whether the change we
have observed is due to a modification of the existing TNF
receptor by the induction of a new receptor peptide
similar to the one reported (Creasy et al. 1987) to be
associated with TNF cytolysis susceptibility remains to be
determined.

RESULTS AND DISCUSSION

Using a modified in vitro cytotoxicity assay and purified recombinant TNF-α, we have tested the sensitivity of NIH 3T3 cells, Fisher baby rat kidney (BRK) cells, and several of their oncogene-transfected derivative cells to TNF. Table 1 summarizes our previous finding (Chen et al., 1987).

Table 1. Oncogene Expression and Susceptibility to Cytolysis by TNF

Parental cell line	Oncogenes transfected	Sensitivity
NIH 3T3	none	-
"	v-src	-
"	polyoma middle T	-
"	polyoma large T	-
"	c-src	-
"	c-src + v-myc	-
"	c-src + c-myc	-
"	c-myc	-
"	T24 ras	-
"	c-Ha-ras	-
"	c-src + Ad2/5 E1A	+
NIH 3T3	Ad2/5 E1A (12S + 13S)	+
"	Ad2/5 13S E1A	+
"	Ad2/5 12S E1A	+
"	Ad12 E1A (12S + 13S)	+
Fisher BRK	Ad2 E1A (12S + 13S)	+
"	Ad2 12S E1A	+

Both the 12S and the 13S encoded adenovirus E1A proteins, either in conjunction with c-src or acting alone, can induce TNF cytolytic susceptibility. Table 1 also shows that ras and several other nuclear oncogenes which share some functional similarity with adenovirus E1A, can not sensitize NIH 3T3 cells to TNF. Interestingly, we also find that, although the parental NIH 3T3 cells are not sensitive to TNF, they are sensitive to TNF in the presence of cycloheximide. In addition, the E1A transfected cells are at least ten times more sensitive to cycloheximide (data not shown). It seems that

E1A and cycloheximide have an additive effect and the two might share a common pathway in exerting their effect on TNF susceptibility.

Because activated macrophages also kill E1A expressing cells (Cook et al, 1986, 1987), and TNF-α is produced mainly by monocytes upon activation, it is possible that TNF is a major cytolytic factor responsible for the killing of E1A expressing cells by activated macrophages. We have tested and found a close correlation between the sensitivity of E1A expressing cells to TNF and their sensitivity to activated macrophages. Cell lines more sensitive to TNF are also more sensitive to activated macrophages (Table 2). Presently, antibodies to native TNF are being used to assess the contribution of TNF in the killing of the E1A sensitized cells by activated macrophages.

Table 2. Correlation of Cytolysis Suceptibility of E1A Expressing NIH 3T3 Cells to TNF and Activated Macrophage

Cell Lines [E1A expressed]	TNF sensitivity	aMø sensitivity[§]
NIH 3T3	–	13.5%[*] (1.3%[#])
NIH(pE1Awt/pSV2neo/cos)A [13S+12S]	+++	66.5% (3.0%)
NIH(p13Swt/pSV2neo/cos)A [13S]	+++	66.5% (3.7%)
NIH(p13Swt/pSV2neo/cos)B [13S]	+++	69.6% (3.2%)
NIH(p13Swt/pSV2neo/cos)C [13S]	++	38.5% (2.9%)
NIH(p12Swt/pSV2neo/cos)A [12S]	+	26.8% (3.7%)
NIH(p12Swt/pSV2neo/cos)B [12S]	+++	59.6% (4.9%)
NIH(p12Swt/pSV2neo/cos)C [12S]	+	16.6% (1.9%)

[§] Hamster activated macrophage and cytolysis assays were performed as described (Cook, J. L. et al. 1987). Each value of the mean and the standard deviation was obtained from at least 8 separate experiments.
[*] The mean value.
[#] The standard error of the mean.

In order to determine if TNF receptor is altered by

E1A expression, we performed receptor binding assays on
the parental and the E1A transfected NIH 3T3 cells with
^{125}I labeled TNF. Figure 1A shows the results of a
receptor binding experiment with NIH 3T3 cells, 12S, and
13S E1A gene transfected NIH 3T3 cell lines. The binding
constants were derived from the Scatchard plots shown in
Figure 1B. The extremely sensitive 13S E1A expressing
line, NIH(p13Swt/pSV2neo/cos)A, appears to have a single
class of TNF receptors with a binding affinity constant
(K_d, 1.47 nM) substantially higher than that of the
parental NIH 3T3 cell receptor (K_d, 0.66 nM). The 12S
E1A expressing line, NIH(p12Swt/pSV2neo/cos)A, which is at
least 20 fold less sensitive (data not shown) appears to
have two classes of TNF receptors; one with higher
affinity and one with lower affinity for TNF. Competition
assays using cold ligand also suggested the existence of
two classes of TNF receptors on this cell line (data not
shown).

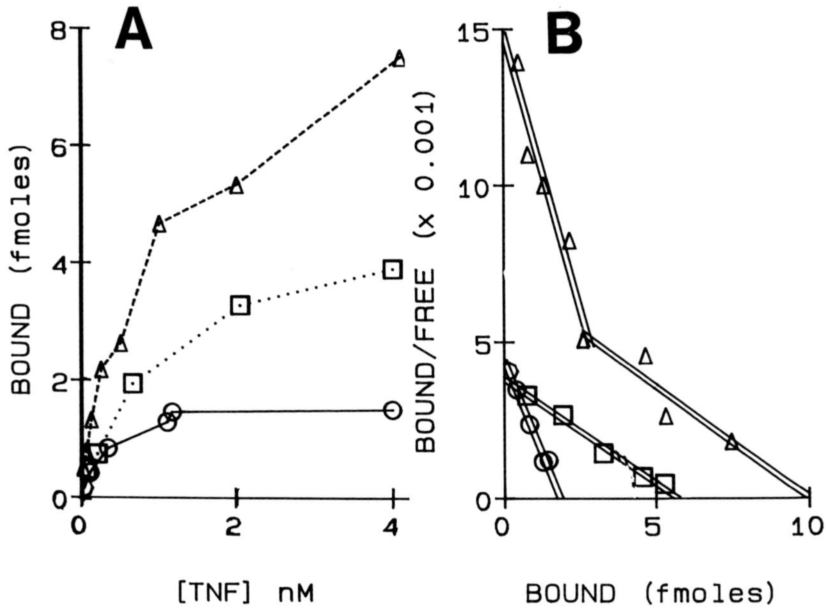

Figure 1. TNF receptor binding assays (1A) and Scatchard

Table 3 summarizes the results of the receptor binding experiments. In addition, it also shows that a small population of resistant L929 cells, L929R, selected from the sensitive parental cells by repeated treatment with TNF, also possesses a class of TNF receptor with lower affinity than those of the sensitive parental L929 cells.

Table 3. Receptor Binding Constants of TNF Resistant and Sensitive Cell Lines

Cell line	K_{d1} (nM)	K_{d2} (nM)	No
TNF sensitive			
L929	1.36 ± 0.15		5
NIH(p13Swt/pSV2neo/cos)A[1]	1.47 ± 0.14		3
NIH(p12Swt/pSV2neo/cos)A[2]	2.58 ± 1.24	0.23 ± 0.05	2
TNF resistant			
L929R[3]	0.88 ± 0.03		3
NIH 3T3	0.66 ± 0.07		3

K_d : Concentration of TNF which gave half maximal binding

No : Number of experiments performed

[1]NIH 3T3 cells expressing the 13S mRNA coded adenovirus E1A protein

[2]NIH 3T3 cells expressing the 12S mRNA coded adenovirus E1A proteins

[3]L929R cells are a resistant population of L929 cells

analysis (1B) of NIH 3T3 and E1A transfected NIH 3T3 cells. o-o (NIH 3T3), Δ-Δ (NIH(p12Swt/pSV2neo/cos)A, ▬ (NIH(p13Swt/pSV2neo/cos)A. TNF was labeled with ^{125}I by the Iodogen method and binding assays were performed in 6-well culture dish with 1×10^6 cells per well. Binding assays were done at 4° for 2 hours.

selected after repeated treatment with TNF.
     Our data on these limited number of cell lines
suggested that a clsss of higher affinity TNF receptors on
the parental NIH 3T3 cells may be converted into a class
of lower affinity receptors associated with TNF cytotoxic
susceptibility. With the 13S E1A expressing cells, the
conversion appears to be complete. In the case of 12S E1A
expressing cells, the conversion appears to be partial,
which might account for their lower sensitivity to TNF.
Receptor binding assays on a larger number of E1A
expressing cells are needed to further substantiate this
preliminary finding. Crosslinking experiments may reveal
change(s) in the TNF receptor peptides induced by the E1A
expression.

REFERENCES

Chen, M.-J., Holskin, B., Strickler, J. et al. (1987)
   Induction by E1A oncogene expression of cellular
   susceptibility to lysis by TNF. Nature 330, 581-583.
Cook, J. L., Walker, T. A., Lewis, A. M. JR., Ruley, H.
   E., Graham, F. L., and Pilder, S. H., (1986) Expression
   of the adenovirus E1A oncogene during cell
   transformation is sufficient to induce susceptibility to
   lysis by host inflammatory cells. Proc. Natl. Acad. Sci.
   83, 6965-6969.
Cook, J. L., May, D. L., Lewis. A. M. JR., and Walker, T.
   A. (1987) Adenovirus E1A gene induction of
   susceptibility to lysis by natural killer cells and
   activated macrophages in infected rodent cells. J.
   Virol. 61, 3510- 3520.
Creasy, A. A., Yamamoto. R., and Vitt, C. R. (1987) A high
   molecular weight component of the human tumor necrosis
   factor receptor is associated with cytotoxicity. Proc.
   Natl. Acad. Sci. USA 84, 3293-3297.
Moran, E., and Mathews, M. B. (1987) Cell 48, 177-178.
Shalloway, D., Johnson, P. J., Freed, E. O., et al. (1987)
   Transformation of NIH 3T3 cells by cotransfection with
   c- src and nuclear oncogenes. Mol. Cell. Biol. 7, 3582-
   3590.
Sugarman B. J. et al. (1985) Recombinant human tumor
   necrosis factor-α : Effects on proliferation of normal
   and transformed cells in vitro. Science 230, 943-945.

Section V. Cytokine Activities and Interactions In Vitro

Monokines and Other Non-Lymphocytic Cytokines, pages 251–260
© 1988 Alan R. Liss, Inc.

BIOLOGICAL ACTIVITIES AND PRODUCTION OF TNF-α

Grace H.W. Wong and David V. Goeddel

Department of Molecular Biology, Genentech,
Inc., 460 Point San Bruno Boulevard, South
San Francisco, California 94080

INTRODUCTION

Tumor necrosis factor alpha (TNF-α) is an important
cytokine released by activated macrophages. In addition
to its known anti-tumor activity, it has pleiotropic
effects on a variety of cell types involved in inflammation, hematopoiesis and immunity. Here we describe some of
the biological properties of TNF-α. We also compare the
regulation of TNF-α mRNA synthesis with regulation of mRNA
synthesis for another cytokine, interleukin-1 (IL-1$_\beta$).

BIOLOGICAL ACTIVITIES OF TNF-α

a) Antiviral activities

In some cells, TNF-α alone is capable of inducing
cellular resistance against infection with RNA and DNA
viruses measured by inhibition of viral replication and
inhibition of cytopathic effects mediated by the virus
(Wong and Goeddel, 1986a; Mestan et al., 1986). In these
cases the antiviral activity of TNF-α is not mediated by
the induction of known interferons (IFNs), because
pretreatment of cells with TNF-α did not produce
detectable levels of IFN-α, -β, or -γ mRNA, and antibodies
against IFN-α, -β, and -γ did not abolish the antiviral
activity of TNF-α (Wong and Goeddel, 1986a).

In most cells tested TNF-α significantly enhances the
antiviral activity of IFN-γ (Wong and Goeddel, 1986a,b;

Goeddel et al., 1986; Wong et al., 1988). In addition to
IFN-γ, TNF-α also enhances the antiviral activity of
IFN-αA and IFN-β (Fig. 1).

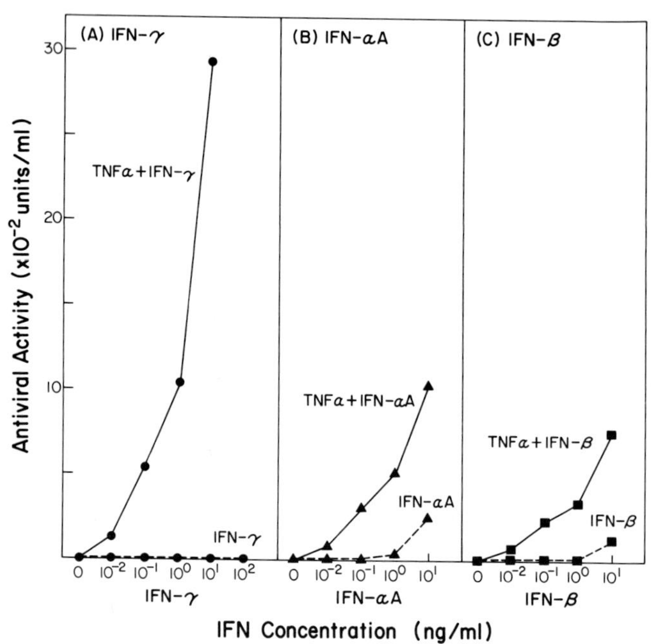

Figure 1. TNF-α enhances the antiviral activity of IFNs.
A549 cells were treated with pure recombinant human IFN-γ
(A), IFN-αA (B) and IFN-β (C) giving the indicated concentrations with or without 0.1 μg/ml TNF. Samples were
then serially diluted 2-fold. After 24 hr, cells were
infected with vesicular stomatitis virus (VSV) at a
multiplicity of infection of 10. After 24 hr the
cytopathic effect was determined by staining the cells
with crystal violet and the titer was quantitatively
monitored using the microelisa autoreader (MR 580,
Dynatech) or visually. The antiviral titer is expressed
as the reciprocal of the dilution inhibiting 50 percent of
the cytopathic effect. At all concentrations tested, no
detectable cytokine-associated cytotoxic activity was
observed on A549 cells in the absence of virus during the
24-48 hr incubation.

The combination of TNF-α and IFN-γ can protect
uninfected HUT 78 and RPMI 1788 cells against HIV
infection, as indicated by the inhibition of production of
HIV mRNA, core protein p21 and infectious HIV (Wong
et al., 1988). Furthermore, TNF-α and IFN-γ can
selectively kill virus-infected cells (Wong and Goeddel,
1986a; Wong et al., 1988). Thus, a major function of
TNF-α may be to synergize with the interferons in
antiviral defense and potentiation of the immune response.

b) <u>Cytotoxic activities of TNF-α</u>

If the cytotoxic activity of TNF-α is mediated by the
generation of reactive oxygen species, addition of
anti-oxidant enzymes might be expected to inhibit TNF-α
mediated killing. Surprisingly, the anti-oxidant enzyme
catalase enhances, rather than inhibits, the cytotoxic
activity of TNF-α (Fig. 2). The effect of the phenolic
anti-oxidant butylated hydroxytoluene (BHT) on TNF-α
killing was also examined. BHT, unlike the anti-oxidant
enzymes, completely blocked TNF-α cytotoxicity in human
cervical carcinoma ME-180 cells (Fig. 2a). When ME-180
cells were exposed to TNF-α, catalase and BHT at the same
time no inhibition was observed (Fig. 2a). Catalase
enhanced TNF-α killing of ME-180 cells more than 20-fold
in the presence or absence of BHT (Fig. 2a). Similar
results were observed when mouse fibrosarcoma L-M cells
were tested (Fig. 2b). However, catalase did not render
fibroblasts susceptible to TNF-α killing. Cell lines
tested included NIH-3T3 (murine fibroblast), NRK (normal
rat kidney), rat-1 (rat fibroblast), Vero (monkey kidney
fibroblast), and primary fibroblast cultures derived from
normal murine lungs or kidneys. Thus the enhancing
cytotoxic effect of TNF-α by catalase appears to be
selective for neoplastic cells.

The synergism between hydrogen peroxide (H_2O_2) and
TNF-α in killing ME-180 and L-M cells (Table I) and the
observed failure of H_2O_2 to inactivate TNF-α in vitro
(data not shown) appear to rule out the possibility that
the catalase acts by stabilizing TNF-α through the
scavenging of H_2O_2. Because both H_2O_2 and
catalase enhance the cytotoxicity of TNF-α, the enhancing
effect of catalase is unlikely to be associated with

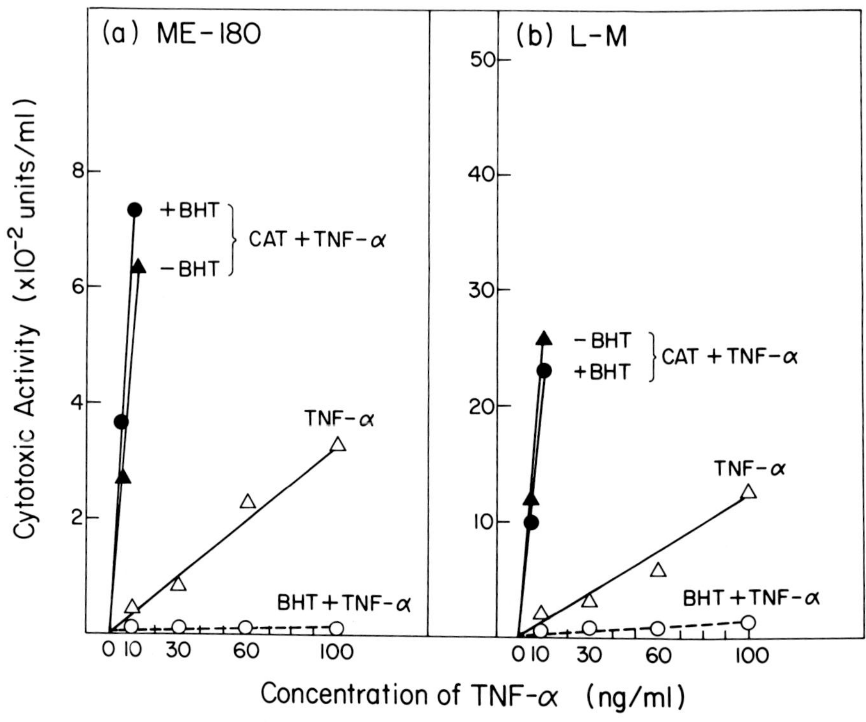

Figure 2. Effect of BHT on the cytotoxic activity of TNF-α in the presence or absence of catalase (CAT). ME-180 (a) or L-M (b) cells (2-3×10^4 cells/well) were incubated with TNF-α (10-100 ng/ml) in the presence or absence of catalase (10 μg/ml, Sigma) or BHT (1 μg/ml, Sigma) alone or in combination. The assay conditions and quantitation of cytotoxic activity were described previously (Kramer and Carver, 1986).

H_2O_2 scavenging activity. It is unclear how catalase specifically potentiates TNF-α cytotoxicity. It will be important to determine the relevance of this _in vitro_ finding to the tumoricidal effect of TNF-α _in vivo._

REGULATION OF CELLULAR GENES BY TNF-α

TNF-α not only enhances the antiviral activity of IFN-γ, it also synergizes with IFN-γ to induce or inhibit

TABLE I. H2O2 Enhances TNF-α Cytotoxicity

	Cell Viability (percent)	
	ME-180	L-M
Control	94	96
H2O2	87	85
TNF-α	51	64
H2O2 + TNF-α	0	0

2×10^5 cells/ml were pretreated with H2O2 (0.003 percent) or TNF-α (0.1 ng/ml) or both for 1 hr, washed and further incubated for 7 hr. Cell viability was determined by trypan blue exclusion.

the expression of many cellular genes. Induced genes include class I and class II MHC (Pujol-Borrell et al., 1987; Wong and Goeddel, 1987), MHC-associated β2-microglobulin (Fig. 3) and 2',5' oligoadenylate synthetase (Wong and Goeddel, 1986a). In some cases, TNF-α alone induces gene expression and synergy with IFN-γ is not observed. Examples are metallothionein-II and the IFN-α inducible 6-16 mRNA (Wong and Goeddel, 1987). In contrast, TNF-α and IFN-γ suppress the levels of c-Ha-ras and transforming growth factor-β (TGF-β) mRNA in ME180 cells (Wong and Goeddel, 1987).

TGF-β was found to inhibit the induction of class II MHC induction by IFN-γ in Hs 294T human melanoma cells (Czarniecki et al., 1987). However, it did not significantly suppress HLA-DR mRNA induced by the combination of TNF-α and IFN-γ in A172 human glioblastoma cells (Fig. 3). TNF-α, IFN-γ or TGF-β alone or in combination had no effect on mRNA level for lipocortin (Fig. 3), which is known to be an endogenous inhibitor of phospholipase A2 inducible by glucocorticoids (Foeller et al., 1986).

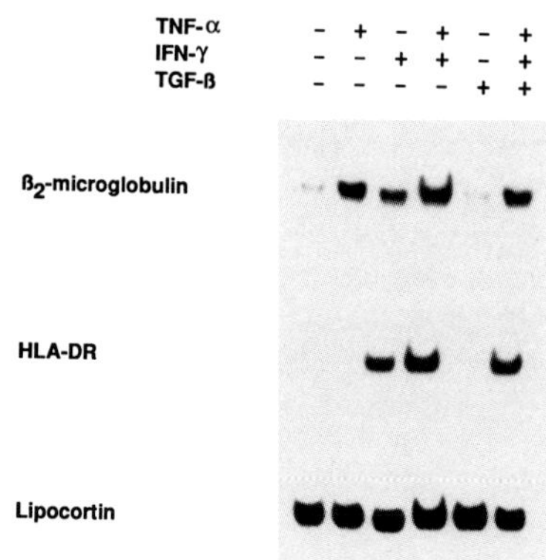

Figure 3.   Regulation of β2-microglobulin, HLA-DR and
lipocortin mRNA by TNF-α, IFN-γ, and/or TGF-ß.   Cytoplasmic
RNA was extracted from confluent A172 human glioblastoma
cells after exposure to TNF-α (1 µg/ml), IFN-γ (1 µg/ml),
TGF-ß (100 ng/ml) alone or in combination for 48 hr.
PolyA[+] RNA (2 µg/lane) was hybridized with synthetic DNA
probes corresponding to the published sequences (Suggs et
al., 1981; Larhammar et al., 1982; Foeller et al., 1986).

REGULATION OF TNF-α SYNTHESIS

    In response to antigens or mitogens, macrophages
produce TNF-α.   The expression of TNF-α mRNA is transient
(Fig. 4).   The level of TNF-α mRNA in the PU5 murine
macrophage cell line is maximal at 2-4 hr after induction
with phorbol myristate acetate (PMA) and drops to basal
level at 24 hr.   Cycloheximide, a protein synthesis
inhibitor, further enhances the accumulation of TNF-α mRNA
(Goeddel et al., 1986).   A combination of PMA and
lipopolysaccharide (LPS) gives stronger induction than
either alone (Goeddel et al., 1986).   Virus infection or
treatment with polyI:polyC can also induce TNF-α mRNA
(Wong and Goeddel, 1986a,b).   Glucocorticoids can inhibit

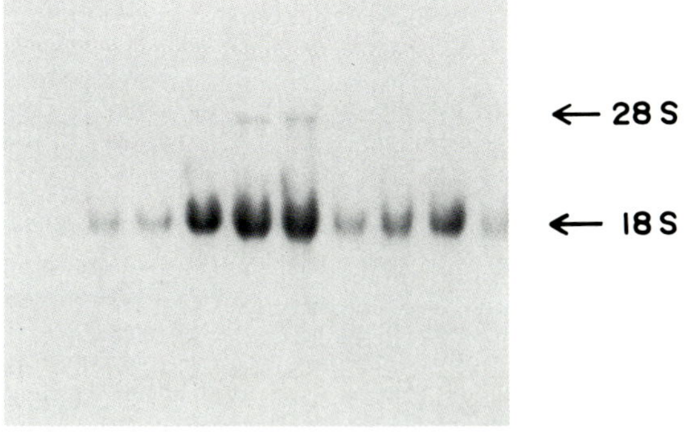

Time after exposure to PMA (hrs)

Figure 4. Transient expression of TNF-α mRNA. The murine
macrophage cell line PU5-1.8 (1×10^6/ml) was treated with
PMA (50 ng/ml) for the times indicated. Three μg of
poly(A)$^+$ RNA was used per lane for hybridization with
^{32}P-labeled TNF-α cDNA insert (Pennica et al., 1984).
The TNF-α hybridizing band migrates at 18S and the arrows
indicate the locations of the 28S and 18S ribosomal RNA.

the induction of TNF-α mRNA (Goeddel et al., 1986). Indomethacin, a cyclooxygenase inhibitor, enhances the
production of TNF-α (Wong and Goeddel, 1987). Prostaglandin E$_2$ (PGE$_2$), but not histamine, inhibit both
TNF-α and IL-1$_\beta$ mRNA induced by a combination of PMA and
LPS (Fig. 6). Interestingly, PGE$_2$ alone induced high
level of IL-1$_\beta$ mRNA PU5 cells (Fig. 5). TGF-β has been
reported to inhibit the production of TNF-α activity in
response to mitogen (Espevik et al., 1987), yet it did not
inhibit the TNF-α mRNA induced by LPS and PMA in the PU5
cells (Fig. 6). Similarly, TGF-β did not suppress the
levels of IL-1$_\beta$ mRNA in the PU5 cells (Fig. 6). Lack of
inhibition was not due to the absence of the TGF-β
receptor on these cells because TGF-β suppressed their
induction of Ia antigens by murine IFN-γ (data not
shown). Thus inhibition of TNF-α by TGF-β is unlikely to
be acting at the transcriptional level.

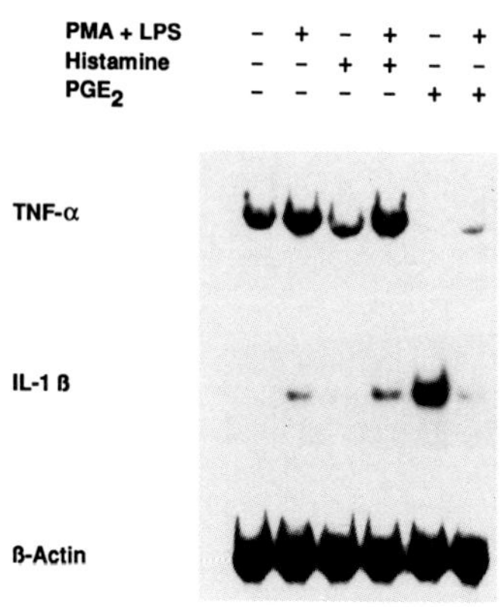

Figure 5. Effect of histamine and PGE2 on induction of TNF-α and IL-1$_\beta$ mRNA by PMA and LPS. PU5-1.8 cells (1x10^6/ml) were treated with PMA (50 ng/ml) and LPS (100 µg/ml) in the presence or absence of histamine (10 µg/ml, Sigma) or PGE2 (50 ng/ml, Sigma) for 4 hr before RNA extraction. Four µg of poly(A)$^+$ RNA per lane was hybridized to murine TNF-α (Pennica et al., 1985), murine IL-1$_\beta$ (Gray et al., 1986) or β-actin (Ponte et al., 1984) probes.

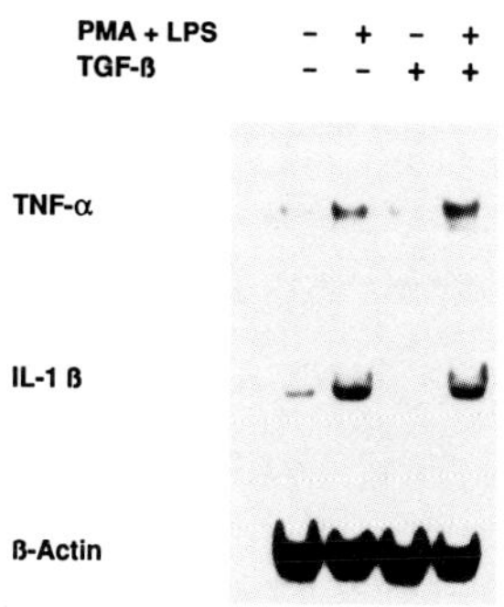

Figure 6. TGF-β does not inhibit induction of TNF-α and IL-1$_\beta$ mRNA by PMA and LPS. PU5-1.8 cells were exposed to PMA and LPS with or without TGF-β (100 ng/ml) for 3 hr. Four µg per lane of poly(A)$^+$ RNA was hybridized to TNF-α, IL-1$_\beta$ or β-actin probes.

PRODUCTION OF TNF-α AND IL-1$_\beta$ mRNA BY MAST CELLS

Activated macrophages are not the only cellular sources of TNF-α. Mast cells are also capable of producing TNF-α in response to mitogenic stimulation.

Like macrophages, the production of TNF-α mRNA is transient, peaks at 2 hr and drops to undetectable levels at 24 hr (data not shown). Likewise, there is a transient peak of IL-1$_\beta$ mRNA in stimulated mast cells. It will be of interest to examine whether the regulation of these cytokines is coordinately controlled. Neither TGF-β nor histamine inhibits the production of TNF-α or IL-1$_\beta$ in PU5 macrophages. We wondered whether these mediators affect the production of TNF-α or IL-1$_\beta$ in mast cells. In mast cells the production of TNF-α or IL-1$_\beta$ induced by PMA and LPS is not affected by TGF-β or histamine. Both histamine and PGE2 are products of mast cells; however, PGE2 but not histamine feedback down-regulates the production of TNF-α.

Substance P (SP) has been reported to induce TNF-α and IL-1 production in macrophages (Cozens and Rowe, 1987). We tested whether SP can induce mRNA production of these cytokines in mast cells. SP was found to increase the levels of both TNF-α and IL-1$_\beta$ mRNA in mast cells. Thus SP, which is present in high levels in diseases such as asthma and arthritis, may mediate some of its inflammatory effects by inducing local production of these cytokines.

Virus infection has been shown to induce TNF-α production in macrophages (Wong and Goeddel, 1986a,b; Aderka et al., 1985). Infection of mast cells with viable but not heat-killed virus caused production of both TNF-α and IL-1$_\beta$ mRNA (unpublished). Thus virus infection not only triggers the production of IFNs but also the production of TNF-α, IL-1$_\beta$ and possibly other cytokines.

CONCLUSIONS

Cellular production of TNF-α is not constitutive, but is tightly regulated. TNF-α production can be induced by mitogens or pathogens. TNF-α potentiates the MHC-inducing and antiviral activities of IFN-γ. Thus TNF-α actively participates in the initiation, regulation and expression of the immune response. TNF-α can induce and suppress many cellular genes. It is not clear whether changes in the expression of these genes is the direct cause or a consequence of TNF-α action. It remains to be seen how many other as yet unknown genes are regulated by TNF-α.

Cloning and characterization of genes regulated by TNF-α
will provide insight into the mechanism of action of TNF-α
and its synergism with other cytokines.

ACKNOWLEDGMENTS

We thank the Process Development and Manufacturing
Group at Genentech for producing purified recombinant
human TNF-α, IFN-γ, and TGF-β, and Jeanne Arch for typing
the manuscript.

REFERENCES

Aderka D et al. (1985). Cell Immunol 92:218-225.
Cozens PJ, Rowe PM (1987). Immunobiol 175:7.
Czarniecki C et al. (1987). Interferon Res 7:699
   (abstract).
Espevik T et al. (1987). J Exp Med 166:571-576.
Foeller C et al. (1986). Nature 320:77-81.
Goeddel DV et al. (1986). In Cold Spring Harbor Symposia
   on Quantitative Biology 51:597-609.
Gray P et al. (1986). J Immunol 137:3644-3648.
Kramer SM, Carver, ME (1986). J Immunologic Methods
   93:201-206.
Larhammar D et al. (1982). Proc Natl Acad Sci USA
   79:3687-3691.
Mestan J (1986). Nature 323:816-819.
Muesing MA et al. (1985). Nature 313:450-458.
Pennica D et al. (1984). Nature 312:724-729.
Pennica D et al. (1985). Proc Natl Acad Sci USA
   82:6060-6064.
Ponte P et al. (1984). Nucl Acids Res 12:1687-1695.
Pujol-Borrell R et al. (1987). Nature 326:304-306.
Suggs SV et al. (1981). Proc Natl Acad Sci USA
   78:6613-6617.
Wong GHW, Goeddel DV (1986a). Nature 323:819-822.
Wong GHW, Goeddel DV (1986b). In "The Biology of the
   Interferon System," Boston: Martinez-Nijhoff, pp
   273-277.
Wong GHW, Goeddel DV (1987). In Mani JC (ed):
   "Proceedings of the 18th International Conference on
   Leucocyte Culture," Palais des Congres La Grande Motte,
   in press.
Wong GHW et al. (1988). J Immunol, in press.

Monokines and Other Non-Lymphocytic Cytokines, pages 261–266

ACTIONS OF IL-1 AND TNF ON HUMAN OSTEOBLAST-LIKE CELLS : SIMILARITIES AND SYNERGISM

Maxine Gowen

Department of Human Metabolism and Clinical Biochemistry, University of Sheffield Medical School, Beech Hill Road, Sheffield S10 2RX, UK

INTRODUCTION

It is now widely accepted that cytokines have a role in the local regulation of bone turnover. Many factors including IL-1, TNF, TGF beta and PDGF have been shown to have effects on various bone cell types in vitro. We have demonstrated that IL-1 is a potent stimulator of bone resorption (Gowen et al, 1983), osteoblast proliferation (Gowen et al, 1985), and the production of prostaglandins by human osteoblast-like cells (Gowen et al, 1984). Others have shown that TNF is also a stimulator of bone resorption (Bertolini et al, 1986). We have also demonstrated effects of IL-1 (Beresford et al, 1984) and TNF (Smith et al, 1987) on the synthesis of bone matrix proteins.

IL-1 and TNF share many of their activities on a variety of cell targets (Nathan, 1987) and this would also seem to be the case in bone. We have now directly compared the actions of recombinant human IL-1 alpha and recombinant human TNF alpha on human trabecular bone cells in vitro. In addition we have demonstrated a marked synergism between these factors when used in combination.

METHODS

Materials

Recombinant human IL-1 alpha (specific activity 2 x 10^7 U/ml) was kindly donated by Dr. P.T. Lomedico, Hoffman

La Roche, NJ, and recombinant human TNF alpha (specific
activity 6 x 10^7U/ml) was a generous gift of Dr. G.R.
Adolf, Boehringer Ingelheim, Vienna. All tissue culture
materials were obtained from Gibco Europe, Paisley,
Scotland.

Cell culture

     Human bone cells were obtained by outgrowth from
fragments of trabecular bone cultured as described
previously (Gowen et al, 1985). These cells exhibit all
osteoblastic characteristics demonstrable in vitro
(Beresford et al, 1983; Beresford et al, 1986; MacDonald
et al, 1986). After reaching confluence they were passaged
once into multiwells for experimental use.

Cell proliferation

     Cells were seeded at a density of 10^4 per cm^2 and
cultured in Eagles Minimal Essential Medium (MEM) with 3%
heat-inactivated fetal calf serum (FCS). After 48 hours the
cells were washed once with serum-free MEM and fresh medium
was added containing 1 uM indomethacin and cytokines as
shown. After 66 hours 1 uCi of $[^3H]$-thymidine was added
to each well and the incubation was continued for a further
six hours. Cell layers were washed thoroughly with
phosphate buffered saline and the cold TCA-insoluble
material was prepared for liquid scintillation counting.

Prostaglandin production

     Cells were cultured as described above with the
indomethacin omitted from the medium. Culture medium was
harvested and assayed immediately for prostaglandin (PG)
content using a commercially available antiserum (Steranti
Research, UK), specific for PGE_2 (100%) with cross-
reactivity with PGE_1 (50%) and negligible cross-reactivity
with other prostanoids.

RESULTS

     In a direct comparison of the effects of IL-1 and TNF
on human osteoblast-like cells, IL-1 was seen to be both
more potent and more powerful at eliciting a response.
Figure 1 shows that IL-1 had an ID_{50} of 0.1-1pM, whereas
the ID_{50} was not reached even when TNF at 1 nM was used.

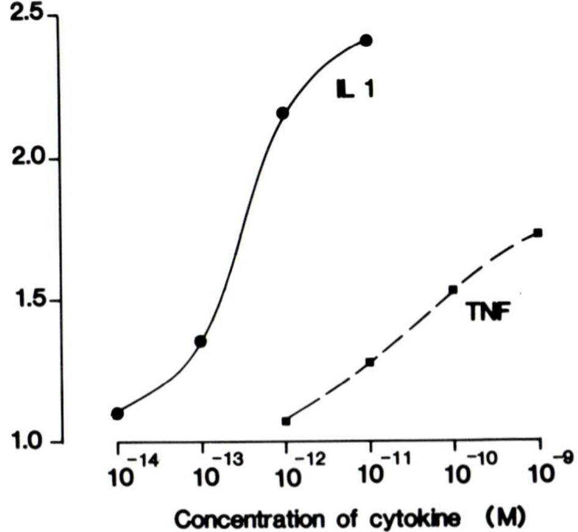

Figure 1.   Stimulation of the proliferation of human bone
cells by IL 1 and TNF.

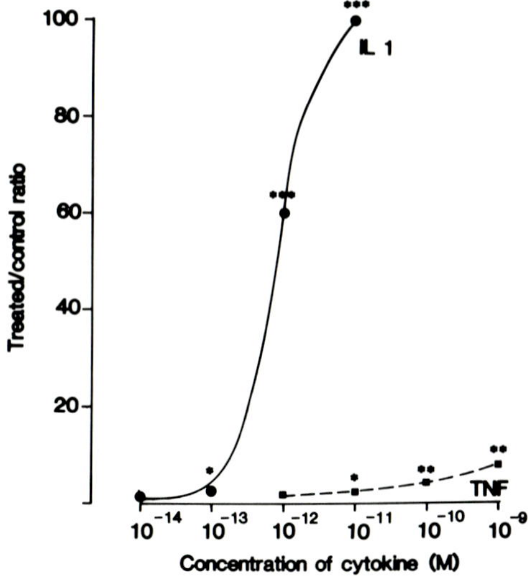

Figure 2.   Stimulation by IL 1 and TNF of the production of
prostaglandins by human bone cells.

Similarly, IL-1 was much more effective at stimulating the
production of prostaglandins than was TNF (Figure 2). We
have demonstrated previously that both TNF and IL-1 inhibit
the production of the osteoblast markers osteocalcin and
alkaline phosphatase (Beresford et al 1984; Gowen et al -
manuscript submitted). Table 1 summarises all of these
actions and shows that in all cases, IL-1 is a more potent
agent than TNF.

TABLE 1.   Actions of IL-1 and TNF on human osteoblasts

	Minimum active concentration (M)	
	IL-1	TNF
Increases proliferation	10^{-12}	10^{-10}
Increases PGE production	10^{-13}	10^{-12}
Decreases osteocalcin	10^{-11}	10^{-9}
Decreases alkaline phosphatase	10^{-11}	10^{-9}

When added to bone cells in combination TNF and IL-1
exhibited a marked synergism both in stimulating cell
proliferation (Table 2) and prostaglandin production (Table
3). Extremely low concentrations of cytokines, eg 10^{-14}M
IL-1 plus 10^{-11}M TNF, were effective in markedly
stimulating the osteoblast-like cells.

TABLE 2.   Actions of IL-1 and TNF in combination on
            osteoblast proliferation.

(nM)		cpm $[^{3}H]$-thymidine incorporation
IL-1	TNF	(control incorporation subtracted)
0.01	–	370
–	1	255
0.01	1	876
–	10	1114
0.01	10	2816
–	100	2074
0.01	100	6651

DISCUSSION

The IL-1 and TNF molecules appear to be members of a
family of factors with an extraordinary range of activities.

TABLE 3. Effects of IL-1 and TNF in combination on
osteoblast prostaglandin production.

(nM)		PGE (pg/100 ul)	
IL-1	TNF	mean $\pm$ SE	
0.01	–	< 5	
0.1	–	12	6
–	1	< 5	
–	10	< 5	
–	100	12	1
0.01	1	< 5	
0.01	10	20	4
0.01	100	2200	60
0.1	1	< 5	
0.1	10	16	2
0.1	100	513	145

Their molecular dissimilarity to one another is puzzling and
they certainly appear to act via separate specific
receptors. Their overlapping actions extend to those in
connective tissue cells, and while these appear to be
identical, IL-1 is consistently a great deal more potent,
and usually stimulates a response of greater magnitude than
TNF. It is possible that this difference in potency is a
guide to the relative importance of the two cytokines
in modulating bone cell function. However, it is important
to bear in mind the relative amounts of the factors produced
in a local microenvironment, and a direct comparison has yet
to be made.

Local production of IL-1 and TNF in bone is another
important aspect of this work. It is likely that the two
cytokines would be produced in concert and the results
presented here show that this can dramatically alter the
sensitivity of the cells to the factors. We have
demonstrated the production of TNF and IL-1 by human
osteoblast-like cells, at concentrations of 10^{-10}M and
10^{-13}M respectively (M. Gowen, D. Hughes – unpublished
observations). This suggests that the cytokines may play a
role in the physiological remodelling of bone.

Bone remodelling consists of a complex series of
cellular events occurring in a tightly controlled sequence,
both temporally and spatially. Locally produced
intercellular factors acting in a paracrine and/or

autocrine manner are likely to be important in this control.
Two such factors are IL-1 and TNF, which have now been shown
to have actions on bone resorbing and bone forming cells at
a very low concentration, and to be produced by bone cells
themselves.

REFERENCES

Baron R, Vignery A, Horowitz M (1983). Lymphocytes,
  monocytes and bone remodelling. Peck WA (ed). Bone and
  Mineral Metabolism, Vol. 2.
Beresford JN, Gallagher JA, Poser JW, Russell RGG (1983).
  Production of osteocalcin by human bone cells in vitro.
  Metab Bone Dis & Rel Res 229-234.
Beresford JN, Gallagher JA, Gowen M, Poser, JW, Wood DD,
  Russell, RGG (1984). The effects of monocyte-conditioned
  medium and interleukin-1 on the synthesis of non-
  collagenous proteins by mouse bone and human bone cells in
  vitro. Biochem Biophys Acta 801: 58-65.
Beresford JN, Gallagher JA, Russell RGG (1986). 1,25-
  dihydroxyvitamin D$_3$ and human bone-derived cells in
  vitro : effects on alkaline phosphatase, type I collagen
  synthesis and proliferation. Endocrinol 119: 1776-1785.
Bertolini BR, Nedwin GE, Bringman TS, Smith DD, Mundy GR
  (1986). Stimulation of bone resorption and inhibition of
  bone formation in vitro by human tumor necrosis factors.
  Nature 319: 516-521.
Gowen M, Wood DD, Ihrie EJ, McGuire MKB, Russell, RGG
  (1983). An interleukin-1 like factor stimulates bone
  resorption in vitro. Nature 306: 378-380.
Gowen M, Wood DD, Ihrie EJ, Russell RGG (1984). Stimulation
  by human interleukin-1 of cartilage breakdown and
  production of collagenase by human chondrocytes but not by
  human osteoblasts in vitro. Biochim Biophys Acta 797:186.
Gowen M, Wood DD, Russell RGG (1985). Stimulation of the
  proliferation of human bone cells in vitro by human
  monocyte products with interleukin-1 activity. J Clin
  Invest 5: 1223-1239.
MacDonald BR, Gallagher, JA, Russell RGG (1986).
  Parathyroid hormone stimulates DNA synthesis by cells
  derived from human bone. Endocrinol 118: 2445-2449.
Nathan CS, (1987). Secretory products of macrophages. J
  Clin Invest 79: 319-326.
Smith DD, Gowen M, Mundy GR (1987). Effects of interferon
  gamma and other cytokines on collagen synthesis in fetal
  rat bone cultures. Endocrinol 120: 2494-2499.

Monokines and Other Non-Lymphocytic Cytokines, pages 267–272

INHIBITED STEROID INDUCTION OF PEPCK IN HEPATOMA CELLS
TREATED WITH HurIL-1 AND HurTNF

R.E. McCallum, M.R. Hill and R.D. Stith

Departments of Microbiology and Immunology
(R.E.M., M.R.H.), and Physiology and Biophysics
(R.D.S.), University of Oklahoma Health Sciences
Center, Oklahoma City, OK 73190

INTRODUCTION

Monocytic cells respond during acute infection and
inflammation with the release of immunoregulatory
monokines, including interleukin-1 (IL-1) and tumor
necrosis factor/cachectin (TNF) (Dinarello and Mier,
1987). TNF plays a pivotal role in the pathophysiology
of endotoxin shock (Bauss et al., 1987; Beutler and
Cerami, 1987) and we have shown that, during endotoxin
shock in mice, IL-1 down regulates hepatic glucocorticoid
receptors, correlating with impaired hormonal induction
of the rate-limiting gluconeogenic enzyme, phosphoenolpyruvate carboxykinase (PEPCK) (Hill et al., 1986; Hill
et al., 1987; Stith and McCallum, 1983).

Over a decade ago "tumor-necrosis serum", elicited
in BCG-infected mice challenged with endotoxin, was shown
to contain a factor(s) which partially blocked the
steroid induction of PEPCK in hepatoma cells. This
inhibitor, glucocorticoid antagonizing factor (GAF), was
partially characterized by Berry et al. (1980) and was
also produced by macrophages incubated in vitro with
endotoxin. The purpose of this study was to utilize
recombinant IL-1 and TNF in rat hepatoma cells to
determine if immunomodulatory hormones (monokines)
interact with conventional hormonal inducers of enzyme
synthesis. We present evidence that IL-1 and TNF act
synergistically to block both dexamethasone and cAMP
induction of PEPCK in hepatoma cells. This effect most
likely occurs at the transcriptional level.

MATERIALS AND METHODS

Human recombinant IL-1α (Lot. SM-46, specific
activity = 1 x 10^7 LAF U/mg) was kindly provided by Dr.
P.T. Lomedico (Hoffmann-La Roche, Nutley, NJ). Human
recombinant TNFα (Lot. 3056-55, specific activity = 5.02
x 10^7 U/mg) was kindly provided by Dr. H.M. Shepard
(Genentech, South San Francisco, CA). Both of these
preparations contained ≤ 0.125 endotoxin units/ml (LAL
assay).

Reuber H35 (HII4E) rat hepatoma cells were cultured
in Iscove's medium containing 10% fetal bovine serum and
gentamicin (50 μg/ml) at 37°C in a humidified 5% CO_2
incubator. Serum was removed from the medium 24 hr
before the cells were used. Four hr after the
simultaneous addition of hormonal inducers and monokines
cells were harvested, homogenized, and centrifuged at
435,000 x g for 10 min at 4°C. The cytosol fraction was
assayed radiometrically for phosphoenolpyruvate
carboxykinase (PEPCK) activity by the incorporation of
$^{14}CO_2$ into oxalacetate, as described previously (Hill et
al., 1987). Units of activity are expressed as nmol of
oxalacetate formed per 15 min per mg cytosol protein.

RESULTS AND DISCUSSION

The activity of PEPCK in the H4IIE rat hepatoma cell
line was measured four hr after addition of inducers.
The optimal concentration of dexamethasone was 2 μM,
increasing PEPCK activity from 293 ± 19 units to 495 ± 41
units. The optimal concentration of db-cAMP was 0.5 mM,
causing 76.5% enzyme induction. Theophylline (0.1 mM)
was added to inhibit phosphodiesterase activity when
db-cAMP was employed.

Treatment of hepatoma cells with HurIL-1 or HurTNF
for 4 hr inhibited the hormonal induction of PEPCK to
less than one-half the activity measured in control cells
(TABLE 1.). The dose response was very narrow, however,
with 9 units/ml (≈5 x 10^{-11} M) of HurIL-1 and 7,530 and
753 units/ml (≈9 x 10^{-9} and 9 x 10^{-10} M) of HurTNF the
only doses causing a significant inhibition of the
hormonal induction of PEPCK. This narrow window has been
observed with some of the immune effects of monokines.

TABLE 1. Effect of HurIL-1 and HurTNF on Induction of
PEPCK by Dexamethasone and db-cAMP in Rat Hepatoma Cells

Treatment (dose)	PEPCK Activity (units/mg)	% Induction
Uninduced control	187 ± 11^{a}	0
Induced control[b]	333 ± 13	78.1
HurIL-1 (units/ml)		
900	317 ± 14	69.5
90	328 ± 71	75.4
9	257 ± 10^{c}	37.4^{c}
0.9	302 ± 15	61.5
HurTNF (units/ml)		
75,300	319 ± 11	70.6
7,530	269 ± 12^{c}	43.9^{c}
753	264 ± 15^{c}	41.2^{c}
75.3	341 ± 14	82.4

[a] Mean ± SEM, obtained from 6-8 determinations.

[b] Inducers added simultaneously with IL-1 or TNF (2 μM
dexamethasone, 0.5 mM db-cAMP, and 0.1 mM theophylline.

[c] Significantly different from induced control (P≤0.05),
determined by Student's t-test.

The combination of HurIL-1 (9 units/ml) + HurTNF
(753 units/ml) caused a greater inhibition of induction
than either of the monokines alone (P≤0.05)(FIGURE 1.).
The induced control cells exhibited approx. 112 units
above basal activity, whereas, the combined monokine
treatment reduced PEPCK activity to 8 units below basal
activity. HurIL-1 or HurTNF had no effect on the basal
(uninduced) activity of PEPCK. The effects of monokine
treatment on PEPCK activity, therefore, represent
inhibited induction, rather than accelerated degradation.

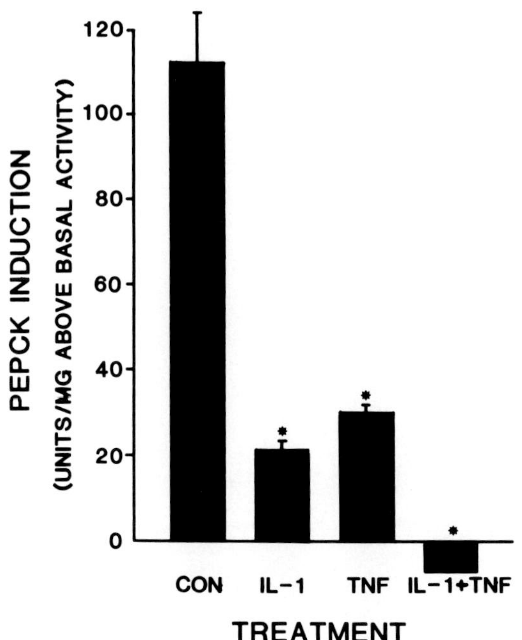

FIGURE 1. Effect of HurIL-1 (9 units/ml), HurTNF (753 units/ml), on Hormonal Induction of PEPCK in Rat Hepatoma Cells. *Significantly less than control value (P≤0.05).

Additional experiments were performed in which the monokines were reduced 10-fold to concentrations (HurIL-1, 5 x 10^{-12} M; HurTNF, 9 x 10^{-11} M) at which no effect on PEPCK induction was observed when the monokines were added alone (TABLE 1.). HurIL-1 and HurTNF, in combination, however, significantly reduced both dexamethasone induction and db-cAMP induction of PEPCK (FIGURE 2A. and FIGURE 2B.).

The results indicate that HurIL-1 and HurTNF inhibit the hormonal induction of PEPCK, a key hepatic gluconeogenic enzyme. Furthermore, the monokines act synergistically to reduce dexamethasone and cAMP induction of enzyme activity. Recent data show that IL-1 and TNF act synergistically in a variety of biological responses, including tumor necrosis, the local Shwartzman reaction, hypotension, inflammatory reactions, and bone resorption (Dinarello and Mier, 1987; Ruggiero and Baglioni, 1987; Stashenko et al., 1987).

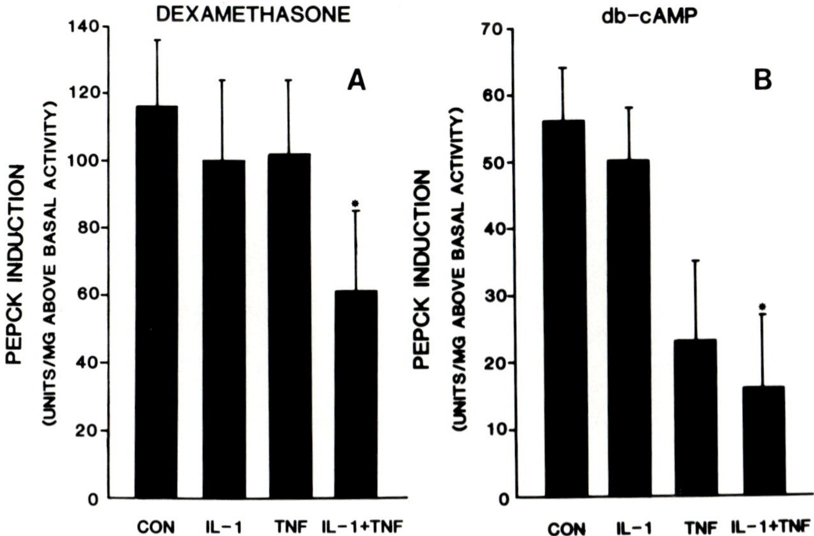

FIGURE 2. Synergistic Inhibition of Dexamethasone (A) and db-cAMP (B) Induction of PEPCK in Rat Hepatoma Cells Treated with HurIL-1 (0.9 units/ml) and HurTNF (75.3 units/ml). *Significantly less than control value (P≤0.05).

The hormonal regulation of hepatic PEPCK gene expression occurs at the transcriptional level and is exceedingly complex (Granner et al., 1986; Wynshaw-Boris et al., 1986). Our results suggest that IL-1 and TNF act at the molecular level to down regulate gene expression of enzyme proteins essential for host survival following shock and trauma. TNF/cachectin has been shown to alter gene expression of several adipocyte proteins (Torti et al., 1985; Beutler and Cerami, 1987), and IL-1 appears to suppress lipoprotein lipase synthesis in adipocytes by affecting gene expression (Price et al., 1986). Studies using molecular probes are currently underway in our laboratory to elucidate the mechanism of IL-1/TNF impaired gene expression of PEPCK.

ACKNOWLEDGMENTS

This study was supported by NIH grants AI20322 and DK37428. The excellent technical assistance of David McDonald is gratefully acknowledged.

REFERENCES

Bauss F, Dröge W, Männel (1987). Tumor necrosis factor
  mediates endotoxic effects in mice. Infect Immunity
  55:1622-1625.
Berry LJ, Goodrum KJ, Ford CW, Resnick G, Shackleford GM
  (1980). Partial characterization of glucocorticoid
  antagonizing factor in hepatoma cells. In Schlessinger
  D (ed): "Microbiology-1980", Washington, DC: American
  Society for Microbiology, pp 77-81.
Beutler B, Cerami A (1987). The endogenous mediator of
  endotoxic shock. Clin Res 35:192-197.
Dinarello CA, Mier JW (1987). Lymphokines. New Eng J
  Med 317:940-945.
Granner DK, Sasaki K, Andreone T, Beale E (1986).
  Insulin regulates expression of the phosphoenolpyruvate
  carboxykinase gene. Recent Prog Horm Res 42:111-141.
Hill MR, Stith RD, McCallum RE (1986). Interleukin 1: A
  regulatory role in glucocorticoid-regulated hepatic
  metabolism. J Immunol 137:858-862.
Hill MR, Stith RD, McCallum RE (1987). Monokines mediate
  decreased hepatic glucocorticoid binding in endotoxemia.
  J Leukocyte Biol 41:236-241.
Price SR, Mizel SB, Pekala PH (1986). Regulation of
  lipoprotein lipase synthesis and 3T3-L1 adipocyte
  metabolism by recombinant interleukin 1. Biochim
  Biophys Acta 889:374-381.
Ruggiero V, Baglioni C (1987). Synergistic
  anti-proliferative activity of interleukin 1 and tumor
  necrosis factor. J Immunol 138:661-663.
Stashenko P, Dewhirst FE, Peros WJ, Kent RL, Ago JM
  (1987). Synergistic interactions between interleukin
  1, tumor necrosis factor, and lymphotoxin in bone
  resorption. J Immunol 138:1464-1468.
Stith RD, McCallum RE (1983). Down regulation of hepatic
  glucocorticoid receptors after endotoxin treatment.
  Infect Immunity 40:613-621.
Torti FM, Deickmann B, Beutler B, Cerami A, Ringold GM
  (1985). A macrophage factor inhibits adipocyte gene
  expression: An in vitro model of cachexia. Sci
  229:867-869.
Wynshaw-Boris A, Short JM, Loose DS, Hanson RW (1986).
  Characterization of the phosphoenolpyruvate
  carboxykinase (GTP) promoter-regulatory region. I
  Multiple hormone regulatory elements and the effects of
  enhancers. J Biol Chem 261:9714-9720.

Monokines and Other Non-Lymphocytic Cytokines, pages 273–279
© 1988 Alan R. Liss, Inc.

INDUCTION OF IL-2 RECEPTOR EXPRESSION BY INTERLEUKIN-1 AND TUMOR NECROSIS FACTOR ON YT CELLS

J.C. Lee, A. Truneh, M.F. Smith, M.-J. Chen and
K.Y. Tsang
Depts. of Immunology (J.C.L., A.T.) and Molecular
Genetics (M.-J.C.), Smith Kline & French
Laboratories, Philadelphia, PA 19101; Temple
University Medical School (M.F.S.), Philadelphia,
PA 19140; and Medical University of South
Carolina (K.Y.T.), Charleston, SC 29425

ABSTRACT

Tumor necrosis factor (TNF-α) and interleukin-1
(IL-1) share between them many biological properties in
their effects on different cell types. It has not been
firmly established whether TNF has an effect on lymphoid
cells. Therefore, the effect of human recombinant TNF-α
and IL-1ß on interleukin-2 receptor (IL2R) expression on a
human leukemia cell line (YT) was examined. IL2R
expression was assessed by flow cytometric analysis using
a monoclonal antibody to IL2R (anti-TAC). TNF-α, like
IL-1ß, induced increased levels of IL2R expression on YT
cells with similar kinetics of induction. Maximum
induction occurred at 20 to 30 hours. RNA isolated from
TNF-α or IL-1ß treated YT cells contained increased
levels of IL2R specific mRNA by Northern blot analysis
using an IL2R specific cDNA probe. Kinetic and IL-1ß mRNA
expression studies indicated that the TNF effect was
direct. None of the three classes of interferon, alone or
in the presence of TNF-α, appreciably induced IL2R. The
effect of combined treatments with IL-1 and TNF-α was
additive while IL-2 and TNF-α had synergistic effects.
Since IL2R expression is known to be associated with
lymphocyte activation, the present results suggest that
TNF-α may play a role in the regulation of immune
responses, at least at the level of IL2R induction.

INTRODUCTION

Interleukin 2 (IL-2) is a T cell product which
regulates the growth and function of T cells as well as
non-T cells (i.e., B cells and NK cells) (Cantrell and
Smith, 1984). Cellular proliferation and other
physiologic responses result from the interaction of this
molecule with its specific, high affinity cell surface
receptors (Robb et al., 1984). The cell surface receptor
for IL-2 was initially identified by the monoclonal
antibody anti-TAC (Uchiyama et al., 1984) as a 55,000
dalton glycoprotein with two external domains, a short
transmembrane and an intracytoplasmic segment (Leonard et
al., 1983). Interleukin-1, a macrophage product is
thought to to play a major role in the direct activation
of T cells through the induction of IL-2 secretion and
IL-2R expression (Lowenthal et al., 1986). Despite its
similarity to IL-1 in terms of its biological activity
profile as a proinflammatory molecule (Dinarello, 1984),
TNF has not been demonstrated to have any effect on T or B
lymphocytes. We now present evidence that recombinant
human TNF-α enhances IL2R expression on a lymphoblastic
null-cell leukemia cell in a fashion similar to that of
IL-1.

RESULTS AND DISCUSSION

The human leukemia cell line, YT has been well
characterized as an NK-like cell (Yodoi et al., 1985). We
examined the comparative effects of TNF, IL-1, IL-2 and
the three types of interferon to induce IL2R expression on
YT cells. Human recombinant IL-1ß was a potent inducer of
IL2R expression. Recombinant IL-2, however, was only
weakly active and the interferons were inactive. Human
recombinant TNF-α, was also a potent inducer of IL2R
expression, an observation not previously reported. The
kinetics of IL2R expression induced by TNF and IL-1 were
also examined (Figure 2). Maximum expression of IL2R was
observed at 20 to 30 hours and declined with time. In
contrast, the expression of IL2R induced by IL-2 did not
reach a maximum level until 48 hours. Except for the
difference in the level of IL2R expression, there was no
discernible difference in the kinetics between IL-1ß and
TNF-α.

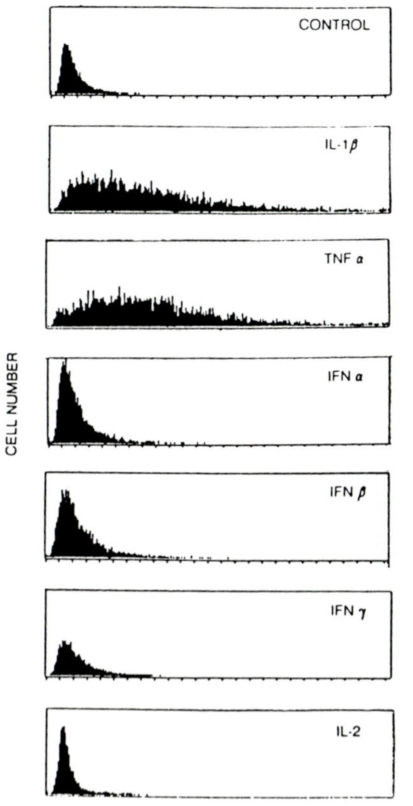

Figure 1. FACS analysis of IL2R expression in YT cells. 100 units of the respective test cytokines were added to 10^5 YT cells for 20 hr. The cells were incubated with FITC conjugated anti-IL2R monoclonal antibody for 30' at 4°C. The cells were washed and analyzed on an EPIC V flow cytometer. The result represents linear histograms depicting distribution of cells in each green fluorescent channel. Dead cells were excluded from analysis by propidium iodide staining, and FITC conjugated isotype control antibody was also included in the experiment.

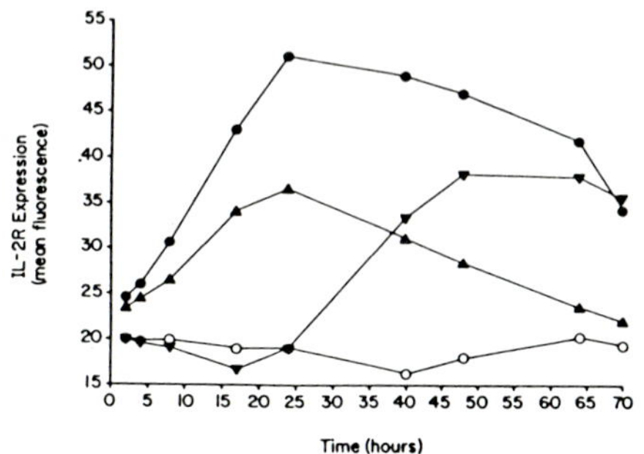

Figure 2. Time course of IL2R expression. YT cells were cultured alone (o---o) or in the presence of 100 units of TNF-α (▲---▲), IL-2 (▼---▼) or 10 units of IL-1ß (●---●) and analyzed for IL2R expression at intervals indicated (reproduced by permission of J. Immunol.).

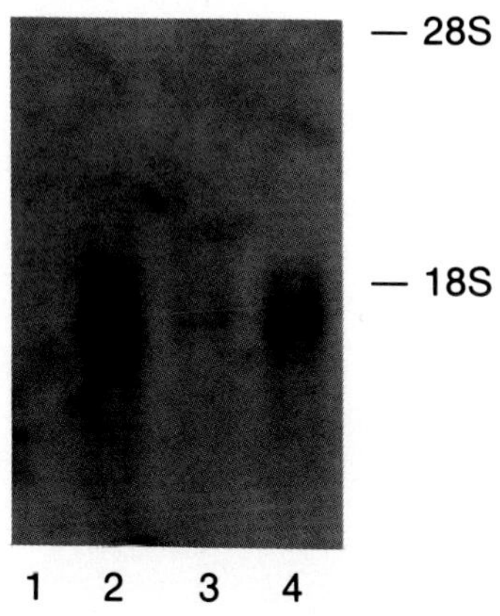

Figure 3. Northern blot analysis of IL2R mRNA in treated YT cells. Lane 1, control YT RNA; Lane 2 to 4, IL-1ß; IL-2, and TNF-α treated YT RNA, respectively (reproduced by permission of J. Immunol.).

In order to ascertain that the increase of IL2R expression in TNF-treated YT cells, as determined by FACS analysis, was a result of newly synthesized mRNA encoding for IL2R, the control and treated cells were examined for the presence of IL2R-specific transcripts by Northern blot analysis. A labelled IL2R cDNA probe encompassing 0.9 Kb of the human IL2R gene (Leonard et al., 1984) was used in the hybridization experiments. As shown in Figure 3, only RNA obtained from TNF, IL-1, and IL-2 treated YT cells showed increased hybridization.

The results obtained from the kinetic experiment suggest that TNF directly induces IL2R expression and does not act via an indirect mechanism. One possible indirect mechanism was the induction of of IL-1 synthesis by TNF-α, which in turn induced the expression of IL2R. In fact, TNF-α has been shown to induce the production of IL-1 in other cell types (Dinarello et al., 1986). To exclude this possibility, we examined the expression of IL-1ß message in TNF treated YT cells. Using the IL-1ß specific cDNA probe isolated from a LPS-stimulated monocyte cDNA library in a Northern blot analysis, we could not detect any change in the extent of hybridization of the radiolabelled IL-1ß probes to treated YT cell RNA (Lee et al., 1987). The lack of induction of newly synthesized IL-1ß message in TNF treated cells indicated that TNF enhanced IL2R expression on YT cells in a direct manner. Similarly, we could not demonstrate the induction of IL-1α message (data not shown). In addition, under no circumstance did we detect IL-1 activity in YT cell

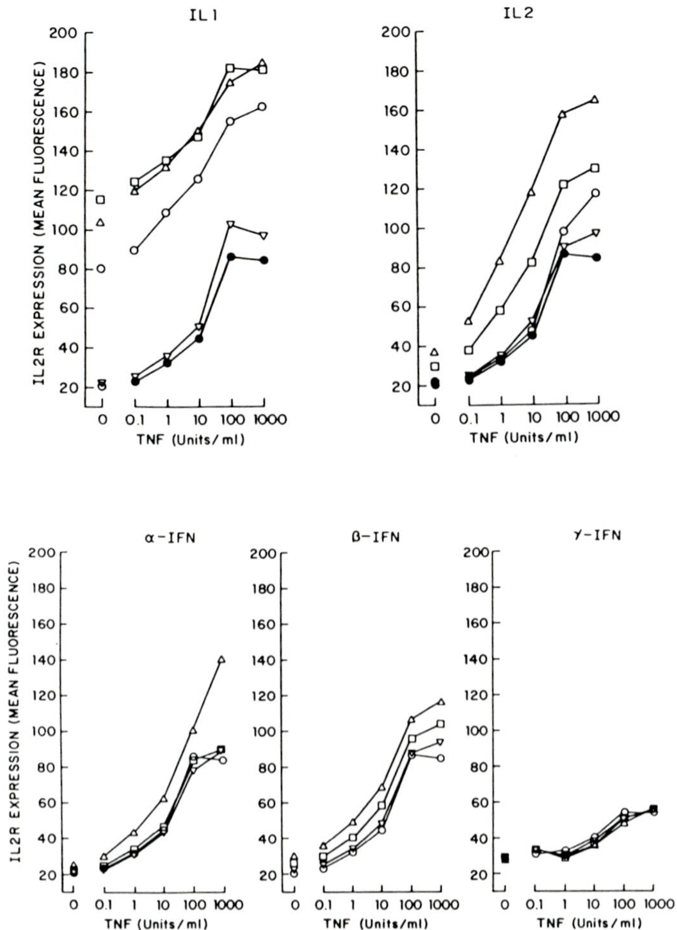

Figure 4. Differential effects of cytokines on TNF induced IL2R expression in YT cells. Interleukin-1, interleukin-2, interferon α, ß and γ at various concentrations (Δ---Δ, 100 units, □---□, 10 units, o---o, 1 unit, ∇---∇, 0.1 unit) were added to YT cell cultures in the presence of varying concentrations of TNF. Control TNF dose response curve is indicated by ●---●. The effects of the cytokines alone (without TNF) at the above indicated concentrations are shown to the left of each frame.

culture supernatant and/or cell associated IL-1 as
measured by the EL-4/IL-2 bioassay (Simon et al., 1985,
unpublished observation).

The interaction between the various cytokines and TNF
in the induction of IL2R in YT cells was also examined
(Figure 4). Only additive effect was observed when the
cells were treated with IL-1 in combination with TNF.
IL-2, on the other hand demonstrated synergistic effects
with TNF, while the interferons had little or no effect.
The additive effect seen in TNF and IL-1 treated cells
indicated that the activation pathways of the two
cytokines are separate while the IL-2 and TNF action are
related. While TNF upregulated IL2R by its own right, it
may also downregulate the turnover rate of IL2R. Such
possibilities are currently under investigation.

To date, TNF has not been shown to be active in the
murine thymocyte co-stimulator assay or in any other
bioassays designed to measure the lymphocyte activating
activity of IL-1. The finding that TNF, a macrophage-
derived molecule distinct from IL-1, enhances IL2R
expression on YT cells is potentially important and could
have major implications for the understanding of the role
of TNF in immunoregulation. In view of that, work is in
progress to examine the effects of TNF on normal T
lymphocytes as well as its interactive role with other
defined lymphokines/cytokines in cell-mediated immune
responses.

REFERENCES

Cantrell DA, Smith K (1984). The interleukin 2 T cell
  system: a new cell growth model. Science 224:1312-1316.
Dinarello CA (1984). Interleukin 1. Rev Infect Dis
  6:51-95.
Dinarello CA, Cannon JG, Wolff SM, Bernheim HA, Beutler B,
  Cerami A, Figari IS, Palladino Jr MA, O'Connor JV
  (1986). Tumor necrosis factor (cachectin) is an
  endogenous pyrogen and induces production of interleukin
  1. J Exp Med 163:1433-1450.
Lee JC, Truneh A, Smith Jr MS, Tsang KY (1987). Induction
  of interleukin 2 receptor (TAC) by tumor necrosis factor
  in YT cells. J Immunol 139:1935-1938.

Leonard WJ, Depper JM, Robb RJ, Waldmann TA, Greene WC (1983). Interleukin 2 receptor gene expression in normal human T lymphocytes. Proc Natl Acad Sci USA 80:6957-6961.

Leonard WL, Depper JM, Crabtree GR, Rudikof S, Pumphre JJ, Robb RJ, Kronke M, Suetlik PB, Peffer NJ, Waldmann TA (1984). Molecular cloning and expression of cDNAs for the human interleukin 2 receptor. Nature 311:626-631.

Lowenthal JW, Cerottini J-C, MacDonald HR (1986). Interleukin 1-dependent induction of both interleukin 2 secretion and interleukin 2 receptor expression by thymoma cells. J Immunol 137:1226-1231.

Robb RJ, Greene WC, Rusk CM (1984). Low and high level affinity cellular receptors for interleukin 2. Implications for the level of TAC antigen. J Exp Med 160:1126-1146.

Simon PL, Laydon JT, Lee JC (1985). A modified assay for interleukin 1 (IL 1). J Immunol Methods 84:85-94.

Uchiyama T, Broder S, Waldmann T (1981). A monoclonal antibody (anti-Tac) reactive with activated and functionally mature human T cells. I. Production of anti-Tac monoclonal antibody and distribution of Tac (+) cells. J Immunol 126:1393-1397.

Yodoi J, Teshigawara K, Nikaido T, Fukui K, Noma T, Honjo T, Takigawa M, Sasaki M, Minato N, Tsudo M, Uchiyama T, Maeda M (1985). TCGF (IL-2)-receptor inducing factor(s). I. Regulation of IL-2 receptor on a natural killer-like cell line (YT cells). J Immunol 134:1623-1630.

Monokines and Other Non-Lymphocytic Cytokines, pages 281–284

INTERLEUKIN 1 EFFECTS ON MONOCYTE RECEPTOR EX-PRESSION

William P. Arend, J. Timothy Ammons and Brian
L. Kotzin
Division of Rheumatology, Department of Medi-
cine, University of Colorado Health Sciences
Center, Denver, CO   80262

INTRODUCTION

Culture of human monocytes in interferon-γ (IFN-γ)
has been reported by many investigators to up-regulate the
expression of an Fc receptor that avidly binds monomers of
murine IgG2a (reviewed in Arend et al., 1987). Bacterial
lipopolysaccharides (LPS) have been reported to be inhibitory to some Fc-dependent monocyte functions. However,
the mechanisms of these alterations and the direct effects
of LPS on Fc receptor function have not previously been
described. In addition, recent studies from our laboratory
have demonstrated the presence of nuclear antigens on the
surface of a subset of human monocytes (Holers and Kotzin,
1985). These nuclear antigens are recognized by monoclonal
antibodies and represent the binding of nuclear material to
specific receptors (Bennett et al., 1987; Kotzin et al., manuscript in preparation). The effects of LPS on expression of
the receptor for nuclear antigens has not been examined.

The objectives of our studies were to examine the effects of LPS on Fc receptor and nuclear antigen expression
on human monocytes and to explore the possibility that LPS
effects are mediated through the induction of interleukin 1
(IL 1) production.

MATERIALS AND METHODS

Human peripheral blood mononuclear leukocytes were
obtained from the blood of normal donors, as recently de-

scribed, and monocytes were isolated by adherence (Arend et
al., 1987). Monocytes were cultured for 24 hr in LPS-free
RPMI medium with 10% FCS in the presence of various a-
mounts of recombinant IFN-γ, LPS or recombinant IL 1β.
Fc receptor expression and nuclear antigen expression on
monocytes were determined by cytofluorographic analysis.
The binding of irrelevant murine IgG2a or IgG2b monoclonal
antibodies detected the two major Fc receptors (Arend et
al., 1987). Murine monoclonal antibodies specific for human
DNA or histones were used to quantify nuclear antigen
bound to receptors on human monocytes (Holers and Kotzin,
1985). In either set of experiments, bound murine monoclonal antibodies were detected with a specific fluorescein-
ated anti-mouse Ig as the second step reagent. Both percent positive cells and receptor density per cell (median
channel fluorescence) were determined.

RESULTS AND DISCUSSION

Effects of LPS and IL 1 on Fc Receptor Expression

The results of initial experiments indicated that 24 hr
culture of adherent monocytes in 1 to 100 U/ml IFN-γ led
to a progressive increase in receptors for murine IgG2a
without any effect on IgG2b binding (Arend et al., 1987).
These values increased from less than 3% monocytes positive
for IgG2a binding in the absence of added IFN-γ to 20%,
65% and 75% Fc receptor-positive cells after culture in 1, 10
and 100 U/ml IFN-γ, respectively. In addition, the density
of Fc receptors per cell increased 3.5-fold during culture in
IFN-γ. In contrast, monocytes incubated in 100 U/ml IFN-γ
and 0.01 to 2 ng/ml LPS displayed a progressive inhibition
in IgG2a binding to 25% of levels seen with IFN-γ alone.
This was accompanied by a 3-fold reduction in Fc receptor
density (Arend et al., 1987).

The results of additional experiments indicated that the
mechanism of LPS inhibition of IFN-γ-induced Fc receptor
expression may involve stimulation of IL 1 production in the
cultured monocytes. The reduction in Fc receptor expression with increasing doses of LPS correlated with first the
intracellular and then the extracellular appearance of IL 1
activity. Furthermore, culture of monocytes with increasing
doses of purified IL 1 or recombinant IL 1β led to a progressive decline in IFN-γ-induced Fc receptors (Arend et al.,

1987). These results indicate that exogenous IL 1 simulates the inhibitory effects of LPS on Fc receptor expression.

Effects of LPS and IL 1 on Nuclear Antigen Expression

Similar experiments were performed measuring nuclear antigen expression on cultured human monocytes. It was observed that freshly-isolated monocytes were ≈10% positive for the presence of nuclear antigens. Culture for 18 hr in standard RPMI medium with 10% FCS (which contained ≈2 ng/ml LPS) led to the appearance of nuclear antigen on 40–45% of the monocytes. This effect appeared to be due to the presence of contaminating LPS in the standard medium. Thus, cells cultured for 18 hr in LPS-free conditions displayed no change in expression of nuclear antigens. The addition of increasing amounts of LPS from 0.01 to 1 ng/ml during the culture led to a progressive increase in the expression of the receptors for nuclear antigens. Peak expression was achieved with doses as low as 0.2 ng/ml LPS. Furthermore, the addition of 0.1 to 5.0 units/ml of recombinant IL 1β simulated the effects of LPS on inducing the appearance of nuclear antigen receptors on monocyte surfaces over 18 hr culture. 0.2 ng/ml LPS and 5.0 units/ml recombinant IL 1β increased nuclear antigen expression from 13% of monocytes to 44% and 40%, respectively. In contrast to effects on Fc receptor expression, the addition of IFN-γ to the culture did not stimulate nuclear antigen expression or inhibit LPS-induced expression.

The effects of IFN-γ, LPS and IL 1 on monocyte receptor expression are summarized in Table 1.

Table 1: Regulation of receptors on human monocytes

Stimulating material	Fc receptor expression	Nuclear antigen receptor expression
IFN-γ	Increased	No change
LPS	Decreased	Increased
IL 1	Decreased	Increased

SUMMARY

Induction of Fc receptor expression on human monocytes specific for binding of murine IgG2a was induced by culture in IFN-γ. A progressive inhibition of IFN-γ-induced Fc receptors was observed with the addition of either LPS or IL 1 to the culture. In contrast, induction of a receptor for nuclear material on human monocytes was observed to be dependent upon the presence of LPS in the culture whereas IFN-γ had no effects on this receptor. Exogenous IL 1 also induced the appearance of the nuclear antigen receptor on cultured monocytes. These results suggest that IL 1 may either inhibit (Fc) or stimulate (nuclear antigen) the expression of specific receptors on human monocytes.

REFERENCES

Arend WP, Ammons JT, Kotzin BL (1987). Lipopolysaccharide and interleukin 1 inhibit interferon-γ-induced Fc receptor expression on human monocytes. J Immunol 139:1873-1879.

Bennett PM, Kotzin BL, Merritt MJ (1987). DNA receptor dysfunction in systemic lupus erythematosus and kindred disorders. Induction by anti-DNA antibodies, anti-histone antibodies and anti-receptor antibodies. J Exp Med 166: 850-863.

Holers VM, Kotzin BL (1985). Human peripheral blood monocytes display surface antigens recognized by monoclonal antinuclear antibodies. J Clin Invest 76:991-998.

Monokines and Other Non-Lymphocytic Cytokines, pages 285–290
© 1988 Alan R. Liss, Inc.

In TNF Mediated Cytolysis Apoptosis Can Occur in the Absence of Nuclear Disintegration.

Scott M. Laster*, Mary Scanlon[+], John G. Wood[+], and Linda R. Gooding.*

Departments of Microbiology and Immunology* and Anatomy and Cell Biology[+], Emory University School of Medicine, Atlanta, Georgia 30322.

INTRODUCTION

Tumor necrosis factor (TNF) is a cytokine produced by macrophages which can induce a variety of diverse cellular responses including; proliferation, differentiation, and cytotoxicity. In this report we will focus solely on the cytotoxic activity of TNF. Recently, it has been reported that the cytolysis of MCF-7 cells, a spontaneously sensitive target, is accompanied by the phenomena known as nuclear disintegration (Dealtry, _et al_., 1987). Nuclear disintegration is believed to be an early step in the process of cell lysis known as apoptosis, or programmed cell death. Apparently, in some cells, TNF can induce an endogenous "suicide" program leading to cell death. Lymphotoxin (LT), a closely related cytokine has also been shown to cause nuclear disintegration in L929 cells (Schmid _et al_., 1986).

Most cell types are not, however, spontaneously sensitive to lysis by TNF. For example, in human foreskin fibroblasts, a resistant target, TNF induces the expression of at least two novel proteins (Kirstein and Baglioni, 1986). It is believed that these proteins protect these cells from lysis since pretreatment with inhibitors of transcription or translation will result in cell lysis upon subsequent exposure to TNF. In this report, we have investigated whether the lysis of a resistant target (C3HA) treated with cycloheximide (CX) also involves nuclear disintegration and apoptosis. Our results show that while C3HA cells do indeed undergo apoptosis, they do not undergo nuclear disintegration.

MATERIALS AND METHODS

Reagents. All cells were grown in Dulbecco's Modified Eagles
Medium (Gibco) with 10% fetal calf serum (Hyclone). Cycloheximide was purchased from Sigma Corp. and was used at 25
ug/ml in all experiments. rTNF was obtained from Cetus Corp.
and used a 100 U/ml in all experiments.

Cytotoxicity Assays. ^{51}Cr and ^{3}H-THD-release assays were
performed as described previously (Chapes and Gooding, 1985,
and Duke et al., 1983). Triton x-100 was used to dissolve
plasma membranes to count low M. W. DNA in the ^{3}H-THD assay.

Microscopy. Light microscopy as performed on a Leitz Epivert
microscope. Microfilaments were stained using TRITC-labeled
phalloidin (Sigma) following treatment with TNF and/or CX.
Fluorescence was observed on a Leitz Laborlux 12 microscope
fitted with a Wild MPS 51S automatic photography system.

RESULTS

F17 cells. The cell line F17 is an adenovirus transformed
rat cell line which is spontaneously sensitive to lysis by
TNF (Courtesy of W. Wold, University of St. Louis). F17
cells die by a classical form of apoptosis and have been
included as a positive control. Some 12-24 hours after the
addition of TNF the cytoplasm of these cells begins to boil.
The surface of the cell literally explodes with large blebs
or apoptic bodies (Fig. 1a). In F17 cells this process is
accompanied by nuclear disintegration. Fragments of degraded
genomic DNA appear in cytoplasm of apoptic cells. For this
reason ^{3}H-THD can be used effectively as a radioactive marker
to measure cell death (Table 1).

C3HA cells. The cell line C3HA is a 3T3-like cell line
produced in this laboratory. C3HA cells are not spontaneously sensitive to lysis by TNF but can be killed by TNF
when treated with inhibitors of transcription or translation
(i.e., actinomycin D or cycloheximide). C3HA cells also die
by an apoptic process (Fig. 1b), however, apoptosis in C3HA
is not accompanied by nuclear disintegration (Table 1).
Fragments of genomic DNA are not released into the cytoplasm.
When analyzed by electrophoresis, the DNA from dead C3HA
cells also reveals no fragmentation (data not shown). As a
result, ^{3}H-THD cannot be used as a marker to measure cell
death in this cell line (Table 1).

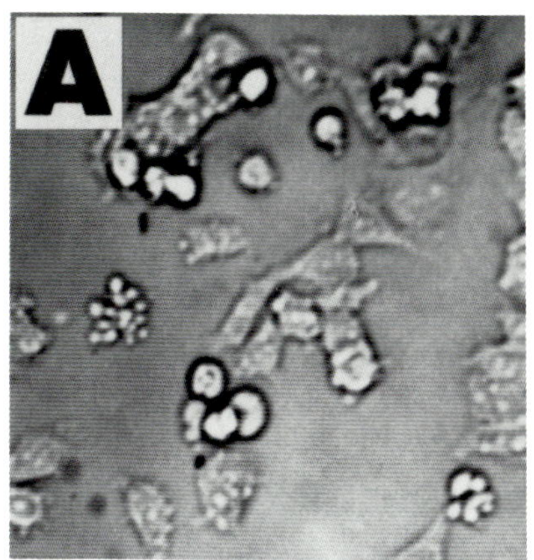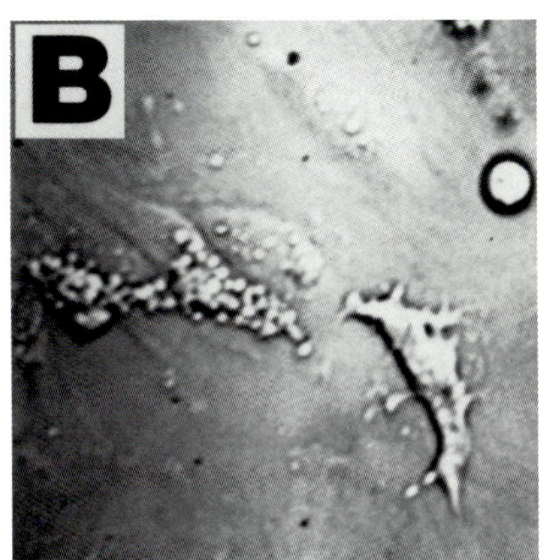

Figure 1. Photomicrographs of cells undergoing lysis mediated by TNF. (A) F17 cells and (B) C3HA cells.

TABLE 1. Cytolysis of F17 and C3HA Cells with TNF

Target	Additions	Recent Specific Radiolabel Release	
		^{3}H-THD	^{51}Cr
F17	TNF	66±5	39±3
C3HA	CX	0±0	9±2
	TNF	−1±1	4±3
	TNF + CX	1±2	86±6

Since apoptosis in C3HA cells does not involve nuclear
disintegration, we have begun to examine the changes in
cytoplasmic structure which lead to cell death. The major
structural component of C3HA cytoplasm (and other 3T3-like
cells) are large bundles of actin filaments known as stress
fibers (Fig. 2a). We hypothesized that any change in the
structure of C3HA cytoplasm should involve a degenerative
change in structure of the stress fibers. Indeed, we find
that changes in stress fiber morphology do precede apoptosis
(Fig. 2b). The disappearance of stress fibers begins first
in the perinuclear area and then spreads progressively
towards the extremities of the cell. Interestingly, although
stress fibers disappear, the actin in apoptic cells still
stains with phalloidin indicating that it remains in the f-
actin form.

DISCUSSION

Apoptic cell death has been observed in a variety of
cellular systems. T lymphocytes treated with glucocorticoids
die by apoptosis (Wyllie and Morris, 1982). Apoptosis or
nuclear disintegration has also been observed in several
systems of immune mediated cytolysis; including the cytolysis
induced by T lymphocytes, LT (Schmid, et al, 1986) and TNF
(Dealtry et al, 1987). From these reports it has been
possible to reconstruct the sequence of degenerative changes
in cell structure which lead to cell death (reviewed by
Willey, 1985). The first change in cell structure which has
been observed is the disintegration of the chromosomal DNA
into 220 bp, nucleosome sized fragments. Presumably, this
represents the activation of an endogenous nuclease. After
this, the nuclear membrane breaks down and fragments of DNA
are released into cytoplasm. Only then do changes in
cytoplasmic structure begin. The cytoplasm boils, followed
by a loss in cell volume and finally, lysis of plasma
membrane. This is precisely the sequence of events we have
observed in F17 cells. It is not, however, the sequence of
events we have observed in C3HA cells. These cells undergo
cytoplasmic apoptosis without nuclear disintegration suggesting that with TNF nuclear disintegration is neither the cause
of, nor obligate for apoptosis to occur.

What then is the cause of cytoplasmic degeneration in these
cells? Changes in microfilament structure accompanying lysis
induced by LT have been reported previously (Leopardic et

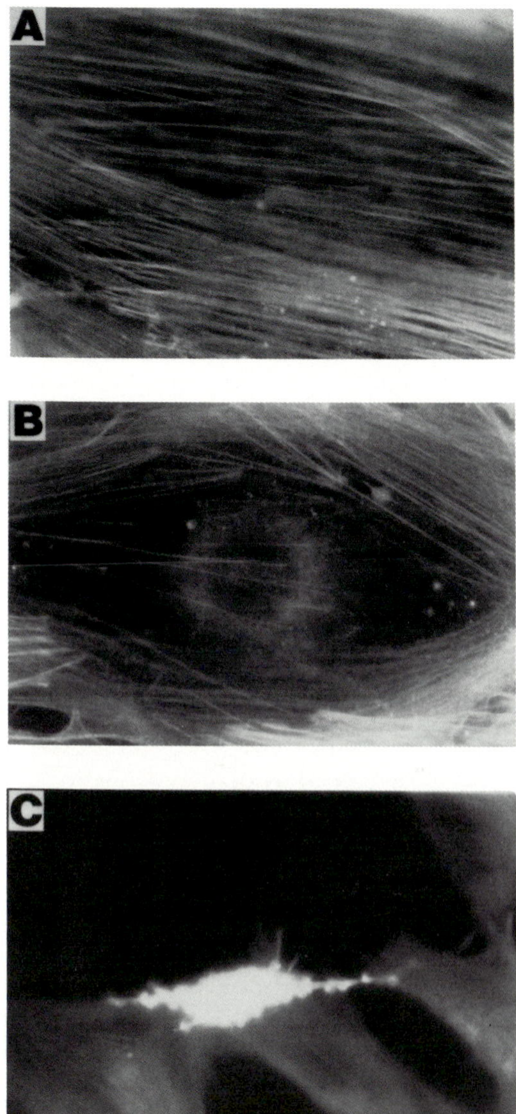

Figure 2. C3HA cells stained with phalloidin undergoing apoptosis mediated by TNF + CX. (A) before treatment (B) after one hour incubation, and (C) after two hours incubation.

al., 1984). We also observed changes in microfilament
structure accompanying lysis by TNF. Furthermore, our
results shown clearly that the degeneration of stress fibers
precedes cytoplasmic apoptosis. In the future we hope to
determine whether the degeneration of this cytoskeletal
component is indeed the cause of cytoplasmic apoptosis or
merely one of many cellular structures which degenerate in
response to TNF.

This work was supported by grants CA40266 (L.R.G.)
and NS17731 (J.G.W.). S.M.L. was supported as a
trainee by grant AI07265.

REFERENCES

Chapes S. K. and Gooding L. R. (1985). Evidence for the
    involvement of cytolytic macrophages in rejection of SV40-
    induced tumors. J. Immunol. 135:2192-2198.
Dealtry G B, Naylor M S, Fiers W and Balkwill F R (1987).
    DNA fragmentation and cytotoxicity caused by tumor necrosis
    factor is enhanced by interferon-gamma. Eur. J. Immunol.
    17:689-693.
Duke R C, Chervanak R, and Cohen J J (1983). Endogenous
    endonuclease-induced DNA fragmentation:An early event in
    cell-mediated cytolysis. Proc. Natl. Acad. Sci. USA
    80:6361-6365.
Kirstein M and Baglioni C (1986). Tumor Necrosis Factor
    Induces Synthesis of Two Proteins in Human Fibroblasts. J.
    Biol. Chem. 261:9565-9567.
Leopardi E, Friend D S and Rosenau W (1984). Target Cell
    Lysis: Ultrastructural and Cytoskeletal Alterations. J. of
    Immunol. 133:3429-3436.
Schmid D S, Tite J P and Ruddle N H (1986). DNA fragmenta-
    tion: manifestation of target cell destruction mediated by
    cytotoxic T-cell lines, lymphotoxin-secreting helper T-cell
    clones, and cell-free lymphotoxin-containing supernatant.
    Proc. Natl. Acad. Sci. USA 83:1881-1885.
Wyllie A H, and Morris R G (1982). Hormone-Induced Cell
    Death:Purification and Properties of Thymocytes Undergoing
    Apoptosis After Glucocorticoid Treatment. Amer. J. Path.
    101:78-87.
Wyllie A H (1985). The Biology of Cell Death in Tumours.
    Anticancer Res. 5:131-136.

POTENTIATING EFFECTS OF TUMOR NECROSIS FACTOR ON INTERLEU-
KIN-1 MEDIATED PANCREATIC BETA-CELL TOXICITY

Thomas Mandrup-Poulsen, Klaus Bendtzen, Charles
A. Dinarello and Jørn Nerup
Steno Memorial Hospital, Gentofte (T.M.-P., J.N.)
and University Hospital of Copenhagen, Copenhagen, Denmark (K.B.) and Tufts University School
of Medicine, Boston, MA 02111 (C.A.D.)

INTRODUCTION

Insulin-dependent diabetes mellitus (IDDM) is believed
to be caused by an immune-mediated selective destruction
of pancreatic beta-cells. The destructive mechanism is unknown. The role of islet cell antibodies and MHC-restricted
Tc-cells in the early events of the destructive process
has been questioned (Nerup et al., 1987). Pathoanatomically
the islets in IDDM are infiltrated first by macrophages
and Th-cells (Sibley et al., 1985, Kolb et al., 1986), and
later by virtually all lymphocyte subsets (Bottazzo et al.,
1985). Interaction between mononuclear cells in immune infiltrates may lead to high local concentrations of cytokines. This concept prompted us to investigate the effects
of cytokines on pancreatic islets in vitro. We have previously reported that the monokine IL-1 has profound effects on islet beta-cells in culture (Mandrup-Poulsen et
al., 1986, 1987b, Spinas et al., 1986, 1987, Bendtzen et
al., 1986, Table 1).

TABLE 1. Effects of exposing isolated islets to IL-1 for > 24 h.

	≤ 0.5 U/ml	≥ 1.0 U/ml	REF
GLUCOSE-STIMULATED INSULIN RELEASE	↑	↓	1,2,3
INSULIN CONTENT	↑	↓	1,2,3
PROINSULIN TO INSULIN CONVERSION	–	↓	4
(PRO)INSULIN BIOSYNTHESIS	↑	↓	4
PREPROINSULIN M-RNA	↑	↓	4
TOTAL PROTEIN BIOSYNTHESIS	↑	↓	4
GLUCOSE OXIDATION	↑	↓	5
OXYGEN CONSUMPTION	–	↓	5
ISLET DNA	–	↓	5,6
SELECTIVE LM/EM DESTRUCTION OF BETA-CELLS	–	+	7

Although the activity of crude cytokine preparations
on beta-cells is abolished by anti-IL-1 antibody (Bendtzen et al., 1986), we were interested in investigating possible modulatory effects of other cytokines on IL-1 mediated beta-cell toxicity.

METHODS

Rat islets isolated, precultured, and cultured as described previously (Mandrup-Poulsen et al., 1986) were incubated with or without the following human recombinant
cytokines, either alone or in combinations: IL-1a, IL-1b,
TNFa, TNFb, IFNg (for details see Mandrup-Poulsen et al.,
1987a). After 6 or 7 days culture medium was assayed for
insulin by RIA.

RESULTS & DISCUSSION

Fifty percent inhibition of glucose stimulated insulin
release (IR) was obtained with approximately 0.3 U/l of
rIL-1b and 10 U/ml of rIL-1a. This IL-1 induced inhibition
of IR was previously demonstrated to be parallelled by decreases in insulin content and electron-microscopic (EM)
evidence of beta-cell destruction (Mandrup-Poulsen et al.,
1986, 1987b). rTNFa (but not rTNFb or IFNg) at concentra-

tions $\geq$ 5,000 U/ml (25 ng/ml) caused an inhibition of max. 40% (Fig. 1), but this effect was not accompanied by decreases in insulin content (Bendtzen et al., 1986) or LM or EM morphological changes (Mandrup-Poulsen et al., 1987b).

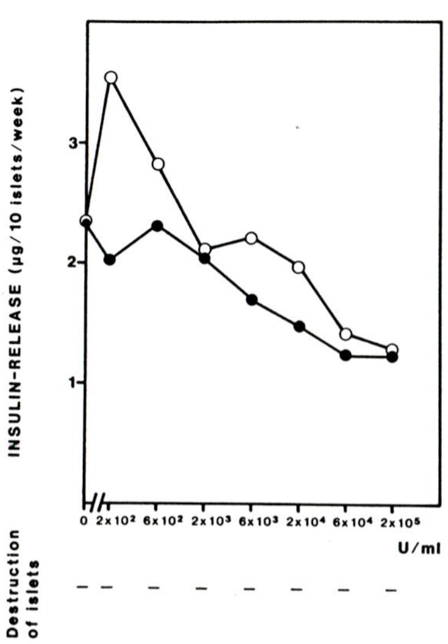

Figure 1. Glucose stimulated insulin release (µg/10 islets/week) and LM destruction score of rat islets incubated with varying concentrations of TNFa (2×10^{8} U/mg) for 7 days. Two independent experiments in duplicate.

rTNFa at concentrations $\leq$ 500 U/ml (2.5 ng/ml) did not affect insulin release (Figs. 1 and 2). However, the addition of 500 U/ml of rTNFa before, concomitantly to or after the addition of 1 U/ml of rIL-1b caused a marked potentiation of IL-1 induced inhibition of IR (Fig. 2, Mandrup-Poulsen et al., 1987a).

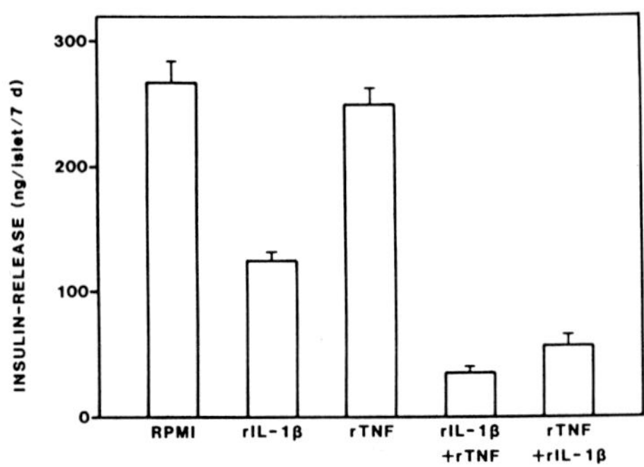

Figure 2. Effects of control medium, rIL-1b/rTNFa alone
or rIL-1b + rTNFa/rTNFa + rIL-1b (addition separated by
60 min.). Means $\pm$ SEM of 7 experiments; RPMI vs. rIL-1b:
2a = 0.02, RPMI vs. rTNFa: NS. rIL-1b vs. rIL-1b + rTNFa
or rTNFa + rIL-1b: 2a = 0.02; rIL-1b + rTNFa vs. rTNFa
+ rIL-1b: 2a = 0.02 (paired Wilcoxon's test). Data from
Mandrup-Poulsen et al., 1987a reproduced with permission
from The Journal of Immunology.

The addition of 500 U/ml of TNFa to varying doses
of rIL-1a or b shifted the dose responses curve 10 times
to the left (Mandrup-Poulsen et al., 1987a). IFNg or TNFb
were ineffective, and TNFa did not potentiate the LAF activity of rIL-1a or b. However, experiments with rodent
cytokines are needed before excluding modulatory effects
of IFNg and TNFb on IL-1 mediated beta-cell inhibition,
and of TNFa on the LAF activity of IL-1 on murine thymocytes.

These observations raise the possibility that IDDM
may be caused by immunologically mediated mechanisms involving IL-1 and TNFa, produced in the islet inflammatory
infiltrate by e.g. macrophages or NK-cells.

REFERENCES

Bendtzen K, Mandrup-Poulsen T, Nerup J, Nielsen JH, Dinarello CA, Svenson M (1986). Cytotoxicity of human pI
   7 interleukin-1 for pancreatic islets of Langerhans.
   Science 232:1545-1547.
Bottazzo GF, Dean BM, McNally JM, MacKay EH, Swift PGF,

Gamble DR (1985). In situ characterization of autoimmune phenomena and expression of HLA molecules in the pancreas in diabetic insulitis. N Engl J Med 313:353-360.

Kolb H, Kantwerk G, Treichel U, Kürner T, Kiesel U, Hoppe T, Kolb-Bachofen V (1986). Prospective analysis of islet lesions in BB-rats. Diabetologia 29:559 A.

Mandrup-Poulsen T, Bendtzen K, Nerup J, Dinarello CA, Svenson M, Nielsen JH (1986). Affinity-purified interleukin-1 is cytotoxic to isolated islets of Langerhans. Diabetologia 29:63-67.

Mandrup-Poulsen T, Bendtzen K, Dinarello CA, Nerup J (1987a). Human tumor necrosis factor potentiates human interleukin-1 mediated rat pancreatic b-cell cytotoxicity. J Immunol (in press).

Mandrup-Poulsen T, Egeberg J, Nerup J, Bendtzen K, Nielsen JH, Dinarello CA (1987b). Ultrastructural studies of time course and cellular specificity of interleukin-1 mediated islet cytotoxicity. Acta Pathol Microbiol Immunol Scand (C) 95:55-63.

Nerup J, Mandrup-Poulsen T, Mølvig J (1987). The HLA-IDDM association: implications for etiology and pathogenesis of IDDM. Diab Metab Rev 3:779-802.

Sibley RK, Sutherland DER, Goetz F, Michael AF (1985). Recurrent diabetes mellitus in the pancreatic iso - and allograft. Lab Invest 53:132-144.

Spinas Ga, Mandrup-Poulsen T, Mølvig J, Bæk L, Bendtzen K, Dinarello CA, Nerup J (1986). Low concentrations of interleukin-1 stimulate and high concentrations inhibit insulin release from isolated islets of Langerhans. Acta Endocrinol 113:551-558.

Spinas GA, Hansen BS, Linde S, Kastern W, Mølvig J, Mandrup-Poulsen T, Dinarello CA, Nielsen JH, Nerup J (1987). Interleukin-1 dose-dependently affects the biosynthesis of (pro)insulin in isolated rat islets of Langerhans. Diabetologia 30:474-480.

Monokines and Other Non-Lymphocytic Cytokines, pages 297–300
© 1988 Alan R. Liss, Inc.

INFLUENCE OF INTERLEUKIN 1 ON HUMAN BONE MARROW BLAST PROGENITOR CELLS IN VITRO

Jan Moreb, James Zucali, Mary Ann Gross
and Charles A. Dinarello
Department of Medicine, (J.M., J.Z., M.A.G.)
University of Florida, Gainesville, FL 32610
and Division of Geographic Medicine, (C.A.D.)
Tufts-New England Medical Center, Boston, MA 02111

INTRODUCTION:

The hierarchy of hematopoietic colony-forming cells in human bone marrow places the undifferentiated CFU-blast (CFU-bl) colony forming cell as the earliest progenitor cell so far studied in clonal culture. The growth of the CFU-Bl has been shown to be dependent on the presence of different conditioned media from either PHA-treated human leukocytes, human bladder carcinoma cell line 5637 or hairy cell leukemia Mo cell line (Rowley et al., 1987; Leary and Ogawa, 1987). The identification of such CFU-Bl has been based on the dispersity of translucent and agranular cells within the colony, the morphological appearance of primitive undifferentiated cells when stained, and the ability of these cells to produce secondary colonies including single and multi-lineage colonies on replating.

METHODS:

Non adherent human bone marrow mononuclear cells from normal donors were treated with 4-Hydroperoxycyclophosphamide (4-HC), 100ug/ml, in the presence of a 5-10% suspension of RBCs according to the method described by Rowley et al. (1987). These bone marrow cells were cultured in the presence of 5637 conditioned medium (5637 CM) and erythropoietin. CFU-Bl were identified, scored and replated between day 14 and 28 of culture. At this time, about half of the colony was replated in the same conditions as described above while half was cytocentrifuged and slides prepared for morphology studies. The secondary colonies were scored after 12-14 days of culture.

In order to determine the effect of IL-1 on CFU-Bl colony formation, bone marrow cultures were initiated with 5637 CM which had been previously incubated with antibody to IL-1. Measurements of IL-1 in 5637 CM were determined using the cloned murine helper T cell line D.10.G4.1 (Dinarello et al., 1986).

RESULTS AND CONCLUSIONS:

The CFU-Bl in culture were identified as a homogeneous population of round, translucent, agranular cells as shown in figure la. Upon morphological examination, blast cell colonies consisted of undifferentiated blast cells with nucleoli present and they possessed basophilic cytoplasm (Figure lb).

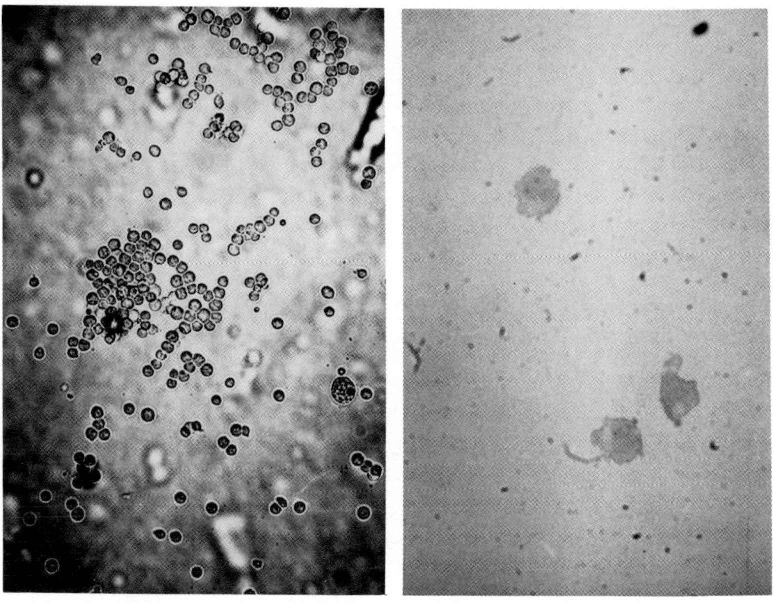

Fig. la   Fig. lb

Figure la. Human blast cells from CFU-Bl at 18 days of culture. (400x)

Figure lb. Morphology of cells obtained from human blast cell colony stained with Wrights-Giemsa. (1000x)

Upon replating (Table 1), secondary colonies of erythroid, granulocytic, monocytic, mixed granulocyte-monocyte and mixed erythroid, granulocyte, monocyte and megakaryocyte colonies were seen. Antibody to IL-1 reduced the IL-1 content of 5637 CM from 802±89 pg/ml to nondetectable levels (<50pg/ml). The addition of 5637 CM treated with antibody to IL-1 reduced the number of CFU-B1 seen at 15 days of culture from 23±5 to 5±5 and the number of CFU-B1 seen at 22 days of culture from 37±14 to 8±1 (Figure 2).

Table 1. CYTOLOGICAL ANALYSIS OF SECONDARY COLONIES SEEN IN REPLATING OF BLAST CELL COLONIES

E	G	M	GM	MIX	No. of SECONDARY COLONIES
	+	+			3
+	+				7
	+			+	2
+		+		+	6
+			+		2
+			+		25
+			+		2
			+		1
			+	+	5

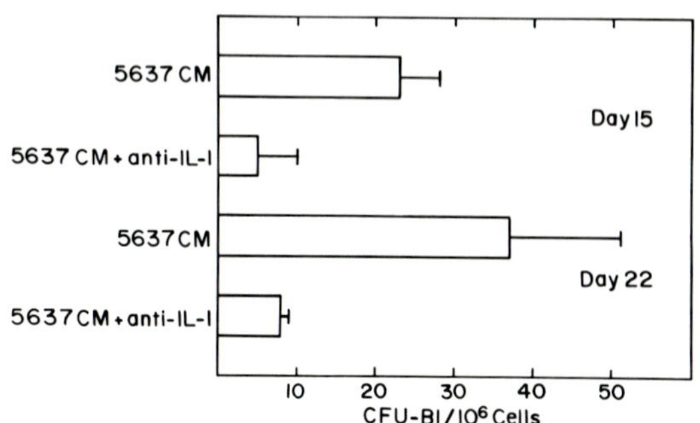

Figure 2. Effect of anti-IL-1 on CFU-B1 Colony Formation.

We conclude that CFU-Bl contain early progenitors which are able to give rise to secondary colonies upon replating. In addition, IL-1 appears to be necessary for the growth of these undifferentiated blast cell colonies. Whether the effect of IL-1 is directly on the blast colony-forming cell or through an accessory cell population needs further investigation.

REFERENCES

1.   Rowley SD, Sharkis SJ, Hottenburg C, Sensenbrenner LL (1987). Culture from human bone marrow of blast progenitor cells with an extensive proliferative capacity. Blood 69: 804-808.

2.   Leary AG, Ogawa M (1987). Blast cell colony assay for unbilical cord blood and adult bone marrow progenitors. Blood 68: 953-956.

3.   Jones RJ, Zuehlsdorf M, Rowley SD, Hilton J, Santos GW, Sensenbrenner LL, Calvin OM (1987). Variability in 4-Hydroperoxycyclophosphamide activity during clinical purging for autologous bone marrow transplantation. Blood 70: 1490-1494.

4.   Dinarello CA, Cannon JG, Mier JW, Bernheim HA, Lo Preste G, Lynn DL, Love RN, Webb AC, Auron PE, Reuben RC, Rich A, Wolff SM, Putney SD (1986). Multiple biological activities of human recombinant interleukin 1. J Clin Invest 77: 1734-1739.

Monokines and Other Non-Lymphocytic Cytokines, pages 301–306
© 1988 Alan R. Liss, Inc.

RECOMBINANT HUMAN MONOCYTE SPECIFIC COLONY–STIMULATING FACTOR STIMULATES BOTH IMMATURE AND MATURE CELLS OF HUMAN MONOCYTE LINEAGE

K. Motoyoshi, K. Yoshida, K. Hatake, N. Yanai,
T. Kawashima, M. Saito, Y. Miura, G.G. Wong,
M. Fujisawa, A. Yuo, T. Okabe and F. Takaku

Jichi Medical School (K.M., K.H., M.S., Y.M.),
Kawachi-Gun, Tochigi-Ken, 329-04, Japan,
Morinaga Milk Industry (K.Y., N.Y., T.K.),
Genetics Institute (G.G.W.) and University of
Tokyo (M.F., A.Y., T.O., F.T.)

INTRODUCTION

Two colony-stimulating factors (CSFs) had been found and purified from human urine. One is CSF-1 which has an apparent molecular weight of 45 KD (Das, 1981). The other is human monocyte specific CSF (hM-CSF) which has an apparent molecular weight of 85 KD (Motoyoshi, 1982). Genes encoding both factors have been cloned (Kawasaki, 1985; Wong, 1987), and recombinant factors have been produced from media conditioned by CHO cells introduced with each of the genes. In this paper, we describe in vitro actions of native and recombinant hM-CSF on immature progenitor cells and mature cells of human monocyte lineage.

MATERIALS AND METHODS

Native hM-CSF had been purified from human urine concentrate by the procedures reported previously (Hatake, 1985), and had a specific activity of 2×10^8 U/mg protein in the standard mouse assay system (Motoyoshi, 1978). Recombinant hM-CSF has been purified to a homogeneous protein from serum free medium conditioned by CHO-3ACSF-69 cells using the same procedure. Monolayer agar culture system was employed to measure human active colony-stimu-lating activity (CSA), as reported previously (Motoyoshi,

1982). To estimate if hM-CSF stimulates human monocytes to
produce monokines, $2x10^6$/ml human peripheral blood monocytes
were cultured in a liquid medium in the absence or presence
of hM-CSF, as reported previously (Ishizaka, 1986).
Supernatant fluid (Mo-CM) was collected and assayed for
human active CSA using a monolayer agar culture containing
$1x10^5$/ml phagocyte-depleted human bone marrow cells. Histoc-
hemical analysis of colonies was performed after double
esterase staining as described previously (Motoyoshi, 1983).
Interleukin 1 (IL-1) activity and interferon (IFN) activity
were measured using thymocyte-costimulating assay and
inhibition of cytopathic effect, respectively, as reported
previously (Kasahara, 1985). To evaluate what kind of CSA
is contained in Mo-CM, anti-hG-CSF serum and anti-hGM-CSF
serum were used.

RESULTS

Purified native hM-CSF at a dose of up to 248 ng did
not stimulate colony formation when added in a monolayer
agar culture containing human phagocyte-depleted bone marrow
cells, but it stimulated human adherent cell-depleted bone
marrow cells to form macrophagic colonies in a dose
dependent manner (Table 1).

TABLE 1. Effect of purified hM-CSF on colony formation by
phagocyte-depleted and adherent cell-depleted human bone
marrow cells

	Number of colonies	
	Phagocyte-depleted	Adherent cell-depleted
Medium	0	0
hM-CSF 3.1 ng/ml	0	2.5 ± 0.7
6.2 ng/ml	0	5.5 ± 0.7
62.0 ng/ml	0	18.0 ± 1.4
248.0 ng/ml	0	37.0 ± 0

Human adherent cell-depleted ($1x10^5$/ml) and phagocyte-
depleted ($1x10^5$/ml) bone marrow cells were cultured for 14
days in a monolayer agar culture containing medium or 3.1-
248 ng/ml purified native hM-CSF. All of the formed colonies
were macrophagic.

Although monocytes obtained from peripheral blood of a healthy volunteer produced a small amount of human active CSA (37.5 ± 11.3 colonies/0.1 ml CM), they produced a large amount of human active CSA in the presence of 62 ng/ml hM-CSF (91.5 ± 0.7 colonies/0.1 ml CM) or the same amount of rhM-CSF (104.5 ± 26.2 colonies/0.1 ml CM). Monocytes did not produce IL-1 nor IFN irrespective of the presence or absence of hM-CSF (Table 2).

Table 2. Monokine production of human peripheral blood monocytes stimulated by hM-CSF.

Stimulator	Human CSA (Colonies/0.1ml)	IL-1 activity (U/ml)	IFN activity (U/ml)
Medium	37.5 ± 11.3	<1	0
hM-CSF 62 ng/ml	91.5 ± 0.7	<1	0
rhM-CSF 62 ng/ml	104.5 ± 26.2	<1	0

Conditioned media (CM) were prepared from liquid cultures of 2×10^6/ml human monocytes obtained from a healthy volunteer in the presence of medium, or 62 ng/ml of purified native or recombinant hM-CSF.

To evaluate what kind of human CSF is contained in Mo-CM, it was preincubated for 36 hours with normal rabbit serum, anti-hG-CSF serum or anti-hGM-CSF serum. Human monocytes produced a small amount of human active CSA (39 ± 6 colonies/ 0.1 ml CM), which was partially neutralized by the addition of anti-hG-CSF serum (10 ± 1 colonies/0.1 ml CM), but not by the addition of anti-hGM-CSF serum (35 ± 1 colonies/0.1 ml CM)(Table 3). On the other hand, the same monocytes produced a larger amount of human active CSA in the presence of hM-CSF (74 ± 6 colonies/0.1 ml CM) or rhM-CSF (59 ± 1 colonies/ 0.1 ml CM), which was partially neutralized by the addition of anti-hG-CSF serum (24 ± 1 or 22 ± 9 colonies/0.1 ml CM) or of anti-hGM-CSF serum (32 ± 1 or 27 ± 2 colonies/0.1 ml CM). In the control experiments, it was confirmed that the same amount of anti-hG-CSF serum completely neutralized 250 U hG-CSF, but did not neutralize hGM-CSF and that the same amount of anti-hGM-CSF serum completely neutralized 50 U hGM-CSF, but did not neutralize hG-CSF. These results indicate that human monocytes mainly produce hG-CSF in the absence of hM-CSF and produce both hG-CSF and hGM-CSF in the presence of hM-CSF.

Table 3. Effect of normal, anti-hG-CSF and anti-hGM-CSF sera
on CSA in Mo-CM, hM-CSF-Mo-CM and rhM-CSF-Mo-CM.

	Normal serum (x100 dil.)	Anti-hG-CSF serum (x100 dil.)	Anti-hGM-CSF serum (x50 dil.)
Mo-CM	39 ± 6	10 ± 1	35 ± 1
hM-CSF-Mo-CM	74 ± 6	24 ± 1	32 ± 1
rhM-CSF-Mo-CM	59 ± 1	22 ± 9	27 ± 2

CM were prepared from liquid cultures of human monocytes
(2×10^6/ml) obtained from a healthy volunteer.

DISCUSSION

Recently human genes encoding GM-CSF, G-CSF, CSF-1 and
IL-3 have been cloned (Clark, 1987), and a large amount of
recombinant factor has been prepared from bacterial and
mammarian cells introduced with such a gene. We have focused
attention on purification, characterization and clinical
application of hM-CSF (Motoyoshi, 1982; Hatake, 1985;
Ishizaka, 1985; Motoyoshi, 1986). We and others have been
interested in whether hM-CSF and CSF-1 were the same glycoprotein with microheterogeneiety in carbohydrate moiety,
because both were found in human urine, both had strong
mouse M-CSA and weak human M-CSA and both were eluted from
a DEAE cellulose column at approximately the same cl^- ion
concentration. On the other hand, recent results of ours and
others demonstrated that hM-CSF and CSF-1 had different
actions on human monocyte lineage (Ishizaka, 1986; Warren,
1986). Although hM-CSF directly stimulated human monocytes
to produce hG-CSF, CSF-1 was reported not to directly stimulate human monocytes. We have also demonstrated that hM-CSF
and CSF-1 had different molecular weights and hM-CSF had an
additional amino acid sequence from 150th to 447th residues
that was not found in CSF-1 (Motoyoshi, 1987; Wong, 1987).
Our previous observation that hG-CSF stimulated human
monocytes to produce hG-CSF (Ishizaka, 1986), was confirmed
by the present study using anti-hG-CSF serum (Table 3).
We have also demonstrated that human monocytes produced
hGM-CSF when stimulated by hM-CSF (Table 3). Table 4 shows
the differences in molecular and biological characteristics
between hM-CSF and CSF-1.

Table 4. Differences between hM-CSF and CSF-1.

	CSF-1	hM-CSF
Molecular weight		
Native form	45 KD	85 KD
Subunit form	22 KD	42 KD
Protein core	15-17 KD	27 KD
Pro-factor	26 KD	61 KD
Size of mRNA	1.5-2 kb	4 kb
cDNA	pcCSF-17	p3ACSF-69
Biological activities		
Mouse M-CSA	++	++
Human M-CSA	+	+
Human monocyte- stimulating activity	−	++

We are now conducting clinical phase II/III studies
on hM-CSF to evaluate whether the administration of hM-CSF
accelerate the recovery from leukocytopenia after anticancer chemotherapy or bone marrow transplantation.

REFERENCES

Clark SC, Kamen R (1987). The human hematopoietic colony-
stimulating factor. Science 236:1229-1237.

Das SK, Stanley ER, Guilbert LJ, Forman LW (1981). Human
CSF-1 radioimmunoassay: Resolution of three subclasses
of human CSFs. Blood 58:630-641.

Hatake K, Motoyoshi K, Ishizaka Y, Takaku F, Miura Y (1985)
Purification of human urinary colony-stimulating factor
by high performance liquid chromatography. J Chromato
344:339-344.

Ishizaka Y, Motoyoshi K, Hatake K, Saito M, Takaku F, Miura
Y (1986). Mode of action of human urinary colony-stimulating factor. Exp Hemato 14:1-8.

Kasahara T, Mukaida N, Hatake K, Motoyoshi K, Kawai T,
Shioiri-Nakano K (1985). IL-1-dependent lymphokine produc-

tion by human leukemic T cell line HBS. 2 subclones. J Immunol 134:1682–1689.

Kawasaki ES, Ladner MB, Wang AM, Arsdell JV, Warren MK, Coyne MY, Schweickart VL, Lee MT, Wilson KJ, Boosman A, Stanley ER, Ralph P, Mark DF (1985). Molecular cloning of a cDNA encoding human CSF-1. Science 230:291–296.

Motoyoshi K, Takaku F, Mizoguchi H, Miura Y (1978). Purification of human urinary colony-stimulating factor from human urine. Blood 52:1012–1020.

Motoyoshi K, Kusumoto K, Takaku F, Miura Y (1982). GM-colony stimulating and binding activities of purified human urinary CSF to murine and human bone marrow cells. Blood 60: 1378–1386.

Motoyoshi K, Takaku F, Miura Y (1983). Regulatory mechanism of granulopoiesis in the bone marrow of CSF-producing tumor-bearing nude mice. Blood 62:980–987.

Motoyoshi K, Takaku F, Maekawa T, Miura Y, Kimura K, Furusawa S, Hattori M, Nomura T, Mizoguchi H, Ogawa M, Kinugasa K, Tominaga T, Shimoyama M, Deura K, Ohta K, Taguchi T, Masaoka T, Kimura I (1986). Protective effect of partially purified human urinary colony-stimulating factor on granulocytopenia after antitumor chemotherapy. Exp Hemato 14: 1069–1075.

Motoyoshi K (1987). Purification, gene cloning and clinical application of human monocyte specific colony-stimulating factor. Acta Haemato Jpn 50, (in press).

Warren MK, Ralph P (1986). Macrophage growth factor CSF-1 stimulates human monocyte production of IFN, TNF and CSA. J Immunol 137:2281–2285.

Wong GG, Temple PA, Leary AC, Witek-Gianotti JS, Yang YC, Ciarletta AB, Chung M, Murtha P, Kriz R, Kaufman RJ, Ferenz CR, Sibley BS, Turner KJ, Hewick RM, Clark SC, Yanai N, Yokota H, Yamada M, Saito M, Motoyoshi K, Takaku F (1987). Human CSF-1: Molecular cloning and expression of a 4 kb cDNA encoding the hematopoietin and determination of the complete amino acid sequence of the human urinary protein. Science 235:1504–1508.

Monokines and Other Non-Lymphocytic Cytokines, pages 307–312
© 1988 Alan R. Liss, Inc.

TRANSFORMING GROWTH FACTOR β: A SELECTIVE GROWTH INHIBITOR
FOR HEMATOPOIETIC PROGENITOR CELLS

Francis Ruscetti, Garwin Sing, Larry Ellingsworth,
Sandra Ruscetti and Jonathan Keller

National Cancer Institute (F.R., G.S.), Program
Resources, Inc. (J.K.) Frederick, MD, Collagen
Corp., Palo Alto, CA (L.E.) and National Cancer
Institute, Bethesda, MD (S.R.)

Transforming growth factor β (TGF-β) belongs to a
family of protein growth factors that regulate growth and
differentiation of many cell types (Sporn et. al., 1986).
TGF-β is a 25-Kd disulfide-linked homodimeric protein whose
sequence is remarkedly conserved with only a single amino
acid difference between mouse and man. Recently, a second
form of TGF-β, now known TGF-β2, was identified in bovine
bone (Ellingsworth et. al., 1986). It shares significant
amino acid homology (70%) to the first type of TGF-β, now
known as TGF-β1. TGF-β1 and TGF-β2 have been shown to be
equally potent in a variety of assay systems (Massague,
1986). Immunohistochemical studies using antibodies to the
N-terminus of TGF-β1 showed that TGF-β1 is locally produced
by cells in centers of active hematopoiesis (fetal liver and
bone marrow). Platelets at 2 mg TGF-β/kg and bone at 0.2 mg
TGF-β/kg are the two most abundant sources. These findings
suggest that TGF-β is involved in regulating hematopoiesis.

In general, two techniques have been used to study hemopoietic cell growth and differentiation in vitro: (1) the
measurement of cell number and type in suspension culture
and (2) colony formation by different cell types in semi-
solid media. Both assays depend on adding exogenous humoral
factors for growth stimulation (Burgess and Metcalf, 1980).
Factors used here include granulocyte-macrophage (GM-CSF),
granulocyte (G-CSF) or macrophage (CSF-1) colony stimulating factors, which induce terminal maturation of the cell
types for which they are named, and erythropoietin (Epo),
which induces end-stage erythroid maturation. Also,
interleukin-3 (IL-3), which induces multipotential bone

marrow colony formation (CFU_{GEMM}) consisting of granulocytes, erythroid cells, monocytes and megakaryocytes, was
used. TGF-β1 is a potent inhibitor of IL-3 induced murine
bone marrow proliferation and colony formation but, surprisingly, has little or no effect on the growth and differentiation induced by GM-CSF, G-CSF or CSF-1 (Table 1).
TGF-β1 also inhibits early erythroid differentiation stimulated by Epo in the GEMM assay while Epo-induced terminal
erythroid differentiation is unaffected (data not shown).
Also, IL-3 but not GM-CSF induced granulocyte-macrophage
colonies were inhibited. However, small clusters (5-20
cells) of terminally differentiated pure myeloid colonies
were consistently seen in cultures containing IL-3 and
TGF-β1. These results suggest that TGF-β1 selectively
inhibits early murine hematopoietic progenitor growth and
differentiation but not more mature progenitors (Keller
et al., 1988). These inhibitory effects of TGF-β are at
least partially reversible and non-toxic, since cell
viability was not effected and colony formation was restored by 50% after washing out TGF-β1.

TABLE 1. Effect of TGF-β on Murine Bone Marrow Proliferation
and Colony Formation

Stimulator	Marrow Cell Proliferation (^{3}H-Thymidine Uptake)	Colony Formation GEMM (Colony Number)	GM	G	M
None	0	0	0	0	0
IL-3	+	0	+	+	+
IL-3 + TGF-β	0	0	0	+/-	+/-
IL-3 + EPO	ND	+	+	+	+
IL-3 + EPO + TGF-β	ND	0	0	+/-	+/-
GM-CSF	+	0	+	+	+
GM-CSF + TGF-β	+	0	+	+	+/-
G-CSF	+	0	0	+	0
G-CSF + TGF-β	+	0	0	+	0

Since these data suggest that TGF-β has a selective role in regulating hematopoietic progenitor populations, a variety of IL-3 dependent progenitor cell lines which represent leukemic myeloid cell lines blocked at various stages of differentiation based on phenotype, function, and morphology were tested for their TGF-β sensitivity. In all cases tested, TGF-β1 inhibits the growth of IL-3 induced cell lines such as FDC-P1 and DA-1 (Table 2). The effective dose that resulted in 50% of maximal stimulation (ED-50) was simliar for all cell lines. This inhibitory effect was consistently observed among other IL-3 dependent cell lines regardless of their derivation. In addition to responding to IL-3, one cell line, NSF-60, proliferates in response to GM-CSF, CSF-1, G-CSF, and interleukin-4. Growth factor-induced proliferation of NFS-60 is also inhibited by TGF-β1 in a dose-dependent manner with ED-50's of 6-10 pM. Since normal marrow cell growth and differentiation stimulated by GM-CSF and G-CSF were not inhibited by TGF-β, these results with NSF-60 suggest that the state of differentiation of a cell and not the growth factor responsiveness determines whether TGF-β will have an inhibitory effect.

Table 2. Effect of TGF-β on Proliferation of Myeloid Leukemic Cell Lines

Cells	Stimulator(s)	TGF-β1 Growth Inhibition [ED-50 (pM)]
FDC-P1	IL-3, GM-CSF	8-24
B6 Sut A	IL-3	15-20
DA-1	IL-3	10-20
32D cl 23	IL-3	8-16
NFS-60	IL-3, GM-CSF, IL-4 G-CSF, CSF-1	10-60
Bone Marrow	IL-3	20-40
Bone Marrow	GM-CSF, G-CSF	none

We next sought to extend these observations on the
effect of TGF-β to human bone marrow growth. In contrast to
the mouse, both human IL-3 and GM-CSF promoted the proliferation and differentiation in the presence of Epo of multi-
potent colonies <u>in vitro</u>, CFU$_{GEMM}$. Colony formation assays
were performed to determine if TGF-β had an effect on the
formation of these early hematopoietic colonies (Table 3).
In the presence of TGF-β1, only pure small clusters of either
differentiated granulocytes or monocytes were observed (Sing
et al., 1988).   Therefore, TGF-β1 blocks the growth and differentiation of early human hematopoietic progenitors while
allowing clusters (less than 20 cells) of more differentiated
progeny to develop. Also, GM colony formation induced by IL-3
and GM-CSF was inhibited by TGF-β1. However, as in the mouse,
G-CSF induced colony formation was not inhibited by TGF-β.
In our hands, TGF-β1 and TGF-β2 had identical effects at
similar doses in all these assays. Therefore, TGF-β1 and
TGF-β2 suppress the growth and differentiation of early
growth factor-mediated events but are inactive on late acting
growth factor-mediated myeloid and erythroid responses.

TABLE 3. Effect of TGF-β on Human Bone Marrow Proliferation
and Colony Formation

Stimulator	Marrow Cell Proliferation (^{3}H-Thymidine Uptake)	Colony Formation GEMM (Colony Number)	GM	G	M
None	0	0	0	0	0
IL-3	+	0	+	+	+
IL-3 + TGF-β	0	0	0	+	+
IL-3/GM-CSF + EPO	ND	+	+	+	+
IL-3/GM-CSF + EPO + TGF-β	ND	0	0	+	+
GM-CSF	+	0	+	+	+
GM-CSF + TGF-β	0	0	0	+	+
G-CSF	+	0	0	+	0
G-CSF + TGF-β	+	0	0	+	0

A recent report states that TGF-β1 inhibits IL-3 mediated hematopoietic responses but that TGF-β2 does not (Ohta et al., 1987). Since we had never observed any difference between β1 and β2 in our hematopoietic assays, the biological activty of TGF-β1s and TGF-β2s purified from both bovine bone and porcine platelets were compared. All four purified samples have identical biological potencies in standard TGF-β assays. Under all conditions presented above, TGF-β1 and TGF-β2 were equally potent in selectively inhibiting hematopoiesis.

Thus, the inhibitory effect of TGF-βs on hematopoietic cells appears to be a function of the state of cellular differentiation, such that as erythroid and myeloid cells undergo maturation there is a stage at which they become insensitive to the growth inhibitory effect of TGF-β. The resistance to the inhibitory action of TGF-β1 could be due either to a change in the affinity or the number of TGF-β receptors or a change in the cellular or genetic functions mediated by TGF-β. Experiments have been initiated to distinguish between these possibilities.

Since both murine and human leukemic cells have been shown to maintain growth factor responsiveness in vitro, a loss of negative growth control might contribute to a preleukemic state by permitting the unrestrained growth of factor dependent leukemic clones. Such a process could result in the out-growth of IL-3 dependent myeloid leukemic progenitor cells. In fact, this study indicates that at least in the case of the growth of IL-3 dependent leukemic cells in vitro, myeloid leukemic cells can remain sensitive to TGF-β inhibition. This effect is independent of the growth factor used to signal growth, suggesting that the state of differentiation of a cell determines its sensitivity to TGF-β1. The capacity to selectively inhibit early marrow cell growth could have clinical applications. If TGF-B growth-arrested marrow stem cells are less sensitive to the toxic effects of chemotherapeutic agents particularly cell cycle active drugs, TGF-β could be a valuable component of cancer treatment programs that have dose-limiting myelotoxicity. If some hematopoietic tumors are more sensitive in vivo to actions of TGF-β1 than normal cells, TGF-β could be a useful adjunct to cytoreductive combination chemotherapy. Experiments to evaluate these potential therapeutic applications of TGF-β1 in pre-clinical models are underway.

REFERENCES

Burgess AW, Metcalf D (1980). The nature and action of granulocyte-macrophage colony stimulating factors. Blood 56:947.

Keller JR, Mantel C, Sing G, Ellingsworth LE, Ruscetti SK, Ruscetti FW (1988) Transforming growth factor $\beta 1$ selectively regulates early murine hematopoietic progenitors and inhibits the growth of IL-3 dependent myeloid leukemia cell lines. Submitted.

Massaque J (1987). The TGF-β family of growth and differentiation factors. Cell 49:437.

Ohta M, Greenberger JS, Anklesaria P, Bassols A, Massaque J (1987). Two forms of transforming factor-β distinguished by multipotential haemnopoietic progenitor cells. Nature 329:539.

Seyedin S, Thomas T, Thompson A, Rosen D, Piez K (1985). Purification and characterization of two cartilage inducing factors form bovine demineralized bone. Proc Natl Acad Sci USA 82:2267.

Sing G, Keller JR, Ellingworth LE, Ruscetti FW (1988) Transforming Growth Factor β selectively inhibits normal and leukemic human bone marrow growth in vitro. Submitted.

Sporn MB, Roberts AB, Lalage MW, Assoian MA, (1986) Transforming growth factor-β: Biological function and chemical structure. Science 233:532.

ACKNOWLEDGEMENTS

By acceptance of this article, the publisher or recipient acknowledges the right of the U.S. Government to retain a nonexclusive, royalty-free license in and to any copyright covering the article.

This project has been funded at least in part with Federal funds from the Department of Health and Human Services under contract number NO1-CO-74102. The content of this publication does not necessarily reflect the views or policies of the Department of Health and Human Services, or organizations imply endorsement by the U.S. Government.

Monokines and Other Non-Lymphocytic Cytokines, pages 313–316
© 1988 Alan R. Liss, Inc.

TRANSFORMING GROWTH FACTOR-β INDUCES PERSISTENT AND COORDINATE INCREASE IN COLLAGENS TYPE I AND III AND FIBRONECTIN GENE EXPRESSION

John Varga, Joel Rosenbloom, and Sergio A. Jimenez

Department of Medicine, Thomas Jefferson University (JV and SAJ) and School of Dental Medicine, University of Pennsylvania (JR), Philadelphia, PA

INTRODUCTION

Cytokines are capable of influencing the production of connective tissue macromolecules. For example, interferons inhibit collagen synthesis by cultured dermal fibroblasts (Jimenez et.al., 1974). Other less well characterized factors from activated mononuclear cells have been shown to stimulate or inhibit fibroblast production of connective tissue macromolecules in vitro (Freundlich et al., 1976).

Human fibrotic diseases such as scleroderma are characterized by the excessive tissue accumulation of collagen, fibronectin and other connective tissue macromolecules. Fibroblasts from patients with such diseases continue to synthesize increased amounts of collagen in vitro (LeRoy,1974). Mononuclear cell infiltrates have been frequently demonstrated in areas of active fibrogenesis in patients with fibrotic conditions. Products of inflamatory cells may act as signals to stimulate connective tissue macromolecule production by the neighboring fibroblasts and thus play an important role in the initiation or progression of pathological fibrogenesis (Jimenez, 1983). To date, however, no such stimulatory factor has been definitely identified.

Transforming growth factor-β (TGF-β) is a 25kD peptide widely distributed in different tissues and cells including T cells, monocytes and platelets (Sporn et.al., 1987). TGF-β has profound influences on cell proliferation, differentiation and immune regulation; the mechanism of these actions is currently poorly understood. TGF-β is a potent chemotactic agent for fibroblasts (Postlethwaite et.al.,1987) and causes prompt increase in connective tissue formation and angiogenesis <u>in vivo</u> (Roberts et.al., 1986).

In the experiments described below, we investigated the possibility that TGF-β may be capable of stimulating the production of connective tissue macromolecules by normal human dermal fibroblasts in culture and examined the mechanism of such interactions.

MATERIALS AND METHODS

Highly purified human and porcine platelet-derived TGF-β was used. The production of collagen, fibronectin and glycosaminoglycans by human normal dermal fibroblast cultures was assayed by quantitating the incorporation of radiolabeled precursors into media and cell layer macromolecules and by measuring their mRNA levels. For determination of steady-state mRNA levels, total cellular RNA was extracted and dot-hybridized to specific cloned cDNA probes for Types I and III collagens and fibronectin.

RESULTS AND DISCUSSION

TGF-β caused a dose-dependent stimulation of the production of total protein and collagen by confluent cell cultures independently of proliferation (Fig. 1). Processing of newly synthesized procollagens was accelerated (Varga and Jimenez 1986).

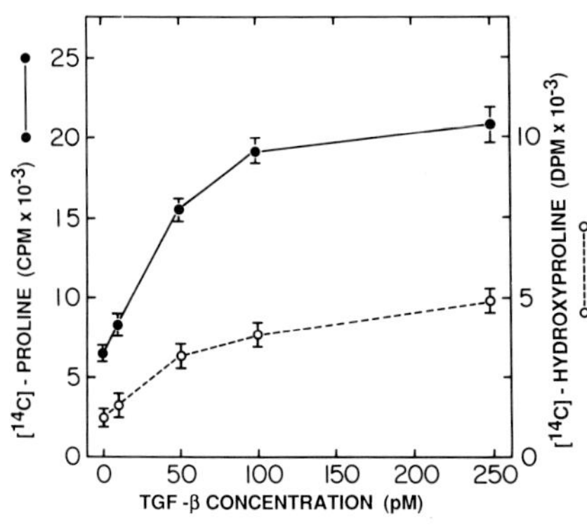

Figure 1. Dose-response of stimulation of fibroblast protein and collagen synthesis.(reproduced by permission)

Fibronectin and glycosaminoglycan synthesis was also increased. Variable but consistent stimulation was noted in the media and cell layer compartments of each of five normal human dermal fibroblast cell lines examined. Stimulation of collagen and fibronectin persisted for at least 72 h following the removal of TGF-β from the cultures. We examined the effect of TGF-β on the steady state amounts of mRNAs for collagens Type I, Type III and fibronectin. Treatment of several normal cell lines with TGF-β resulted in elevated levels of specific RNA transcripts for these macromolecules (Fig. 2). The level of Type I and III collagen mRNAs increased two- to three-fold in a coordinate manner while fibronectin mRNA increased up to eight-fold. The elevated amounts of mRNA for each of these macromolecules persisted for up to 72h following the removal of TGF-β from the cultures (Fig. 3). Our data did not allow us to determine whether stimulation occurs via transcriptional enhancement or post-transcriptional regulation.

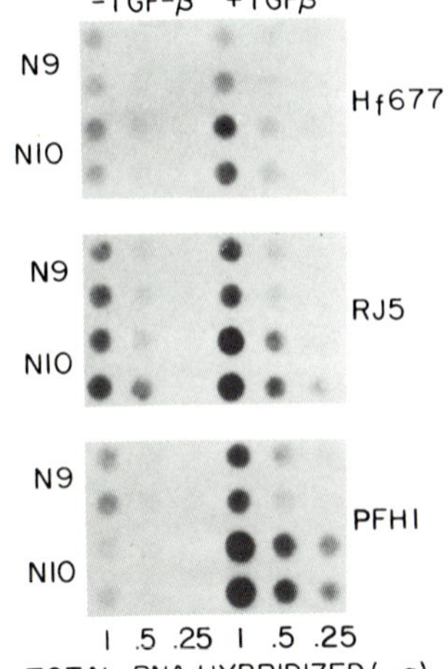

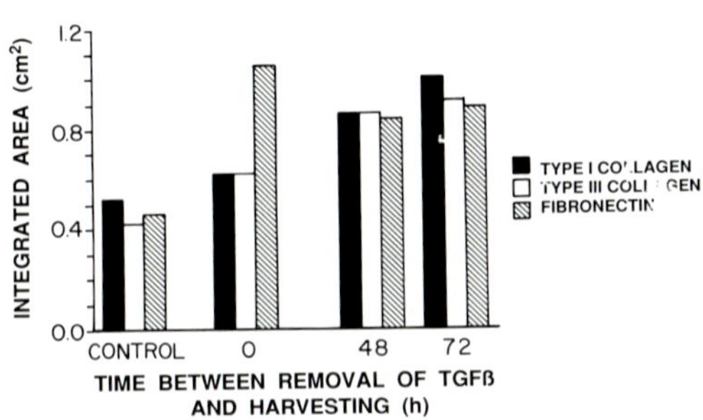

Figure 3. Persistence of elevated steady-state amounts for Types I and III collagen and fibronectin mRNAs after removal of TGF-β. (re-printed by permission)

Figure 2. Dot-blot hybridization with human cDNA probes specific for Type I collagen (Hf 677), Type III collagen (RJ5), and fibronectin (pFH1) of RNA isolated from untreated and TGF-β-treated normal fibroblasts. (reprinted by permission)

TGF-β enhances the formation of extracellular matrix by several mechanisms. We now show that a primary effect of

TGF-β is a potent stimulation of the production of collagen, fibronectin and glycosaminoglycan, as well as accelerated processing of newly synthesized procollagen. We suggest that TGF-β may play a major role in abnormal fibrogenesis associated with human fibrotic diseases.

REFERENCES

Freundlich B, Bomalaski JB, Neilson E, Jimenez SA (1986) Regulation of Fibroblast Proliferation and Collagen Synthesis by Cytokines. Immunology Today. 7:303-307.

Jimenez SA (1983) Cellular Immune Dysfunction and the Pathogenesis of Scleroderma. Semin. Arth. Rheum. 13:104-113.

Jimenez SA, Freundlich B, Rosenbloom J (1984) Selective Inhibition of Human Diploid Fibroblast Synthesis by Interferons. J. Clin. Invest. 74:1112-1116.

LeRoy, EC (1974) Increased Collagen Synthesis by Scleroderma Skin Fibroblasts In Vitro. J. Clin Invest. 54:880-889.

Postlethwaite AE, Keski-Oja J, Moses HL, Kang AH (1987) Stimulation of the Chemotactic Migration of Human Fibroblasts by Transforming Growth Factor-β. J. Exp. Med. 165:251-256.

Roberts AB, Sporn MB, Assoian RK, Smith JM, Roche NS, Wakefield LM, Heine UI, Liotta LA, Falanga V, Kehrl JH, Fauci AS (1986) Transforming Growth Factor Type-b; Rapid Induction of Fibrosis and Angiogenesis in vivo and Stimulation of Collagen Formation in vitro. Proc. Natl. Acad. Sci. USA. 83:4167-4171.

Sporn MB, Roberts AB, Wakefield LM, Assoian RK (1986) Transforming Growth Factor-β; Biological Function and Chemical Structure. Science 233:532-534.

Sporn MB, Roberts AB, Wakefield LM, deCrombrugghe, B (1987) Some Recent Advances in the Chemistry and Biology of Transforming Growth Factor-β. J. Cell Biol. 105:1039-1045.

Varga J, Jimenez SA (1986) Stimulation of Normal Human Fibroblast Collagen Production and Processing by Transforming Growth Factor-β. Biochem. Biophys. Res. Commun. 138:974-980.

Section VI. Cytokine Activities and Interactions In Vivo

Monokines and Other Non-Lymphocytic Cytokines, pages 319–324

INTERLEUKIN 1'S ROLE IN THE INCREASED VASCULAR PERMEABILITY OF INFLAMMATION

Gail S. Habicht and Gregory Beck

Department of Pathology, State University of New York at Stony Brook, Stony Brook, New York 11794

Acute inflammation can be initiated by a variety of stimuli including biological, chemical and physical injury. In the skin, inflammation is characterized by immediate hyperemia and an increase in vascular permeability, mainly in the venules. Margination and adhesion of leukocytes are followed by emigration of these cells into the tissue spaces where neutrophils phagocytose particles and discharge the contents of their granules. Once the injurious stimulus is removed the process of tissue repair begins.

A great diversity of stimuli can initiate the acute inflammatory response. However, the constancy of the response suggests that a common endogenous mediator (or mediators) orchestrates it. We have proposed that interleukin 1 is a major endogenous mediator of the acute inflammatory response. We have previously shown that IL-1 injected into rabbit skin produces an acute inflammatory lesion which was followed by monitoring the migration of ^{51}Cr labeled neutrophils into the inflamed tissue (Habicht and Beck, 1985; Beck, et al., 1986). In this report we show that IL-1 is also capable of producing an increase in vascular permeability, a first step in inflammation.

Classic studies have shown that increased vascular permeability may occur with one of three temporal patterns (Wilhelm, 1973). The immediate transient response occurs within minutes of stimulation, reaches a peak within 10-25 minutes and then wanes. This increase has been shown to be mediated by histamine-like permeability factors. Inflammation, however, is characterized by much longer

periods of increased vascular permeability. In immediate
sustained leakage, vascular permeability increases rapidly
and remains high. This occurs when there is severe tissue
damage such as burns or crushing injuries. In the third
pattern there is an interval between injury and increased
vascular permeability but the leakage may continue for hours
or even days. However, many inflammatory stimuli induce a
combination of the transient and sustained vascular
permeability changes resulting in a biphasic pattern of
increased vascular leakage. While histamine has been shown
to mediate the transient phase, an endogenous mediator of
the sustained phase has not yet been identified.

MATERIALS AND METHODS

     Several different IL-1 containing preparations were
used. Murine IL-1 was partially purified from spirochete
stimulated P388D1 cell supernatants by gel sieve column
chromatography (Habicht, et al., 1985). A crude preparation
of human IL-1 was derived from concentrated, <u>Bacillus
subtilis</u> stimulated U937 supernatants. Natural human alpha
and beta IL-1s were purified by gel sieve chromatography,
chromatofocusing and HPLC gel filtration. Further studies
were done with human recombinant IL-1 alpha and beta
obtained as gifts from the Dainippon Company and Dr. C.A.
Dinarello, respectively. IL-1 was diluted in pyrogenfree
saline and injected intradermally in a volume of 0.1 ml into
shaved rabbit skin. To determine any change in vascular
permeability, BSA, iodinated using Iodobeads and ^{125}I
was injected into the marginal ear vein 15 minutes before
sacrifice as described previously (Habicht and Beck, 1987).
Skin on the back was removed and blood in the large vessels
was expelled by pushing it to the edge. Skins were frozen
at -70 C, lesions were punched out with a 1.5 cm steel
punch, and radioactivity in the tissue sample was
determined.

RESULTS AND DISCUSSION

     Partially purified murine IL-1 (20 U) was injected
intradermally into shaved rabbit backs at various times
ranging from 1 to 255 minutes before sacrifice in order to
determine the kinetics of the inflammatory response as
measured by changes in vascular permeability. Murine IL-1

produced a biphasic response. An increase was seen within 5
minutes which peaked by 25 minutes and then waned. This was
followed by another increase lasting at least 4 hours.
Human IL-1 containing supernatants produced virtually the
same biphasic pattern of increased vascular permeability.
It is unlikely that these changes were due to contaminating
endotoxin in that LPS produced only a single peak of
increased permeability midway between the transient and
sustained peaks.

It has been shown by others that the immediate
transient phase of increased vascular permeability following
an inflammatory stimulus is mediated by histamine or
histamine-like factors (Wilhelm, 1973). In order to
determine the role of histamine in the response to IL-1
injection, rabbits were pretreated with intravenous
injections of 0.1 mg/kg promethazine at 285 and 35 minutes
prior to sacrifice. The response to histamine was totally
abrogated by promethazine. However, in the response to both
murine and human IL-1 containing supernatants only the first
phase of increased vascular permeability was affected by
antihistamine pretreatment.

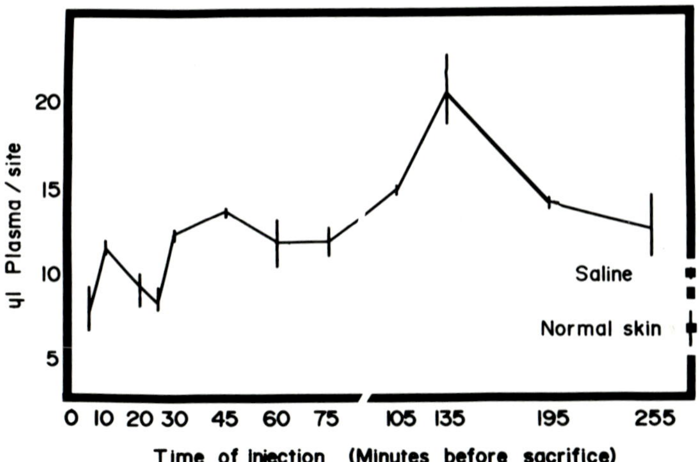

Figure 1. Kinetics of changes in vascular permeability
following intradermal injection of 200 units of human
recombinant interleukin 1 alpha.

We next repeated the studies of altered vascular
permeability using human recombinant IL-1 alpha. Rabbits
were injected with 200 units/site at various times ranging

from 5 to 255 minutes prior to sacrifice. The kinetics of
the response to human recombinant IL-1 alpha are shown in
Figure 1. There was no immediate, transient peak: only the
delayed sustained phase of increased permeability was
observed with a peak at 2 1/4 hours. Thus, local IL-1 alpha
production could account for the sustained phase of
increased vascular permeability in acute inflammation.
However, these data led to the conlusion that a factor other
than IL-1 alpha in the IL-1 containing supernatants was
responsible for the immediate transient phase of increased
vascular permeability.

Both IL-1 beta and TNF are likely to be found in the
monocyte derived IL-1 preparations. To investigate whether
these molecules might be responsible for the transient
phase, rabbits were give intradermal injections of human
recombinant monokines and sacrificed 25 minutes later, a
time at which the transient phase of increased vascular
permeability reaches a peak. Data in Table 1 show that
neither human recombinant IL-1 beta, human recombinant TNF
alpha, nor a combination of IL-1 and TNF could mimic the
monocyte derived preparations of IL-1 in producing the
transient phase. Further studies in which rabbits were
sacrificed at 2 1/4 hours after intradermal injection, the
peak of the delayed, sustained phase of increased vascular
permeability, showed that highly purified natural IL-1 alpha
and beta performed as well as crude IL-1 and recombinant
IL-1 alpha in inducing this phase. Taken together, these
data suggested that while IL-1 mediates the delayed,
sustained phase of increased vascular permeability, another
monocyte derived factor is responsible for the transient
phase. We have shown that such a factor can be isolated
from B. subtilis stimulated U937 supernatants (Beck and
Habicht, this volume). It has a molecular weight of
approximately 40,000 daltons and isoelectric points of 4.9
and 8.0 by chromatofocusing. It has been tentatively called
macrophage derived vasopermeability factor (MVPF). MVPF has
no activity in either IL-1 or TNF bioassays.

We conclude that IL-1 is a major endogenous mediator of
acute inflammation. IL-1 mediates changes in vascular
permeability and is chemotactic for neutrophils in vivo
(Habicht and Beck, 1985; Beck, et al., 1986). There are
several cell types in the skin capable of producing IL-1:
keratinocytes, Langerhans cells, monocytes, macrophages and
endothelial cells (Dinarello, 1985). It may be calculated

that there are sufficient numbers of IL-1 producing cells in
the skin to account for an IL-1 mediated inflammatory
response (Habicht and Beck, 1985). In addition, IL-1
production and release occur rapidly enough to account for
the kinetics of the sustained phase of increased vascular
permeability. Bodel (1970), Matsushima, et al., (1986) and
we (unpublished) have shown that IL-1 can be detected in
macrophage supernatants as early as 30 minutes after
stimulation and that a peak in release occurs at two hours.

TABLE 1. Recombinant Human Monokines Do Not Mediate the
Immediate Transient Phase of Increased Vascular Permeability
in Acute Inflammation

Intradermal injection	ul plasma/site
U937 Supernatant	$111.0 + 1.5^{a,b}$
H r IL-1 alpha	17.4 + 2.4
H r IL-1 beta	18.9 + 0.8
H r TNF alpha	20.0 + 0.4
H r IL-1 beta + TNF alpha	22.2 + 1.6
Saline	19.4 + 3.1
Normal skin	20.1 + 0.4

[a] Mean + S.E.; [b] $p < 0.001$ compared to normal skin.

     IL-1 has several other activities which are consonant
with its being a mediator of local inflammatory changes. It
increases endothelial cell adhesiveness for neutrophils
(Bevilaqua, et al., 1985) and mediates their extravasation.
It is chemotactic for mononuclear cells (Miossec, et al.,
1986). IL-1 may also participate in the resolution of the
inflammatory injury. It promotes tissue remodeling and
repair by stimulating fibroblast proliferation, by causing
collagenase production by these cells and by promoting
vascular smooth muscle growth (Dinarello, 1985).

ACKNOWLEDGMENTS

These studies were supported by NIH Grant AR 36028.

REFERENCES

Beck G, Habicht GS, Benach JL, Miller F (1986). Interleukin
  1: A common endogenous mediator of inflammation and the
  local Shwartzman reaction. J Immunol 136:3025-3031.
Bevilaqua MP, Pober JS, Wheeler ME, Cotran RS, Gimbrone MA
  Jr (1985). Interleukin-1 acts on cultured human vascular
  endothelium to increase the adhesion of polymorphonuclear
  cell leukocytes, monocytes, and related leukocyte cell
  lines. J Clin Invest 76:2003-2011.
Bodel P (1970). Studies on the mechanism of endogenous
  pyrogen production I. Investigation of new protein
  synthesis in stimulated human blood leukocytes. Yale J
  Biol Med 43:145-163.
Dinarello CA (1985) An update on human interleukin-1: from
  molecular biology to clinical relevance. J Clin Immunol
  5:287-297.
Habicht GS, Beck G (1985). IL-1 is an endogenous mediator
  of acute inflammation and of the local Shwartzman reaction
  in The Physiologic, Metabolic, and Immunologic Actions of
  Interleukin-1 Kluger MJ, Oppenheim JJ, Powanda MC, eds.
  Alan R. Liss, Inc., New York pp 12-23.
Habicht GS, Beck G (1987). The role of interleukin-1 in
  increased vascular permeability in inflammation in
  Leukocyte Emigration and Its Sequelae Movat HZ, ed.
  Karger, Basel pp 51-54.
Habicht GS, Beck G, Benach JL, Coleman JL, Leichtling KD
  (1985). Lyme disease spirochetes induce human and murine
  interleukin 1 production. J Immunol 134:3147-3154.
Hurley JV (1983) Acute Inflammation Churchill Livingstone,
  Edinburgh pp 29-63.
Matsushima K, Taguchi M, Kovacs EJ, Young HA, Oppenheim, JJ
  (1986). Intracellular localization of human monocyte
  associated interleukin 1 (IL 1) and release of
  biologically active IL 1 from monocytes by trypsin and
  plasmin. J Immunol 136:2883-2891.
Miossec P, Dinarello CA, Ziff M (1986). Interleukin-1
  lymphocyte chemotactic activity in rheumatoid arthritis
  synovial fluid. Arthritis Rheum. 29:461-470.
Wilhelm DL (1973) Chemical mediators in The Inflammatory
  Process, Vol 2, Zweifach BW, Grant L, McCluskey RT, eds.
  Academic Press, New York pp 251-301.

Monokines and Other Non-Lymphocytic Cytokines, pages 325–328

ISOLATION AND CHARACTERIZATION OF A VASCULAR PERMEABILITY FACTOR FROM STIMULATED U937 CELLS.

Gregory Beck and Gail S. Habicht

Department of Pathology, State University
of New York at Stony Brook, Stony Brook, NY 11794

INTRODUCTION

Acute inflammation is characterized by at least 3
stages: changes in vascular caliber, increased vascular
permeability, and migration of PMNs into extravascular
spaces (Hurley, 1983). We have previously shown interleukin
1 (IL-1) to be a common endogenous mediator of acute
inflammation and the local Shwartzman reaction (Beck et al.
1986). In another study, IL-1 was found to be capable of
causing changes in vascular permeability (Habicht and Beck,
1987). These studies suggested to us that other macrophage
products may be involved in acute inflammation as well. To
this end we have isolated a factor released by stimulated
macrophages that can induce the immediate transient phase of
vascular leakage. We call it macrophage-derived vascular
permeability factor (MVPF).

MATERIALS AND METHODS

Bovine serum albumin (BSA, Sigma, St. Louis, MO) was
iodinated using Iodo-Beads (Pierce Chem. Co., Rockford, IL)
and Iodine-125 (1 mCi, >350 mCi/ml; New England Nuclear,
Boston, MA). The ^{125}I-BSA had a specific activity of 1
uCi/ug. Preparation and handling of rabbits and intradermal
injections of experimental agents and controls for increased
vascular permeability activity were as described in detail
previously (Habicht & Beck, 1987; Beck et al, 1986).
Fifteen minutes before sacrifice ^{125}I-BSA was injected
into the marginal ear vein. The skin on the backs was
removed, and the blood in the large veins was expelled by

pushing it to the edge. The skin was frozen at -70 C and
the lesions were punched out with a 1.5 cm steel punch. A
sample of blood removed 5 min before sacrifice was used to
measure the amount of ^{125}I-BSA in 1 ul of serum.
Samples were assayed for IL-1 activity with thymocytes from
4 to 8 week old BALB/c mice, as previously described (Beck
et al, 1986). In all assays significance of differences was
assessed by Student's t-test.

The human histiocytic tumor cell line U937 (1 X 10^7
cells/ml) was stimulated with sonicated <u>Bacillus subtilis</u>
in RPMI 1640 (10% w/v) in the absence of fetal calf serum.
Forty eight hours later the supernatant was collected by
centrifugation at 3,000 X g, for 15 minutes at 4 C. It was
then concentrated approximately 20 fold with an
ultrafiltration stirred cell equipped with a diaflo
ultrafilter (PM 10, Amicon, Lexington, MA). The crude
concentrate was dialysed against PBS (pH 7.4) which
contained 10 ug/ml of gentamycin.

Samples were applied to an S-200 column (2.6 X 85 cm)
and eluted with PBS at a flow rate of 1.2 ml/min at 4 C.
The effluent was monitored at 280 nm. The samples were
sterilized by filtration (0.22 um; Millipore, Bedford, MA)
and assayed for MVPF activity as described above. Peaks of
activity were pooled and concentrated by ultrafiltration
against a PM 10 ultrafilter. The molecular weight standards
used to calibrate the column were BSA (67,000), ovalbumin
(43,000), chymotrypsinogen A (25,000), and ribonuclease A
(13,700) (Pharmacia, Piscataway, NJ). S-200 column eluates
containing peaks of MVPF activity were applied to a
chromatofocusing column (PBE 94, Pharmacia). The column was
eluted to give a linear pH gradient from pH 8.4 to pH 4.0.
All samples were brought to a pH of approximately 7.2 with
the addition of 4 M Tris base (pH 11). The effluent was
monitored at 280 nm. The column eluates were sterilized by
Millipore filtration (0.22 um) and assayed for IL-1 and MVPF
activity as described above.

RESULTS AND DISCUSSION

Three temporal patterns of vascular leakage during
inflammation have been described. The immediate transient
response occur within minutes, wanes within an hour and is
thought to be due to histamine-like permeability factors.
The immediate sustained reaction is seen after severe

injuries (burns, crushing injuries, chemical agents).
Leakage occurs immediately and may continue unabated for
several hours. The delayed prolonged response is
characterized by delayed leakage. There may be a delay
between injury and leakage, but the leakage can continue for
hours or days (Wilhelm, 1973). Macrophages (and related
cells) found at the site of injuries (Beck et al, 1986)
could contribute to this early phase of inflammation by
releasing factors which mediate changes in vascular
permeability.

When stimulated U937 cell supernatants were
concentrated and injected intradermaly into rabbit backs, a
biphasic pattern of increased vascular permeability was
observed (Figure 1).

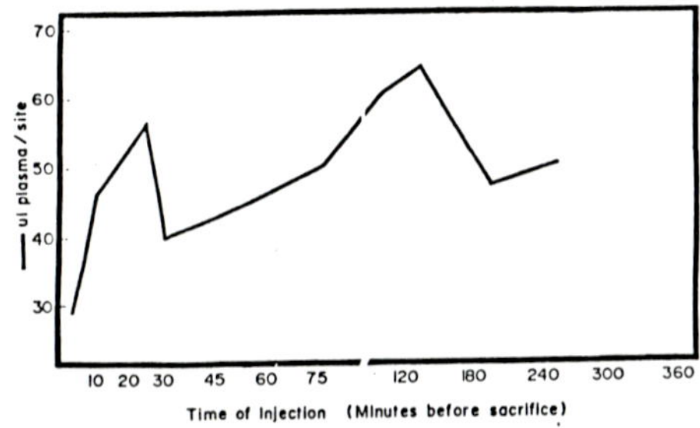

Figure 1. Stimulated U937 cell supernatants caused a
biphasic increase in vascular permeability.

Since these were concentrated supernatants, we were eager to
identify the molecule(s) responsible for this activity. We
found that the second peak of activity was produced by IL-1
(Habicht and Beck, 1987 and Habicht and Beck, this volume).
The material that was found to be active at 20 min (MVPF)
was further characterized. When the supernatants were
fractionated on a gel sieve column, the MVPF activity was
found to have a molecular weight of approximately 40,000.
When the MVPF recovered from the gel sieve column was
concentrated and run over a chromatofocusing column, two
peaks of activity were recovered at pH 8.0 and 4.9.

We were concerned that our samples contained IL-1 that
may have copurified with the MVPF during the chromatography
steps. As seen in Table 1, there was a small amount of IL-1
in the S-200 column fraction, but the activity disappeared
after chromatofocusing.

Table 1. MVPF contains no IL-1 activity

	IL-1 ACTIVITY
	MOUSE THYMOCYTE PROLIFERATION ASSAY
SAMPLE	(^{3}H THYMIDINE; DPM $\pm$ S.E.)

SAMPLE	IL-1 ACTIVITY MOUSE THYMOCYTE PROLIFERATION ASSAY (^{3}H THYMIDINE; DPM $\pm$ S.E.)
RPMI	2,012 $\pm$ 521
S-200 MVPF fraction (m.w. 40,000)	3,876 $\pm$ 321 (a)
S-200 IL-1 fraction (m.w. 20,000)	11,250 $\pm$ 964 (b)
MVPF (pI 8.0)	1,425 $\pm$ 212 (c)
MVPF (pI 4.9)	1,982 $\pm$ 322 (c)

    (a) = p $<$0.2 as compared to RPMI control
    (b) = p $<$0.001 as compared to RPMI control
    (c) = Not significant

The existence of this new monokine shows that
macrophages are able to contribute to the early phases of
the inflammatory response by release of vasoactive agents.
Macrophage induced increases in vascular permeability can
last for up to 6 hrs (MVPF plus IL-1). Studies in progress
show that MVPF is a permeability-increasing substance, and
not a vasodilator. Other activities that this monokine may
possess are currently being investigated.

REFERENCES

Beck G, Habicht GS, Benach JL, Miller F (1986). Interleukin
    1: A common endogenous mediator of inflammation and the
    local Shwartzman reaction. J Immunol 136:3025-3031.
Habicht GS, Beck, G (1987). The role of interleukin 1 in
    increased vascular permeability. In Movat, HZ (ed):
    "Leukocyte Emigration and Its Sequelae,"
    Basel: Karger, pp 51-54.
Hurley JV (1983). "Acute Inflammation." Edinburgh:
    Churchill Livingstone, pp 29-63.
Wilhelm, DL (1973). Chemical mediators. In Zweifach BW,
    Grant L, McCluskey R. (eds): "The Inflammatory Process
    Vol. 2," New York: Academic Press pp 251-301.

Monokines and Other Non-Lymphocytic Cytokines, pages 329–335
© 1988 Alan R. Liss, Inc.

INTERLEUKIN-1 INDUCES CHRONIC GRANULOMATOUS INFLAMMATION

Colin J. Dunn, Marilyn M. Hardee, Anna J. Gibbons,
Nigel D. Staite and Karen A. Richard

Department of Hypersensitivity Diseases Research,
The Upjohn Company, Kalamazoo, Michigan 49001

INTRODUCTION

Several studies indicate that interleukin-1 (IL-1)
induces a transient acute inflammatory response accompanied
by leukocyte accumulation (Beck et al, 1986); Cybulsky et al,
1987), increased vascular permeability (Habicht and Beck,
1987) and an acute phase reaction (Mizel, 1982), which rapidly
resolves. IL-1 has been detected in inflammatory exudates and
shown to be derived from the infiltrating PMN leukocytes
(Yoshinaga et al, 1987). Although IL-1 is also secreted by
mononuclear phagocytes (Mizel, 1982) little information is
available concerning its role in the development of chronic
inflammatory responses, which are characterized by extensive
infiltration of monocytes, activated macrophages, neovascularization and fibrosis.

The studies described below demonstrate that local slow-
release of IL-1 results in the formation of chronic inflammatory granulomatous tissue and suggest that continued micro-
environmental release of this cytokine is sufficient for the
evolution and persistence of chronic inflammatory disease.

METHODS

Female CF-1 mice (25-30 g) from the Upjohn breeding
facility were used throughout.

Slow-release ethylene vinyl acetate (EVA) copolymer
disks were prepared as previously described (Rhine et al,

1980). Recombinant human IL-1 (rhIL-1) was dissolved in
10 mM Tris-glycerol (10%) buffer and incorporated into the
EVA preparation at concentrations of $4x10^2-4x10^4$ U/disk.
Control preparations consisted of buffer alone or bovine
serum albumin (BSA-Sigma) at 2 and 50 mg/disk. rhIL-β was
purified according to Paslay et al, 1987; rhIL-1α was obtained
from Dainippon. Other monokines (rhIL-2; rat rIfnγ Amgen,
CA) were incorporated into EVA at protein concentrations
approximating those for rhIL-1. Specific activities (U/mg
protein) were: rhIL-1α, rhIL-1β=$2x10^7$ U/mg (mouse thymocyte
proliferation); rhIL-2=$0.3x10^7$ U/mg (HT-2 cell proliferation);
rIfnγ=$1x10^7$ U/mg (L-929 cytotoxicity). Endotoxin contamination was assessed using the limulus chromogenic assay
(Whittaker, MD).

Each EVA disk was divided into four and implanted sc.
into the mouse dorsal flank (one quarter disk/mouse).
Implants were removed at different time intervals, fixed in
formalin and stained for histological evaluation. Duplicate
experiments of 4-6 mice/group were carried out.

RESULTS

Lesions induced by sc. EVA-buffer or -BSA (0.5 mg; 12.5
mg/mouse) induced a predominantly fibrotic reaction inter-
spersed with diffuse inflammatory cell infiltrates (fig. 1A).
Endotoxin levels were 15-375 pg for 0.5-12.5 mg BSA.

In contrast, rhIL-1β (10^3-10^4 U/disk) administered sc.
in EVA copolymer resulted in the early formation (4 days)
of inflammatory granuloma tissue consisting of dense monocytic infiltrates mixed with scattered polymorphonuclear
(PMN) leukocytes and neovascularization. This exudative
inflammatory response rapidly developed into well-organized
granulomatous tissue by 7 days, characterized by large vacuolar
activated macrophages, intensification of neovascularization
and diminished PMN accumulation (fig. 1B). These lesions
persisted for at least 21 days at which time scattered
lymphoid cell infiltration and fibrosis was also evident.
Endotoxin levels were 5-50 pg for 10^3-10^4 U rhIL-1β. Although
rhIL-1α induced a similar response it was significantly less
potent than rhIL-1β.

Subcutaneous implantation of EVA-rhIL-2 (10^2-10^4 U/disk)
resulted in the appearance of distinct perivascular lympho-

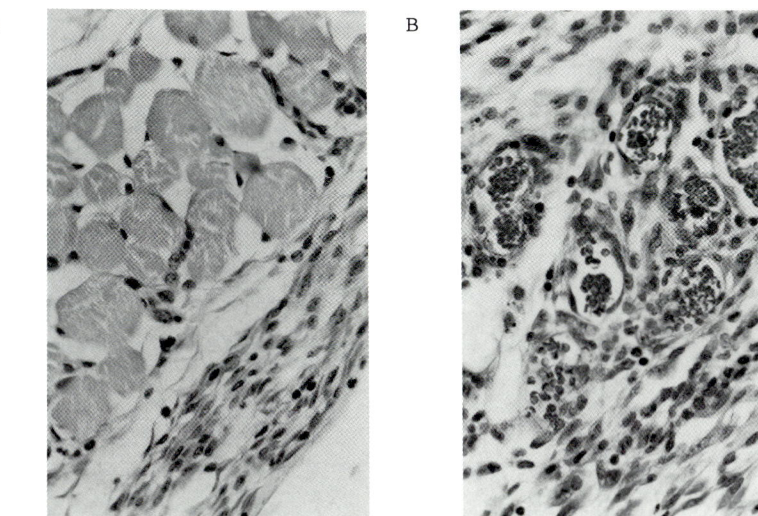

Figure 1. Subcutaneous 7 day lesions induced by EVA-cytokine implants (H&Ex400). A. EVA-BSA (12.5 mg/disk)-note mild fibrotic response with diffuse inflammatory cell infiltrate. B. EVA-rhIL-1β (10^4 U/disk) - development of granulomatous tissue characterized by intense neovascularization, macrophage infiltration and sparse PMN leukocyte accumulation.

cytic foci (4 days) which rapidly progressed by 7 days to a dense "lymphoid" lesion consisting mainly of large lymphocytes, many of which were vacuolar with the appearance of lymphoblasts (fig. 2A). Proliferation, as evidenced by the presence of binucleate cells, was common as was neovascularization. PMN leukocytes were scarce and fibrosis was absent. Multinucleate giant cells bordered the EVA implant.

EVA-rIfnγ (10^3-10^4 U/disk) implants were the least reactive, inducing fibrotic lesions resembling those for EVA-buffer/BSA shown in fig. 1A. Similar responses were observed following EVA-endotoxin (150-1500 pg sc.). The only remarkable feature was the formation of multinucleate giant cells at the tissue-EVA-Ifnγ polymer interface (fig. 2B).

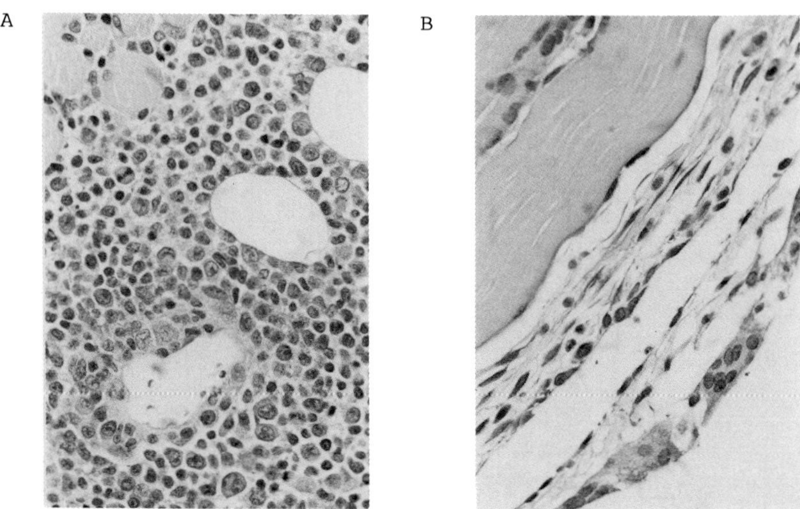

Figure 2. Subcutaneous 7 day lesions induced by EVA-cytokine
implants (H&Ex400). A. EVA-rhIL-2 (10^3 U/disk) - perivascular lymphocytic accumulation associated with dense lymphoid
cell infiltration and large "lymphoblastoid" cells. B. EVA-
rIfnγ (10^4 U/disk) - mild fibrotic response; note presence
of multinucleate giant cells.

DISCUSSION

Although the acute inflammatory effects of IL-1 are well-
established (Beck et al, 1986; Dunn et al, 1987; Cybulsky
et al, 1987) the role of this cytokine has yet to be confirmed
in chronic inflammatory disease. Studies clearly show that
IL-1 is produced by cells involved in chronic inflammation,
such as macrophages (Mizel, 1982) and endothelium (Warner
et al, 1987). In turn, IL-1 augments vascular - leukocyte
adhesion (Dunn and Fleming, 1984) and neovascularization
(Prendergast et al, 1987) via endothelial cell stimulation,
and fibrosis through induction of fibroblast proliferation
(Mizel, 1982). Exudates obtained from chronic inflammatory
disease have been shown to contain significant levels of IL-1
(Wood et al, 1983; Symons et al, 1987; Tracey et al, 1987).
Collectively, these observations suggest that IL-1 has the

potential to induce and perpetuate chronic inflammation.

We have shown that a prolonged local inflammatory reaction
was induced by sc. administration of rhIL-1β from a slow-
release EVA polymer. Predominant monocyte infiltration,
macrophage activation, neovascularization and fibrosis was
observed as early as 4 days post-induction, persisting for
at least 21 days. These features are consistent with those
for chronic granulomatous inflammation and differ markedly
from the acute, PMN-dominated inflammation which resolves
following a single sc. administration of IL-1 (Beck et al,
1986; Cybulsky et al, 1987). The relative paucity of PMN
leukocytes and lack of abcess formation and necrosis indicate
that the response to IL-1 represents true chronic inflammation
rather than "recycling" acute inflammation.

Continual slow-release of IL-1 from EVA polymer was
detected <u>in</u> <u>vitro</u> over a 14 day period (data not shown),
confirming the observations of others (Prendergast et al,
1987). That the response to EVA-rhIL-1β was not due to non-
specific irritation by protein or the EVA copolymer itself
was demonstrated by (i) the mild fibrotic responses to EVA-
buffer and EVA-BSA implants (ii) the dissimilar reactions
induced by rIfnγ (non-inflammatory) and rIL-2 (formation of
lymphoid tissue), monokines of comparable MW and protein
concentration. Also, endotoxin does not appear to have been a
complicating factor since (i) EVA-BSA (12.5 mg/disk) contained
significantly higher levels of endotoxin than EVA-rhIL-1β
but was virtually non-inflammatory (ii) EVA-endotoxin (150-
1500 pg/disk) implants failed to induce significant inflammatory responses.

We conclude that rhIL-1β, and to a lesser degree
rhIL-1α, induces the formation of chronic inflammatory
granulomatous tissue when given in a continual release
form which is qualitatively distinct from lesions induced
by rIfnγ and rIL-2. This model system may be analogous to
prolonged release of endogenous IL-1 by macrophages recruited
to an inflammatory site which determines chronicity of the
lesion. Mechanisms involved could include IL-1 induced
vascular leukocyte adhesion, neovascularization and fibrosis.
IL-1 has recently been shown to stimulate further production
of IL-1 from mononuclear leukocytes (Dinarello et al, 1987)
and endothelium (Warner et al, 1987) which may amplify the
effects of this cytokine and the subsequent development of
chronic inflammation.

REFERENCES

Beck G, Habicht GS, Benach JL, Mille F (1986). Interleukin-1
  A common endogenous mediator of inflammation and the local
  Schwartzman reaction. J. Immun 136:3025-3031.
Cybulsky MI, McComb DJ, Dinarello CA, Movat HZ. Mediation
  by interleukin-1 of neutrophil leukocyte emigration induced
  by endotoxin (1987). In Movat HZ (Ed.) "Leukocyte emigration and its sequelae." Basel, Switzerland: S. Karger, pp
  38-50.
Dinarello CA, Ikejima T, Warner SJC, Orencole SF, Lonnemann
  G, Cannon JG, Libby P (1987). Interleukin-1 induces
  interleukin-1. I. Induction of circulating interleukin-1
  in rabbits in vivo and in human mononuclear cells in vitro
  J. Immun 139:1902-1910.
Dunn CJ, Fleming WE (1984). Increased adhesion of polymorphonuclear leukocytes to vascular endothelium by specific
  interaction of endogenous (interleukin-1) and exogenous
  (lipopolysaccharide) substances with endothelial cells
  in vitro. Eur. J. Rheum Inflam 7:80-86.
Dunn CJ, Schaub RG, Fleming WE, Gibbons AJ (1987). Vascular
  changes induced by interleukin-1 in vivo: scanning electron
  microscopy studies. In Movat HZ (Ed.). "Leukocyte emigration and its sequelae," Basel, Switzerland: S. Karger,
  pp 55-61.
Habicht GS, Beck G. The role of interleukin-1 in vascular
  permeability in inflammation (1987). In Movat HZ, (Ed.)
  "Leukocyte emigration and its sequelae." Basel, Switzerland:
  S. Karger, pp 51-54.
Mizel S. Regulation of immune and inflammatory responses by
  interleukin-1 (1982). Clin Immun Newsletter 3:123-126.
Paslay JW, Yem AW, Carter DB, Tomich C-SC, Curry KA, Tracey
  DE, Deibel MR (1987). Purification and preliminary charact-
  erization of recombinant human interleukin-1β. Fed Proc
  46:(6)2282.
Prendergast RA, Lutty GA, Dinarello CA (1987). Interleukin-1
  induces corneal neovascularization. Fed Proc 46:(4)1200.
Rhine WD, Hsieh DST, Langer R. Polymers for sustained
  macromolecule release: procedures to fabricate reproducible
  delivery systems and control release kinetics (1980). J
  Pharm Sci 69:265-270.
Symons JA, Bundick RV, Suckling AJ, Rumsby MG. Cerebrospinal
  fluid interleukin-like activity during chronic relapsing
  experimental allergic encephalomyelitis. (1987) Clin exp
  Immunol 68:648-654.

Tracey DE, Richard KA, Deibel MR, Hardee MM, Cornette JC, Jeffcoat MK, Williams RC (1987). High levels of interleukin-1 alpha in periodontal crevicular fluids. J. Leuk Biol 42:605.

Warner SJC, Auger KR, Libby P (1987). Interleukin-1 induces interleukin-1. II. Recombinant human interleukin-1 production by adult human vascular endothelial cells. J Immun 139:1911-1917.

Wood DD, Ihrie EJ, Dinarello CA, Cohen PL. Isolation of an interleukin-1 like factor from human joint effusions (1983). Arthritis Rheum 26:975-983.

Yoshinaga M, Goto F, Goto K, Ohkawara S, Kiramura M, Mori S, (1987). Triggering of polymorphonuclear leukocytes to produce interleukin-1 at the inflammatory site. In Movat HZ, (Ed.). "Leukocyte emigration and its sequelae," Basel, Switzerland: S. Karger, pp 169-180.

Monokines and Other Non-Lymphocytic Cytokines, pages 337–342
© 1988 Alan R. Liss, Inc.

INTERLEUKIN-1 AND TUMOR NECROSIS FACTOR DEPRESS CYTOCHROME P-450 DEPENDENT LIVER DRUG METABOLISM IN MICE

Pietro Ghezzi,Riccardo Bertini, Marina Bianchi, Annalaura Erroi, Pia Villa and Alberto Mantovani.

Istituto di Ricerche Farmacologiche "Mario Negri", Via Eritrea 57, Milano,Italy 20157.

INTRODUCTION

Cytochrome P-450-dependent mixed function oxidases, (also known as drug metabolizing enzymes) are a family of enzymes involved in the metabolism of foreign compounds including drugs and environmental chemicals. These enzymes are present in all tissues, but mostly in the liver. Cytochrome P-450-dependent enzymes are also involved in the hydroxylation of endogenous compounds including vitamin D, leukotriene B4 and steroids. Infective and inflammatory diseases,as well as cancer, were reported to cause a decrease in the levels of liver cytochrome P-450 and therefore decrease the ability to metabolize certain drugs. We have studied the role of the immune system, and particularly of monokines, in the depression of liver P-450 in these pathological conditions. For this purpose,we have used bacterial lipopolysaccharide (LPS) as a model inflammatory agent , which is a well known inducer of the acute phase response. We have studied the relative role of interleukin-1 (IL-1) and tumor necrosis factor (TNF) in the depression of liver P-450 induced by LPS in vivo in mice and in vitro in isolated hepatocytes. In an attempt to pharmacologically modulate this effect of LPS, we have pretreated mice with dexamethasone (DEX), a synthetic corticosteroid which inhibits IL-1 and TNF synthesis and has been reported to protect against the lethal effect of LPS. The results reported here clearly indicate that IL-1 depresses cytochrome P-450 both in vivo and in vitro, and that both LPS and TNF also depress liver cytochrome P-450 levels in vivo but their effect is mediated via IL-1 and can be prevented by inhibiting IL-1 synthesis with DEX.

MATERIALS AND METHODS

Recombinant human IL-1-alpha was a gift from Dr. Lomedico, Hoffmann La Roche, Nutley,N.J. Recombinant human TNF was a gift from Dr.Lin,Cetus Corp., Emeryville,CA. LPS (E.coli,O55:B5) was from Sigma. Rabbit antiserum to human natural (alpha and beta) IL-1 was a kind gift from C.A. Dinarello, Boston,MA.Animal treatment and biochemical determinatino were as previously described (Ghezzi et al. 1986a).Hepatocyte and monocyte cultures were performed as previosly described (Ghezzi et al.1986a; Rossi et al.1985)

RESULTS

Role of macrophages in the LPS-induced depression of liver cytochrome P-450. In a first set of experiments we tested the hypothesis that one or more macrophage products might be involved in the effect of LPS on liver ED. Genetically LPS-resistant mice (C3H/HeJ) were treated with either LPS or serum taken from normally responsive mice (C3H/HeN) 90 min after treatment with LPS.While LPS did not effect liver ED in C3H/HeJ mice, a depression was observed when these mice were treated with post-LPS serum from normal mice.After passive transfer of peritoneal macrophages from normal mice, LPS-resistant mice had decreased liver cytochrome P-450 activity after treatment with LPS (Table 1).

TABLE 1. DEPRESSION OF LIVER P-450 IN LPS-RESISTANT MICE BY POST-LPS SERUM AND INDUCTION OF LPS-RESPONSIVENESS AFTER TRANSFER OF PERITONEAL CELLS FROM NORMAL MICE.

Treatment	C3H/HeN	C3H/HeJ
saline control	100%*	100%
LPS (2.5 ug/mouse)	60%	100%
control serum	not done	100%
post-LPS serum	not done	70%
C3H/HeN macrophages	not done	100%
C3H/HeN macrophages + LPS	not done	75%

* ED activity as percent of saline controls.

Role of IL-1 and TNF.

24 h after administration of TNF or IL-1,a depression of liver ED activity was seen (Table 2), suggesting that these two monokines might be equally important in modulating the levels of liver

cytochrome P-450 in LPS-treated mice. However, when tested on hepatocyte cultures,only IL-1, not TNF, depressed ED activity.

TABLE 2. EFFECT OF DIFFERENT CYTOKINES ON DRUG METABOLIZING ENZYMES IN VIVO IN MICE AND IN VITRO IN ISOLATED HEPATOCYTES.

Treatment	IN VIVO(1 ug/mouse)	IN VITRO (100ng/ml)
LPS	40 % decrease	no effect
TNF	30 % decrease	no effect
IL-1	40 % decrease	40 % decrease

This suggested us that TNF depression of liver drug metabolism in vivo might be mediated via IL-1, which was previously reported to be induced by TNF (Dinarello et al. 1986). In fact,as shown in Table 3, when hepatocytes were treated with supernatants fromLPS- or TNF- stimulated monocytes, a depression of ED activity was observed. This effect was not observed when monocytes were cultured with LPS or TNF in the presence of DEX, which inhibits IL-1 synthesis (Snyder and Unanue 1982). Furthermore, treatment of these monocyte supernatants with anti-IL-1 antiserum inhibited by 80-100 % the cytochrome P-450-depressing activity (data not shown).

TABLE 3. EFFECT OF MONOCYTE SUPERNATANTS ON DRUG METABOLIZING ENZYMES IN ISOLATED HEPATOCYTES.

Addition to hepatocytes	ED activity (percent of control)
none	100%
LPS or TNF	100%
Monocytes	100%
Monocytes + LPS	70%
Monocytes + DEX + LPS	100%
Monocytes + TNF	65%
Monocytes + DEX + TNF	100%

We have then returned to the in vivo model and studied the effect of DEX pretreatment on the depression of liver cytochrome P-450 by LPS or TNF. As summarized in Table 4, pretreatment with DEX (30 mg/Kg) completely protected (extent protection > 90%) against the depression of liver ED by LPS or TNF, but was much less effective (extent protection < 50 %) against the effect of IL-1 on liver ED.

TABLE 4. EFFECT OF DEXAMETHASONE PRETREATMENT ON DEPRESSION OF LIVER DRUG METABOLISM IN MICE TREATED WITH LPS, TNF OR IL-1.

Treatment	Without DEX	With DEX
LPS	- 40%*	< 5% decrease
TNF	- 30%	< 5% decrease
IL-1	- 40%	- 25%

*decrease in liver ED activity 24 h after treatment (1 ug/mouse iv of LPS,TNF or IL-1 and 1 mg/mouse ip of DEX 30 min before cytokines)

DISCUSSION

The liver has been shown to be a major target for the cytokines involved in the acute phase response. The changes in liver metabolism elicited during the acute phase response include: increased synthesis of acute phase proteins such as fibrinogen (Kampschmidt et al,1980) and serum amyloid A (Ramadori et al. 1985), induction of metal binding proteins (Kampschmidt,1981), depressed albumin synthesis (Ramadori et al. 1985), impaired response to glucocorticoids (Moore et al. 1978). These effects are not mediated by a single cytokine. For instance, while IL-1 has been shown to mediate the induction of serum amyloid A (Ramadori et al. 1985), other acute phase proteins,such as fibrinogen, are induced via a cytokine termed hepatocyte stimulating factor/interferon-ß2 (Gauldie et al.1987). Therefore,the cytokines directly affecting liver cytochrome P-450 were studied. Altough both IL-1 and TNF have been reported to depress liver drug metabolism in vivo (Ghezzi et al.1986a,1986b), our data indicate that TNF, like LPS, acts through a second mediator, probably IL-1. The impairment of liver drug metabolism observed in LPS- or TNF-treated mice can be prevented by corticosteroids. Our current hypothesis is that corticosteroids acts by inhibiting the synthesis of IL-1 induced by LPS or TNF.

The depression of liver drug metabolism observed with LPS or TNF might be of potential biological relevance. Studies from this laboratory have shown that LPS treatment decreases the capacity of liver enzymes to metabolically deactivate,by omega-hydroxylation,leukotriene B4 (M.Romano et al. manuscript in preparation). More importantly, TNF treatment decreases the clearance of drug metabolized by cytochrome P-450, such as diazepam and aminopyrine (P.Ghezzi,manuscript in preparation).

This altered drug metabolism might either increase the toxicity of drugs by inhibiting their detoxification/elimination, or decrease the efficacy of drugs requiring metabolic activation to exert their pharmacological action (such as cyclophosphamide). It is therefore important to study how such side effects of TNF might be prevented. On the other hand, the experiments with DEX indicate that this experimental model may be useful in studying the pharmacological modulation of IL-1 in vivo by inhibitors of its synthesis or of its action. Furthermore, since tumor bearing animals were reported to have low cytochrome P-450 activity (Garattini et al, 1987), it will be interesting to study whether TNF- or IL-1-like mediators are involved, and whether it is possible to pharmacologically prevent the cancer-associated impairment of liver metabolism.

<u>REFERENCES</u>

Dinarello CA, Cannon JG, Wolff SM, Bernheim HA, Beutler B, Cerami A, Figari IS, Palladino Jr. MA, O'Connor JV (1986). Tumor necrosis factor (cachectin) is an endogenous pyrogen and induces production of interleukin 1. J Exp Med 163:1433.

Gauldie J, Richards C, Harnish D, Landsdorp P, Baumann H (1987). Interferon beta2/B-cell stimulatory factor type 2 shares identity with monocyte-derived hepatocyte stimulating factor and regulates the major acute phase protein response in liver cells. Proc Natl Acad Sci USA 84: 7251.

Garattini S, Ghezzi P, D'Incalci M (1987) Effects of cancer disease on the metabolism of anticancer agents. Pharmacology and Therapeutics, in press.

Ghezzi P, Saccardo B, Villa P, Bianchi M, Dinarello CA (1986a). Role of interleukin-1 in the depression of liver drug metabolism by endotoxin. Infect Immun 54:837.

Ghezzi P, Saccardo B, Bianchi M (1986b). Recombinant tumor necrosis factor depresses cytochrome P450-dependent microsomal drug metabolism in mice. Biochem Biophys Res Commun 136:316

Kampschmidt RF, Pulliam LA, Upchurch HF (1980). The activity of partially purified leukocytic endogenous mediator in endotoxin-resistant C3H/HeJ mice. J Lab Clin Med 95:616.

Kampschmidt RF (1981). Leukocytic endogenous mediator/endogenous pyrogen. In Powanda MC, Canonico PG (eds): "The physiologic and metabolic responses of the host", Amsterdam: Elsevier/North Holland, pp.55-74

Moore RN, Goodrum KJ, Couch Jr. RE, Berry LJ (1978). Elicitation of endotoxemic effects in C3H/HeJ mice with glucocorticoid antagonizing factor and partial characterization of the factor. Infect Immun 17:707.

Ramadori GG, Sipe JD, Dinarello CA, Mizel SB, Colten HR (1985). Pretranslational modulation of acute phase hepatic protein synthesis by murine recombinant interleukin 1 (IL-1) and purified human IL-1. J Exp Med 162: 930.

Rossi V, Breviario F, Ghezzi P, Dejana E, Mantovani A (1985) Prostacyclin synthesis induced in vascular cells by interleukin-1. Science 229:174.

Snyder DS, Unanue ER (1982). Corticosteroids inhibit murine macrophage Ia expression and interleukin 1 production. J Immunol 129:1803.

Monokines and Other Non-Lymphocytic Cytokines, pages 343–348
© 1988 Alan R. Liss, Inc.

AMPLIFICATION OF ANTIBODY MEDIATED GLOMERULONEPHRITIS BY
TUMOUR NECROSIS FACTOR AND INTERLEUKIN 1

Andrew J Rees, Steve Cashman and Nao Tomosugi

Renal Unit, Department of Medicine, The Royal
Postgraduate Medical School, Hammersmith Hospital,
Du Cane Road, London W12 0NN

INTRODUCTION

There is a considerable body of evidence to show that
the development of a localised infection if often associated
with intensification of immunologically mediated injury
elsewhere in the body. These data have been reviewed
recently (Worthen, Henson, Henson and Rees, 1987) and much
derives from the study of glomerulonephritis, either
clinically (Rees, et al 1977) or experimentally (Naruse et
al 1985). Taken together, the data suggest that the effect
is caused by up-regulation of the inflammatory rather than
the immune response; and it is likely to be caused by the
same factors that mediate the acute phase response to
infection.

It is recognised that cytokines such as interleukin-1
(IL-1) (Dinarello 1984), and tumour necrosis factor (TNF)
(Buetler and Cerami, 1986) are responsible for many aspects
of the acute phase response. Genes for both proteins have
been cloned and expressed to produce the recombinant
molecules. The availability of these recombinant molecules
has allowed us to examine their effects experimentally on
induced mediated antibody injury in vivo. The model of
nephrotoxic nephritis (NTN) in rats was chosen for these
studies because injury is caused by passively administered
heterologous antibodies to glomerular basement membrane
(GBM), the mass of antibody binding to the GBM can be
quantified as well as the severity of injury, and thus the
two can be directly correlated.

The experiments reported here were designed to answer three questions : first what are the effects on the kidney of injecting small doses of recombinant IL-1 and TNF; second do these cytokines intensify injury in nephrotoxic nephritis in the same way as bacterial lipopolysaccharide (LPS) and thirdly is there synergism between the cytokines.

Methods

Nephrotoxic Nephritis. Glomerulonephritis was induced in 150-200G Sprague Dawley Rats by injection of rabbit IgG containing high titres of anti-rat GBM antibodies; this reagent is often called nephrotoxic globulin (NTG). NTG was prepared as described previously (Van Zyl Smit, et al 1983). Injury was assessed by measurement of albumin excretion in the 24 hours after injection of NTG as well as from renal morphology by light and electron microscopy.

Experimental Protocols. The reagents used were human recombinant IL-1 (Wingfield et al 1986) and hr-TNF (Marmenout et al 1985). The hr IL-1 was injected as a single intravenous dose (5-5,000 nanogm IV) one hour before injection of NTG. Hr-TNF was injected intraperitoneally (0.4-40µgm I.P.) as a single dose 2 hours before anti-GBM antibodies. Series of rats studied in parallel were given anti-GBM antibodies alone as negative controls and various doses of LPS (0.025-2.5µgm; 055-B5) as positive controls.

Results

(a) Effects of cytokines : Neither hr-IL-1 nor hr-TNF given alone caused constitutional upset in the doses given; and renal morphology was normal by light and electron microscopy 24 hours after administration. However biopsies taken 4 hours after injection of either cytokine showed that increased numbers of neutrophils had marginated in glomerular capillaries. None of the rats given cytokines alone developed proteinuria. Similarly rats injected with 0.025-2.5µgm of LPS showed no evidence of injury.

(b) Amplification of Injury : The results of experiments with NTG as well as TNF on IL-1 were substantially different. Rats injected with LPS intraperitoneally 2 hours before injection of anti-GBM antibodies (9.3mg) had a dose dependent increase in albuminuria compared to rats given anti-GBM antibodies only (NTG alone 13+4mg/24h; NTG + LPS 0.025µgm,

19+10mg/24hrs, NTG + LPS .25, 75±29mg/24hrs, NTG + LPS 2.5, 59±18mg/24hrs). Injection of hr-IL-1 and hr-TNF caused similar dose dependent increases in albuminuria (Fig 1). Kidneys from rats pretreated with LPS had also significantly more glomerular capillary thrombi than rats given anti-GBM antibodies alone; the results were intermediate in rats pre-treated with either cytokine. These results show that injection of hr-IL-1 and hr-TNF cause a considerable amplification of injury in NTN whether assessed functionally or morphologically.

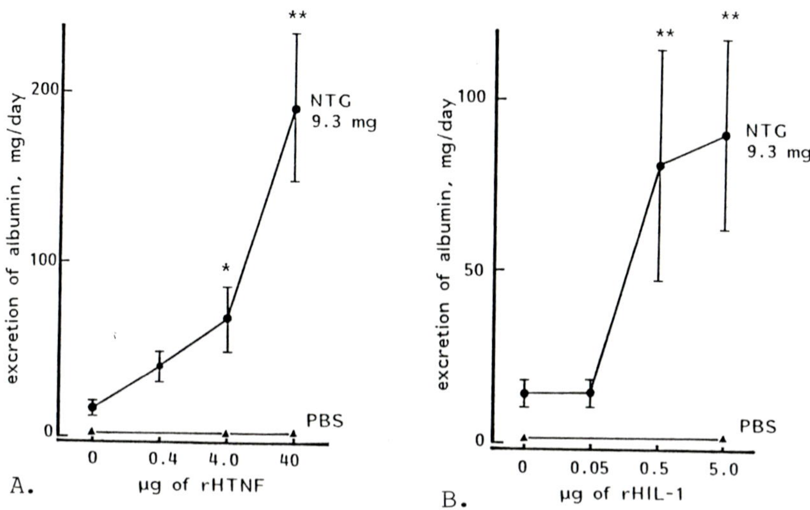

Figure 1. Twenty four hour albumin excretion in groups of rats with nephrotoxic nephritis pretreated with hr-TNF (A) or hr-IL-1 (B). * is p<0.05 and ** is p<0.01 (Wilcoxon).

(c) Synergism between IL-1 and TNF. In the last series of experiments we assessed the combined effects of hr-IL-1 (0.05 or 5.0µgm) and hr-TNF (0.4 or 40µgm). The results show that there was synergism between the effects of the cytokines when suboptimal doses of both cytokines were given. Neither IL-1 (0.05µgm) nor TNF (0.04µgm) alone caused clear cut amplification of injury in contrast to the effect when they were given together. Twenty-four hour albumin excretions were : NTG + IL-1, 14 + 4mg; NTG + TNF, 38 +g mg; NTG + TNF

+ IL-1, 82 + 15mg.   However when the cytokines were given
the optimal dosage TNF (40µgm, and IL-1 (5µgm)), there was no
synergistic effect on albumin excretion. But even in this
situation there was synergistic effect on degree of glomerular
capillary thrombosis.

DISCUSSION

These studies were undertaken in an attempt to try to
understand the reasons why intercurrent infections in
patients and LPS in experimental animals intensify antibody
mediated injury to the kidney. The results show unequivocally
that injection of hr-IL-1 and hr-TNF into rats with nephrotoxic nephritis increase injury in a way analogous to LPS
and suggests that they may be involved. The results raise
three questions : first, how do the cytokines mediate their
effect; second, were the circulating concentrations of
cytokines comparable to those found in natural infections
and thirdly can inhibition of the cytokines reduce injury in
rats injected with NTG alone.

Injury in nephrotoxic nephritis is mediated by
neutrophils and the first stage in an inflammatory response
is adhesion of neutrophils to capillary endothelium
(reviewed by Worthen, Henson, Henson and Rees, 1987). Both
TNF and IL-1 have profound effects on endothelium in vitro;
they change the endothelial surface from being relatively
anticoagulant to being procoagulant (Naworth et al 1986) and
they both increase its capacity to bind neutrophils (Poheman
et al 1986). TNF and IL-1 also effect neutrophils directly
to increase their adhesiveness and their ability to generate
phlogistic molecules (Dinarello 1984, Beutler and Cerami,
1986). Thus the simplest explanation for our finding is that
albuminuria increases and glomerular capillary thrombi result
from analogous changes in vivo. Recent experiments have shown
that TNF and IL-1 both increase the early influx of neutrophils
into glomeruli in rats with nephrotoxic nephritis (Tomosugi,
Cashman and Rees, unpublished).

It is difficult to define a dose of hr-IL-1 that reflects
the effects of naturally synthesised IL-1, many of which are
likely to be local. TNF is more likely to have a hormonal
role and so in preliminary experiments we have measured
serial serum TNF concentrations in rats injected with LPS
0.25µgm LP or with TNF 10µgm I.P. and found them to be almost
identical (Tomosugi, Hay and Rees unpublished). Thus it

appears the doses of TNF that amplify injury in NTN (as
little as 0.4µgm) cause changes in serum concentrations well
within the physiological range.

Lastly and most critically it remains to be seen whether
inhibition of TNF or IL-1 pharmacologically by antibodies will
prevent injury in NTG either alone or amplified by LPS as has
already been reported in mice with cerebral malasia (Grau et
al 1987).

REFERENCES

Beutler B, Cerami A (1986). Cachectin and tumour necrosis
  factor as two sides of the same biological coin. Nature
  320: 584-588.
Dinarello CA (1984). Interleukin-1. Rev Inf Dis 6: 51-95.
Grau GE, Fajardo LF, Piguet P-F, Allet B, Lambert P-H,
  Vassalli P (1987). Tumour necrosis factor (Cachectin) is
  an essential mediator in murine cerebral malaria. Science
  237: 1210-1212.
Marmenout A, Fransen L, Tavernier J, Van der Heyden J,
  Tizard J, Kawashima E, Shaw A, Johnson MJ, Simon R,
  Muller M, Ruysschaert R, Van Vliet A and W Fiers (1985).
  Molecular cloning and expression of human tumour necrosis
  factor and comparison with mouse tumour necrosis factor.
  Eur J Biochem 152: 512.
Naruse T, Tsuchida A, Ogawa S, Yano S, Maekawa T (1985).
  Selective glomerular thrombosis in rats induced by combined
  injections of nephrotoxic antiserum and lipopolysaccharide.
  J Lab Clin Med 105: 146-156.
Nawroth PP, Handley D, Stern DM (1986). The multiple levels
  of endothelial cell - coagulation factor interactions.
  Clinics in Haematol 15: 293-321.
Poheman TH, Stanness KA, Beatty PG, Ochs HD, Harlan JM (1986).
  An endothelial cell surface factor (s) induced in vitro by
  lipopolysaccharide. Interleukin-1 and tumour necrosis
  factor increases neutrophil adherence by a CDW-18 dependent
  mechanism. J Immunol 136: 4548-4553.
Rees AJ, Lockwood CM, Peters DK (1977). Enhanced allergic
  tissue damage in Goodpastures Syndrome by intercurrent
  bacterial infection. Brit Med J 2: 723-726.
Van Zyl Smit R, Rees AJ, Peters DK (1983). Factors affecting
  the severity of injury during nephrotoxic nephritis in
  rabbits. Clin Exp Immunol 54: 366-372.
Wingfield P, Payton M, Tavernier J, Barnes M, Shaw A, Rose K,
  Simona MG, Demczuk S, Williamson K, Kayer J-M (1986).

Purification and characterisation of human IL-1B expressed
in recombinant Escheria coli. Eur J Biochem 160: 491-497.
Worthen GS, Henson PM, Henson J, Rees AJ (1987). Mechanisms
in vascular injury. In Shrier R, Gottochalk CW (eds)
"Diseases of the Kidney". Boston: Little Brown.

Monokines and Other Non-Lymphocytic Cytokines, pages 349–354
© **1988 Alan R. Liss, Inc.**

TNF-α AND IFN-γ HAVE ALTERNATE EFFECTS ON THE IMMUNE SYSTEM
IN VIVO.

Chaim O. Jacob, May Koo and Hugh O. McDevitt

Department of Medical Microbiology, Stanford
University School of Medicine. Stanford, CA
94305

Aberrant expression of class II MHC molecules has
been suggested to be involved in the initiation and
development of autoimmunity (Bottazzo et al., 1983). Since
IFN-γ is the prototype lymphokine which has been shown to
upregulate the expression of MHC class II antigens in many
systems (Wong et al., 1983; Ameglio et al., 1986) we have
tested the in vivo effects of IFN-γ in an autoimmune model
system. Our working hypothesis is that IFN-γ might
upregulate the autoimmune process, while by blocking the
effects of IFN-γ we might downregulate such a process.
This was tested in the (NZB x NZW)F_1 lupus nephritis model
system.

The NZB parental strain develops a mild to moderate
autoimmune hemolytic anemia. Glomerulonephritis is
infrequent and delayed in onset. The NZW parental strain
is phenotypically normal. By contrast, the female F_1
hybrids develop severe glomerulonephritis between 6-7
months of age and by 12 months, 95% of animals die from
renal lesions. Thus, the NZW parent makes a major
contribution in accelerating and worsening the NZB disease.
Backcross experiments have shown that the major genetic
contribution of NZW mice maps within the MHC but may be
separate from the class II loci (Kotzin and Palmer, 1987).

(NZB x NZW)F_1 female mice were treated with
recombinant IFN-γ 5 x 10^4 units/inj/i.p./3 times per week
for a period of 3 months starting at 4 months of age.
Death occured at an earlier age in IFN-γ treated mice
compared to PBS treated controls ($p \leq 0.001$). While PBS-

treated (NZB x NZW)F_1 control mice began to die at around 8 months of age (50% survival, 9.5 months), in the IFN-γ treated group 75-80% were dead by 8 months. No effect of IFN-γ on survival of mice could be seen in an age and sex matched NZW group of mice treated identically.

On the other hand, treatment of (NZB x NZW)F_1 mice with an IgG_1 monoclonal anti rat IFN-γ antibody induced a very significant delay in the development of disease. At the age of 11 months, 80-85% of both control groups (treated with PBS or with a non-relevant IgG_1 monoclonal antibody) were dead, while 95% of mice were alive in the anti IFN-γ treated group. Parallel with the effect on survival, proteinuria and anti-DNA antibody production were modulated by these treatments: i.e., acceleration in IFN-γ treated mice and delay in anti IFN-γ treated mice.

Since TNF has been shown to have similar or additive effects to IFN-γ in some in vitro models (Wong and Goeddel, 1986; Patton et al., 1986; Pujol-Borrell et al., 1987) we have tested the in vivo effects of recombinant murine TNF-α in this model system. (NZB x NZW)F_1 mice were treated with 10μg TNF-α i.p. 3 times per week starting at 4 months of age for a period of 3 months. To our surprise, TNF-α treatment induced a very significant delay in the development of the disease. At the age of 15 months, 8 months after stopping the treatment, 30% of mice are still alive, while all mice in the PBS control group were dead by 12 months.

In parallel with the prolonged survival of TNF-α treated mice, the development of proteinuria was significantly delayed. By 9 months, 65% of control mice have high grade proteinuria, while only 15% of treated mice show proteinuria of this degree. No weight loss was observed in the treated group versus controls.

Since recent cytogenetic studies have shown that TNF-α and TNF-β are tandemly located within the MHC both in man (Dunham et al., 1987) and mouse (Muller et al, 1987) we have further tested the possibility of the involvement of TNF genes in this disease. This was done by restriction fragment length polymorphism (RFLP) analysis.

Indeed a polymorphism could be demonstrated. The NZB mice, similar to Balb/c mice, show a Bam HI fragment of about 10-kb, while NZW mice show an approximately 11.5-kb band using a PVU II fragment of murine TNF-α cDNA probe.

No polymorphism could be demonstrated using a probe from murine TNF-β cDNA and 12 restriction enzymes. Interestingly, the autoimmune mouse strains MRL-+/+, MRL-lpr/lpr, BXSB and NOD show the same TNF-α RFLP pattern as the NZW mice, but some non-autoimmune strains have the same pattern as well.

In order to test whether this polymorphism has any relevance to the function of this gene we have tested the production of TNF-α by peritoneal exudate cells obtained from NZB, NZW, (NZB x NZW)F_1 and Balb/c mice using an in vitro bioassay which quantitates the cytolytic activity of TNF-α (Mukavitz-Kramer and Carver, 1986). NZB and Balb/c mice show very similar cytolytic activities in all experiments (Table 1).

NZW mice, on the other hand, show very low TNF-α biological activity regardless of the method used for activation. The F_1 mice show TNF-α levels much closer to the NZW parent than to the NZB parent.

<u>Table 1</u>   Murine TNF-α production by (5 x 10^5) adherent peritoneal exudate cells from various mouse strains.

Strain		NZB	NZW	(NZB x NZW)F1	Balb/c
Inducing agent(s)			Cytolytic activity		
LPS (μg/ml)	IFN-γ (U/ml)		(U/ml)		
0.01	10	78	14	27	61
-	100	64	15	23	72
0.1	10	92	15	34	104
1	100	126	17	30	121

In view of recent reports (Philip and Epstein, 1986) that LPS and IFN-γ could enhance IL-1 production by cells of monocyte-macrophage lineage, the supernatants of the peritoneal exudate cells from the various strains were assayed for the presence of IL-1. In contrast to the major differences in production of TNF-α, all strains tested produce similar quantities of IL-1. For example, in one experiment 5×10^5 peritoneal adherent cells activated with 100U of IFN-γ and 1 μg of LPS for 16 hours, induced the production of 109 U/ml, 114 U/ml, 98 U/ml and 121 U/ml of IL-1 by NZB, NZW, F_1 and Balb/c mice respectively.

The data presented suggest that the TNF-α gene may be involved in the development of the multigenic lupus-like disease in (NZB x NZW)F_1 mice. We would like to suggest that the NZW parent may contribute to the F_1 disease a TNF-α gene capable of only a low level of TNF production. Thus, replacement therapy with recombinant TNF-α induces a very significant delay in disease development, suggesting that such treatment is supplementing the low TNF production.

There is much data linking cytokines and the development of autoimmunity, but so far a role for TNF has not been established. Rather than having a beneficial effect (as demonstrated here) several previous reports on the involvement of TNF in HLA class II induction on epithelial cells (Pujol-Borrel et al., 1987) and on Graft versus Host Disease (Piquet et al., 1987) as well as its interleukin -1- inducing effect (Dinarello et al., 1986) have implied a deleterious role for TNF in autoimmunity. Most of these studies were done in vitro, and therefore their biological relevance to the homeostasis of the immune system in vivo remains to be determined. The apparent paradoxical opposite in vivo effects of IFN-γ and TNF-α should be considered in the same context.

Both TNF and IFN-γ appear to be part of a network of interactive signals that orchestrate inflammatory and immunological events. It is therefore difficult to interpret the in vivo effects after injection of individual cytokine because of the complex circuitry involved.

Although the role of each cytokine can be studied in defined in vitro systems, the rational use of these compounds as therapeutic agents depends on better understanding of their physiological role and their importance in the pathogenesis of diseases. In this respect, the (NZB x NZW)F_1 system may be an important in vivo model for understanding some of the physiological roles of these agents.

Furthermore, the data presented here suggest a rationale for similar studies in man and may have implications for the treatment of systemic lupus erythematosus in man.

REFERENCES

Bottazzo GF, Pujol-Borrel R, Hanafusa T, Feldman M (1983). Role of aberrant HLA-DR expression and antigen presentation in induction of endocrine autoimmunity. Lancet II:1115-1120.

Wong GHW, Clark-Lewis I, McKinn-Breschin JL, Harris AW, Schrader JW (1983). Interferon-γ induces enhanced expression of Ia and H-2 antigens on B lymphoid, macrophage and myeloid cell lines. J Immunol 131:789-793.

Ameglio F, Tosi R, Tanagaki N, Doley A (1986). Regulation of HLA class II antigen expression. IN: HLA class II antigens. A comprehensive review of structure and function. Solheim BG, Moller E, Ferron S eds. New York, N.Y.

Kotzin BL, Palmer E (1987). The contribution of NZW genes to lupus-like disease in (NZB x NZW)F_1 mice. J Exp Med 165:1237-1251.

Jacob CO, Van der Meide PH, McDevitt HO (1987). In vivo treatment of (NZB x NZW)F_1 lupus-like nephritis with monoclonal antibody to γ-interferon. J Exp Med 166:798-803.

Wong GHW, Goeddel DV (1986). Tumor necrosis factor α and β inhibit virus replication and synergize with interferons. Nature 323:819-822.

Patton JS, Shepard HM, Wilking H, Lewis G et al. (1986). Interferons and tumor necrosis factors have similar catabolic effects on 3T3 L1 cells. Proc Natl Acad Sci USA 83:8313-8317.

Pujol-Borrell R, Todd I, Doshi M, Bottazzo GF, Sutton R, Gray D, Adolf GR, Feldman M (1987). HLA class II induction in human islet cells by interferon-γ plus tumor necrosis factor or lymphotoxin. Nature 326:304-306.

Dunham I, Sargent CA, Twosdale J, Duncan-Campbell R (1987). Molecular mapping of the human major histocompatibility complex by pulse field gel electrophoresis. Proc Natl Acad Sci USA 84:7237-7241.

Muller U, Jongeneel CV, Nedospasov SA, Fischer-Lindahl K, Steinmetz M (1987). Tumor necrosis factor and lymphotoxin genes map close to H-2D in the mouse major histocompatibility complex. Nature 325:265-267.

Mukavitz-Kramer S, Carver ME (1986). Serum-free in vitro
  bioassay for the detection of tumor necrosis factor. J
Immunol Methods 93:201-206.
Piquet PF, Grau GE, Allet B, Vassali P (1987). Tumor
  necrosis factor/cochechtin is an effector or skin and gut
  lesions of the acute phase of graft-vs.-host disease. J
  Exp Med 166:1280-1289.
Dinarello CA, Cannon JG, Wolff SM, Bernheim HA, Beutler B,
  Cerami A, Figari IS, Palladino MA, O'Connor JV (1986).
  Tumor necrosis factor (cachectin) is an endogenous
  pyrogen and induces production of interleukin 1. J Exp
  Med 163:1433-1439.
Philip R, Epstein LB (1986). Tumor necrosis factor as
  immunomodulator and mediator of monocyte cytotoxicity
  induced by itself, γ-interferon and interleukin-1.
  Nature 323:86-89.

ACKNOWLEDGEMENTS:

      We thank Dr. H. M. Shepard for the generous gift of
recombinant IFN-γ and TNF-α. We are very grateful to Dr.
Gail Lewis in Genentech for her contribution, to Peggy
Sullivan for technical help, and Karen Moody for
preparation of the manuscript.

Monokines and Other Non-Lymphocytic Cytokines, pages 355–358

EFFECTS OF RECOMBINANT MURINE INTERLEUKIN-1α ON THE PATHOGENESIS OF MURINE LISTERIOSIS

Charles J. Czuprynski, James F. Brown, Karen M. Young, A. James Cooley and Robin S. Kurtz

Department of Pathobiological Sciences, School of Veterinary Medicine, University of Wisconsin, Madison, Wisconsin 53706

INTRODUCTION

The diverse biological effects of interleukin-1 (IL-1) in inflammation and the immune response led investigators to propose that IL-1 is a key mediator in host resistance to microbial infection (Dinarello, 1984). Until recently direct evidence supporting this hypothesis was unavailable. During the past year, however, investigators have reported that injection of mice with recombinant human or murine interleukin-1α protected them against experimental infection with Pseudomonas aeruginosa and Klebsiella pneumoniae (Ozaki et al., 1987) and Listeria monocytogenes (Czuprynski and Brown, 1987a; Czuprynski and Brown, 1987b), respectively. We have gone on to examine how treatment with IL-1 influences the course of murine listeriosis, with a particular emphasis on the interaction of IL-1 with other cytokines.

RESULTS AND DISCUSSION

Recombinant murine (Lomedico et al., 1984) and human IL-1α were generously provided by P. Lomedico at Hoffmann-La Roche (Nutley, NJ) and used at the activity (in LAF units) designated by the supplier. Mice were infected with L. monocytogenes strain EGD and evaluated by recovery of viable listeriae from the spleen and liver as described previously (Czuprynski and Brown, 1987a). Tissues were also removed for histopathological

evaluation. Sera were obtained for determining circulating levels of other cytokines.

Detailed descriptions of our findings are presented
elsewhere (Czuprynski and Brown, 1987a; Czuprynski and
Brown, 1987b; Czuprynski et al., 1988). We routinely
observed a 1-2 log 10 reduction in the number of viable
listeriae recovered from the spleens and livers of mice at
72 hours after administration of a sublethal dose of
L. monocytogenes. Table 1 summarizes the major points of
these studies.

We have since established that protection is conferred
by similar doses of recombinant human and murine IL-1α
(R. Kurtz and C. Czuprynski, manuscript in preparation).
The protective effects of IL-1α do not appear to require
the presence of a mature cell-mediated immune system as we
have observed enhanced anti-listeria resistance in athymic
(nu/nu) mice treated with IL-1α (Table 2).

TABLE 1. Effects of recombinant IL-1α on murine
listeriosis

	Reference
Protection observed at 100-1000 LAF units (maximal at approximately 1000 units)	1,2
Protection not dependent on LPS	1
Protection reflected in reduced histopathological damage	3
24 to 48 hour lag between IL-1 injection and first signs of protection	1,3
Protection associated with rapid (4 hour) elevation of serum colony-stimulating activity	3
No obvious signs of IL-1 induced toxicity	1,2,3

1 Czuprynski and Brown, 1987a
2 Czuprynski and Brown, 1987b
3 Czuprynski et al., 1988

TABLE 2.   Enhanced anti-listeria resistance of athymic
(nu/nu) mice treated with recombinant human IL-1α

IL-1 (units per mouse)	Mean ± S.E.M. log 10 listeriae per spleen
None	6.9 + 0.27
1000	6.3 + 0.22
1500	6.0 + 0.07

    Because of the diverse biological activities attribut-
ed to IL-1 the mechanisms by which it enhances anti-
microbial resistance are likely to be complex. Recruit-
ment of inflammatory phagocytes may be one mechanism by
which this occurs (Czuprynski and Brown, 1987b). The
early rise in serum colony-stimulating activity after IL-1
administration that we and others have observed (Vogel
et al., 1987; Czuprynski et al., 1988) may also be
important in light of the reported association between
serum colony-stimulating activity and anti-listeria
resistance (Wing et al., 1985). Gamma interferon also has
been shown to increase anti-listeria resistance (Kiderlen,
et al., 1984). We were unable to monitor changes in serum
interferon levels during listeria infection. We have
obtained evidence, however, for enhanced anti-viral
activity in peritoneal macrophages harvested from IL-1α
treated Listeria-infected mice (R. Kurtz and
C. Czuprynski, manuscript in preparation), thus suggesting
that modulation of interferon by IL-1 occurs in vivo.
Future studies in our laboratory will attempt to identify
the interactions of IL-1 with these and other cytokines
during the host response to bacterial infection. It is
hoped that these studies might aid in the eventual
development of cytokine therapy of microbial infections.

    This work was supported by the Office of Naval
Research (N00014-87-K-0318) and United States Public
Health Service Grants AI-21343 and BRSG 05912. We thank
Barb Polce for the preparation of this manuscript.

REFERENCES

Czuprynski CJ, Brown JF (1987a). Recombinant murine
  interleukin-1α enhancement of nonspecific
  antibacterial resistance. Infect Immun 55:2061-2065.
Czuprynski CJ, Brown JF (1987b). Purified human and
  recombinant murine interleukin-1α induced
  accumulation of inflammatory peritoneal neutrophils and
  mononuclear phagocytes: possible contributions to
  antibacterial resistance. Microb Pathogen 3: in
  press.
Czuprynski CJ, Brown JF, Young KM, Cooley AJ, Kurtz RS
  (1988). Effects of murine recombinant interleukin-1α
  on the host response to bacterial infection. J Immunol
  140: in press.
Dinarello CA (1984). Interleukin-1. Rev Infect Dis
  6:51-95.
Kiderlen AF, Kaufman SHE, Lohmann-Mathes ML (1984).
  Protection of mice against the intracellular bacterium
  Listeria monocytogenes by recombinant immune
  interferon. Eur J Immunol 14:964-967.
Lomedico PT, Gubler U, Hellmann CP, Dukovich M, Giri JG,
  Pan YCE, Collier K, Semionow R, Chua, AO, Mizel SB
  (1984). Cloning and expression of murine interleukin-1
  cDNA in Escherichia coli. Nature 312:458-462.
Ozaki Y, Ohashi T, Minami A, Nakamura S (1987). Enhanced
  resistance of mice to bacterial infection by
  recombinant human interleukin-1a. Infect Immun
  55:1436-1440.
Vogel SN, Douches SD, Kaufman EN, Neta R (1987).
  Induction of colony stimulating factor in vivo by
  recombinant interleukin-1α and tumor necrosis
  factors. J Immunol 138:2143-2148.
Wing EJ, Barczynski LC, Waheed A, Shadduck RK (1985).
  Effect of Listeria monocytogenes infection on serum
  levels of colony-stimulating factor and number of
  progenitor cells in immune and nonimmune mice. Infect
  Immun 49:325-328.

Monokines and Other Non-Lymphocytic Cytokines, pages 359–364
© 1988 Alan R. Liss, Inc.

SYNERGISTIC ACTIVITY OF IL-1 WITH TNF AND IL-1 WITH CSF IN
RADIOPROTECTION

Ruth Neta
Armed Forces Radiobiology Research Institute
Bethesda, Maryland 20814
and J. J. Oppenheim
Laboratory of Molecular Immunoregulation, BRMP, NCI
Frederick, Maryland 21701

INTRODUCTION

It is becoming increasingly clear that the modulation
of the immune system proceeds in a two step fashion.
First, exogenous stimulatory signals, immunomodulators,
induce the release of cytokines, primarily by the cells of
the RE system. The cytokines, in turn, act via appropriate receptors to signal RES, immune and hematopoietic
cells to proliferate, differentiate, and to perform host
defense functions.

Numerous immunomodulators were shown to be radioprotective (Ainsworth and Chase 1959, Patchen et al.
1987). Similar degree of radioprotection can be obtained
by administration of IL-1 (Neta et al. 1986 (a), indicating that cytokines may mediate radioprotective effects of
immunomodulators. Consequently, we have used the radioprotection model to determine the role and interaction of
several cytokines, IL-1, TNF, and CSF's. This study shows
that these cytokines act in concert and that their combined administration in appropriate doses may be more
effective than administration of immunomodulators that
induce their in vivo production.

MATERIALS AND METHODS

Mice. B6D2F1 inbred mice were obtained from Jackson
Laboratories, Bar Harbor, Maine. The mice were housed in
the Veterinary Department Facility at the Armed Forces

Radiobiology Research Institute in cages, with Micro-
Isolation unit tops, 10 mice per cage. Female mice, 8-12
weeks of age, were used for all experiments. Standard Lab
chow and HCl acidified water (pH 2.4) were given ad libi-
tum. All cage cleaning procedures and injections were
carried out in a laminar flow unit.

Cytokines. Human recombinant Il-1 was generously
provided by Immunex and by Hoffman-La Roche. The preparations were supplied in PBS at pH7.2 or in 30 mM tris-HCl,
400 mM NaCl, pH 7.8, respectively, and used on a weight
basis. Human recombinant TNF , lot number CP4026P08,
specific activity 9.6×10^6 units per mg in PBS was a generous gift from Biogen. Murine recombinant GM-CSF was
provided by Immunex as a lyophilized powder with sucrose
as a stabilizing agent. Human recombinant G-CSF was a
gift from Amgen. Protein free phenol-water extracted
endotoxin derived from E. Coli K235 (LPS) was obtained
from Dr. S. N. Vogel, Department of Microbiology, Uni-
formed Services University of the Health Sciences. All
reagents were diluted to the desired concentration in 0.5
ml pyrogen-free saline just prior to the single i.p.
injection of mice, 20 hours before irradiation. All cytokine preparations were assayed for LPS contamination in an
LAL assay and determined to contain less than 0.1 ng per
inoculum.

Irradiation. Mice were placed in plexiglass con-
tainers and were given whole body irradiation at 40 rd/min
by bilaterally positioned ^{60}Co elements. The number of
surviving mice was recorded daily for 30 days.

RESULTS

Radioprotection with hrIl-1 and hrTNF

The effect of increasing doses of hrIL-1 and of
hrTNF on protection of lethally irradiated B6D2F1 mice
($LD_{95/30}$=1050 rds) was compared. IL-1 , when administered intraperitoneally 20 hours prior to irradiation in
doses ranging from 75 to 1000 ng protected 80-85% of mice
from death. Although equivalent intraperitoneal doses of
hrTNF had no radioprotective effect, significant radioprotection was obtained with doses ranging from 5 to 10 ug
hrTNF . The degree of radioprotection achieved with the

optimal dose of hrTNF (40-50%) was still significantly
less than that observed with hrIl-1 . Therefore, hrTNF
is a less effective radioprotector in mice than hrIL-1 .
The combination of hrIL-1 and hrTNF resulted in synergistic radioprotective effect, at supralethal doses of
radiation, yielding a greater number of surviving mice
than predicted from the sum of the radioprotective effects
of each cytokine alone (Fig. 1). Furthermore, the effect
of IL-1 and TNF in combination was greater than that
achieved with optimal radioprotective doses of LPS. A
supralethal dose of 1150 rds, rather than the usual dose
of 1050 rds, was used in this experiment in order to
reduce the radioprotective effects of IL-1 and TNF by
themselves, and to better reveal interactions between
these two cytokines. The combination of IL-1 and TNF was
also significantly more radioprotective than a prior
intraperitoneal treatment with optimal doses of LPS (Fig.
1).

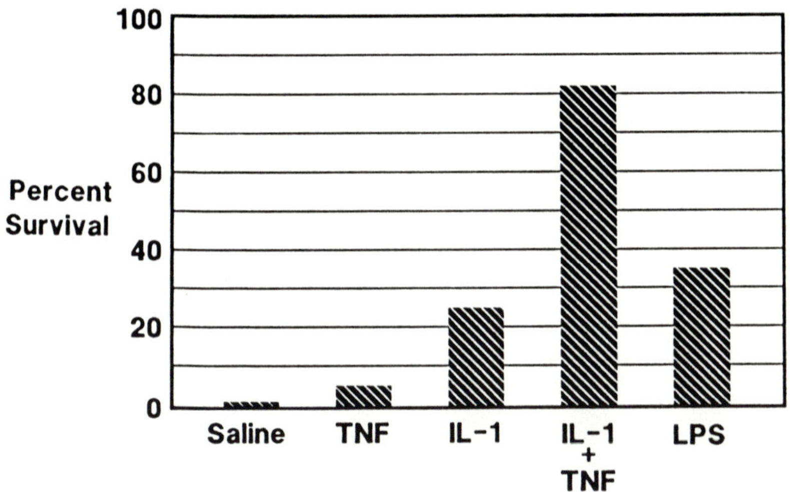

Figure 1. Comparison of radioprotection of B6D2F1 mice
with LPS, IL-1, TNF, and combinations of IL-1 and TNF.
Mice, 8-12 weeks old, received intraperitoneally 0.5 ml
saline (control), 0.1 ug IL-1, 5 ug TNF, or combination of
the two, or LPS, (12.5 ug, determined as optimal dose in
separate study) 20 hrs prior to whole body supralethal
irradiation. The results show the sum of two experiments
consisting of 22 mice in each group.

The Effect of Combinations of IL-1   with GM-CSF or G-CSF

     Administration of radioprotective doses of IL-1
results in cycling of bone marrow cells and, in particular, of cells of myeloid lineage (Neta et al. 1987).
Since in vivo administration of IL-1 induces the production of CSF (Vogel et al. 1987), such cycling may depend
on the action of specific growth factors, CSF's. However,
i.p. administration of GM-CSF 20 hours prior to irradiation, in doses ranging from 1 to 10 ug per mouse, had no
significant radioprotective effects against lethal doses
of radiation (Neta et al. 1986 (b). To further examine
whether CSF's contribute to radioprotection, suboptimal
doses of IL-1   were administered in combination with
GM-CSF or G-CSF. Such combinations greatly enhanced the
survival of mice in comparison to the effect of each
cytokine alone (Fig. 2). The effect of treatment with
combinations of suboptimal doses of IL-1 with GM-CSF (or
G-CSF, results not shown) equals that achieved with optimal doses of IL-1.

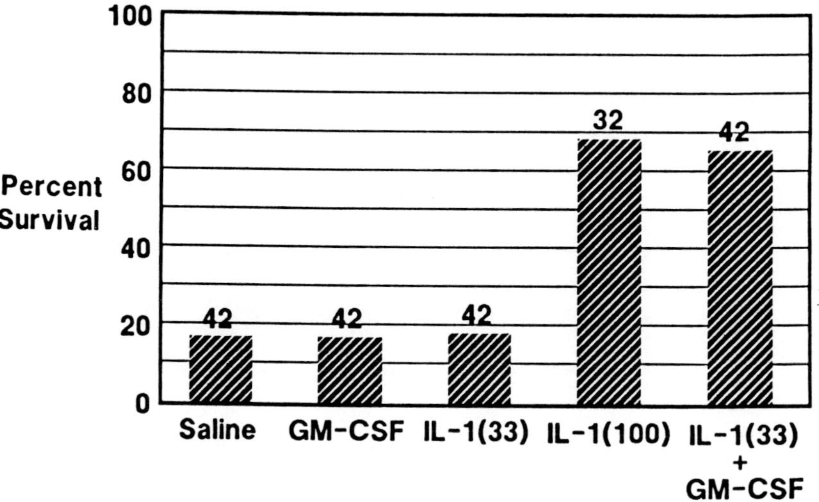

Figure 2. Radioprotection of B6D2F1 mice with combinations of IL-1 and GM-CSF. Mice, 8-12 weeks old, received
intraperitoneally 0.5 ml saline, 1 ug GM-CSF, IL-1 in
doses indicated, or the combination of IL-1 and GM-CSF.
The numbers at the top of the bars indicate the total
number of mice per group.

DISCUSSION

The results presented in this study showing synergistic effects of IL-1 and TNF in radioprotection indicate
that, despite overlapping biological activities, these two
cytokines are not redundant. The synergism of IL-1 and
TNF could be explained in either one of two ways. (a) Two
signals may be required for optimal stimulation of cells
which possess very few receptors for either of the cytokines (10^2 to 10^3 per cell) (reviewed by Nathan, 1987).
(b) Alternatively, different pathways may be triggered by
each of the two cytokines, and therefore their combination
may be more effective in conferring radioprotection.

The finding that IL-1 and TNF in combination are more
effective than optimal doses of LPS (their inducer) suggests that the two cytokines can be administered in more
optimal doses or that toxic effects of LPS itself can be
circumvented by using the purified cytokines.

The lack of radioprotective effects of GM-CSF or
G-CSF when administered alone, and their synergistic
effect when combined with suboptimal doses of IL-1, suggest that this hematopoietic growth factor may be more
effective in the presence of IL-1. This synergy may be
related to the recently described hematopoietin-1 activity
of IL-1 (Moore and Warren, 1987). Since administration of
IL-1 generates CSF, at optimal doses of IL-1 the endogenous levels of CSF may be generated at the requisite
site in the necessary concentration to mediate triggering
of the early hematopoietic progenitor cells. Alternatively, it has been proposed that IL-1, in addition to
inducing CSF, may stimulate the expression of receptors
for CSF on the hematopoietic progenitor cells (Moore and
Warren, 1987).

In summary, the above observations document that
cytokines act in concert and that combined administration
of selected cytokines may present the most effective means
for therapy.

ACKNOWLEDGEMENTS

This work was supported by the Armed Forces Radiobiology Research Institute, Defense Nuclear Agency, under
research work unit MJB3148. The opinions or assertions
contained herein are the private views of the author, no
endorsement by the Defense Nuclear Agency has been given
or should be inferred. The research was conducted according to principles enunciated in the "Guide for the Care
and Use of Laboratory Animals" prepared by the Institute
of Laboratory Animal Resources, National Research Council.

REFERENCES

Ainsworth EJ, Chase HB (1959). Effect of microbial anti-
    gens on irradiation mortality in mice. Proc Soc Exp
    Biol Med 102:483-485.
Moore MAS, Warren DJ (1987). Synergy of interleukin 1 and
    granulocyte colony-stimulating factor: In vivo stim-
    ulation of stem cell recovery and hematopoietic
    regeneration following 5-fluorouracil treatment of
    mice. Proc Natl Acad Sc USA 84:7134-7138.
Nathan CF (1987). Secretory products of macrophages.
    J Clin Invest 79:319-329.
Neta R, Douches SD, Oppenheim JJ (1986). Interleukin 1 is
    a radioprotector. J Immunol 136:2483-2485.
Neta R, Vogel SN, Oppenheim JJ, Douches SD (1986).
    Cytokines in radioprotection. Comparison of the
    radioprotective effects of IL-1 to IL-2, GM-CSF, and
    IFN-gamma. Lymphokine Res 5:s105-s110.
Neta R, Sztein MB, Oppenheim JJ, Gillis S, Douches SD
    (1987). In vivo effects of IL-1. I. Bone marrow
    cells are induced to cycle following administration
    of IL-1. J Immunol 139:1861-1866.
Patchen ML, D'Alesandro MM, Brook I, Blakely WF, MacVittie
    TJ (1987). Glucan: Mechanisms involved in its
    radioprotective effect. J Leuk Biol 42:95-105.
Vogel SN, Douches SD, Kaufman EN, Neta R (1987).
    Induction of colony stimulating factor in vivo by
    recombinant interleukin-1 and recombinant tumor
    necroses factor . J Immunol 138:2143-2148.

Monokines and Other Non-Lymphocytic Cytokines, pages 365–370

EFFECT OF A SYNTHETIC NONAPEPTIDE OF HUMAN IL-1β ON THE CELLULAR IMMUNOREACTIVITY AND IN VIVO GROWTH OF A FIBROSARCOMA OF BALB/C MICE.

Tiziana Musso, Mirella Giovarelli, Cristina Jemma, Guido Forni and the CR Sclavo Peptide Group[A]

Institute of Microbiology, University of Torino, and Centro Ricerche Sclavo, Siena, Italy.

INTRODUCTION

Interleukin 1 (IL-1) has been shown to stimulate various T lymphocyte, NK and macrophage functions and thus play a key regulator role in induction of the immune response (Oppenheim et al., 1986). However, its inflammatory activities restrict its use in man. To overcome this obstacle, the Sclavo Research Center is seeking to identify the minimal structure responsible for IL-1's immunostimulatory activity by synthetizing short peptide fragments and analyzing their biological activities. One peptide corresponding to nine residues of human IL-1β (VQGEESNDK, fragment 163-171, hereafter referred to as 163-171p) has been shown to maintain the capacity of native protein to activate T cell functions in vitro and stimulate the primary and secondary antibody responses to proteins and saccharidic antigens in vivo (Antoni et al.,1986; Nencioni et al., 1987). In this paper we describe a few cell functions modulated by 163-171p in vivo and its ability to impair the growth of a syngeneic tumor.

MATERIALS AND METHODS

Peptides. 163-171p and the peptide 166-174 of human

[A]G.Antoni, D.Boraschi, P.Bossu, S.Censini, P.Ghiara, L.Nencioni, G.Scapigliati, A.Tagliabue, G.F.Volpini.

chorionic somatomammotropin (C166-174) were synthetized by the Sclavo Research Center, Siena, Italy. Both peptides are not toxic over a large dose range (0.5-1000 μg/ml). Their addition to the culture medium does not affect the growth pattern of CE-2 cells nor that of other tumor cell lines (data not shown).

Media. The culture medium used was RPMI-1640 (Flow, Settimo Milanese, Italy) supplemented with 5% fetal bovine serum, penicillin, streptomycin and gentamycin, hereafter referred to as complete medium. All cultures were performed at 37°C in a humidified 5% CO_2 atmosphere.

Mice and tumor. 8-week-old female BALB/c ($H-2^d$) and C57Bl/6 (B6) ($H-2^b$) were purchased from Charles River (Calco, Italy). CE-2 tumor is a poorly immunogenic methylcholanthrene-induced sarcoma of BALB/c (Carbone et al., 1983). Mice were challenged sc with 1 x 10^3 cells. Starting from 4 hr after challenge, a few mice received 163-171p or C166-174 from 0.01 to 2.5 mg/Kg/day (0.2 to 500 μg/mouse) in 0.4 ml of HBSS injected at the challenge site or iv, for the following 10 days. Tumors were measured every three days in the two perpendicular diameters and average value recorded. The YAC-1 lymphoma of A.Wy mice ($H-2^a$) was maintained as a single-cell suspension in complete medium.

Lymphocyte reactivity. Normal mice were injected sc with 0, 50, 500 μg/day of 163-171p or C166-174 for 10 days. Proliferation and IFN production of spleen or lymph node cells were evaluated by culturing 1 x 10^6 lymphoid cells for 16 hr in complete medium supplemented with 5 x 10^{-5} M 2-β-mercaptoethanol in microtiter plates. For proliferation, the cultures were immediately pulsed with 1 μCi of ^{3}HTdR, the ^{3}HTdR uptake was expressed as cpm. The release of IFN was evaluated in the supernatant of parallel cultures.

Assay for IFN activity. IFN-titer in the supernatants was assayed by inhibition of the cytopathic effect of vesicular stomatitis virus on mouse L929 cells in 96-well plates as previously described in detail (Forni and Giovarelli, 1984) and expressed in international units (IU)/ml.

Mixed lymphocyte reaction (MLC) and proliferative response to IL-2. They were performed by using complete medium supplemented with 2-beta-mercaptoethanol. Responder lymphocytes were cultured at 4 x 10^5 cells/well with irradiated stimulator spleen cells at responder/stimulator ratios of 1:2, 1:1 and 2:1. The plates were incubated for 96 hr at 37° C in a humidified 5% CO_2 atmosphere. 16 hr before harvesting, 1 μCi of ^{3}H-TdR (2 Ci/mM) was added to each well and ^{3}H-TdR uptake was expressed in cpm. For proliferative response to IL-2, the responder lymphocytes used in MLC were cultered in the presence of 10, 100, 1,000 U/ml of recombinant IL-2 (Cetus, Emeryville, CA) for 96 hr.

Cytotoxicity assay. Natural killer (NK) cell cytotoxicity was assessed in 4 hr ^{51}Cr release assays carried out in round-bottomed 96-well microtest plates in a volume of 0.2 ml complete medium. 1 x 10^4 ^{51}Cr labelled target cells/well were mixed with effector lymphocytes at various effector-to-target (E:T) cell ratios and cultured for 4 hr. Per cent specific ^{51}Cr release was calculated as previously described (Forni and Giovarelli, 1984).

RESULTS

Ex-vivo experiments showed that daily subcutaneous injection of 50 and 500 μg/mouse of 163-171p for ten days increase weight, spontaneous proliferation, IFN release and NK activity in the spleen (Table 1).

These injections also increase proliferative response to alloantigens and high doses of IL-2 (Table 2). A marginal increase in these parameters is found in both draining and contralateral lymph nodes (Table 1,2). None of the above functions was affected by the injection of the unrelated peptide C166-174 (data not shown).

Another series of experiments, fully performed in vivo, showed that local 163-171p injections significantly inhibit the growth of incipient CE-2 tumor (Table 3). Sublethal irradiation of recipient mice before challenge fully abolishes this inhibitory activity of 163-171p. No tumor inhibition was found following injections of the unrelated peptide.

Table 1. Effect of ten daily sc injections of 163/171p
on spleen and lymph nodes spontaneous reactivity

	163-171p μg/mouse	Weight (mg)	^{3}HtdR cpm $(x10^{-3})$	IFN IU/ml	NK activity E/T 40:1
Spleen	0	97	7	16	2
	50	96	17*	64*	2
	500	110*	15*	32*	19*
Draining lymph node					
	0	3	2	0	0
	50	4	3	2	0
	500	5	3	0	12*
Contralateral lymph node					
	0	3	2	0	0
	50	3	2	2	0
	500	3	3	0	10*

* P <0.05 versus controls.

DISCUSSION

Ex-vivo experiments show that 50 or 500 μg of
163-171p injected repeatedly sc increase spontaneous, IL-2
and alloantigen induced lymphocyte proliferation.
Moreover, they turn on spontaneous IFN release and boost NK
cytotoxicity. The effect of 163-171p is not simply local,
since all these functions are particularly increased in the
spleen, whereas in both draining and contralateral lymph
nodes the increases are less evident. These
immunomodulatory activities are important since 163-171p is
devoid of inflammatory activity (Antoni et al., 1986).
Histological examinations (not shown) indicate, too, that
163-171p repeated sc injections did not induce a
generalized inflammatory reaction in the area of injection
nor in the draining lymph nodes. Rather, selected
lymphocyte functions only are induced.

163-171p is not cytocidal for CE-2 tumor cells in
vitro (data not shown), whereas its in vivo injection
significantly inhibits tumor growth. The fact that host

Table 2. Effect of 163-171p on proliferative responses.

163/171p μg/mouse	Medium only	Stimulator spc B6		Units of IL-2		
				10	100	1000
Spleen 0	12[a]	26	(2)	18	30	64
50	23*	87*	(4)	16	22	60
500	20*	90*	(5)	17	42*	88*
Draining lymph node						
0	9	66	(7)	10	13	81
50	8	84*	(10)	15	18*	117*
500	9	75	(8)	18*	17*	83
Contralateral lymph node						
0	9	64	(7)	11	13	82
50	13	78	(6)	16	18*	103*
500	10	116*	(11)	23*	21*	86

[a]cpm ^{3}H-Tdr uptake x 10^{-3}
* P <0.05 versus controls group.

Table 3. Effect of 163/171p on CE-2 tumor growth.

μg/ mouse	Peptide	Injection route	Surviving/total mice	
0	–	sc	0/40	(0 %)
50	C166-174	sc	0/10	(0 %)
50	163-171P	sc	6/40*	(15 %)
50[a]	163-171p	sc	0/12	(0 %)
500	C166-174	sc	0/10	(0 %)
500	163-171P	sc	5/34*	(15 %)
0	–	iv	1/40	(2.5%)
0.2	C166-174	iv	0/10	(0 %)
0.2	163-171P	iv	4/40	(10 %)

[a]Recipient mice were sublethally irradiated with 4.5 Gy 72 hr before tumor challenge.
*P <0.05 versus controls.

irradiation abolishes this inhibition suggests that it stems from the activation of radiation sensitive immune mechanisms. As 163-171p is able to promote IFN secretion and possibly the secretion of several other unmeasured lymphokines, it is difficult to define whether its inhibitory activity results from a direct action of 163-171p on immune effector functions or an ability to trigger a circuit of cytokine-cell interactions that regulate a multifactorial immunological response (Oppenheim et al.,1986), of which lymphocyte proliferation, boosted NK activity and IFN release are part. We are currently trying to tease apart the immune mechanisms mainly responsible.

ACKNOWLEDGEMENTS

We thank Dr. J. Iliffe for careful review of the manuscript. This work was supported by grants from CNR-Italy PF Oncologia 86.00414.44, MPI 40% and the Italian Association for Cancer Research.

REFERENCES

Antoni G, Presentini R, Perin F, Tagliabue A, Ghiara P, Censini S, Volpini G, Villa L, Boraschi D (1986). A short synthetic peptide fragment of human interleukin 1 with immunostimulatory but not inflammatory activity. J Immunol 137: 3201-3204.
Carbone G, Colombo M, Sensi ML, Cernuschi A, Parmiani G (1983). In vitro detection of cell mediated immunity to individual tumor specific antigens of chemically induced BALB/c fibrosarcomas. Int J Cancer 31: 483-490.
Forni G and Giovarelli M (1984). In vitro reeducated T helper cells from sarcoma-bearing mice inhibit sarcoma growth in vivo. J Immunol 132: 527-533.
Nencioni L, Villa L, Tagliabue A, Antoni G, Presentini R, Perin F, Silvestri S, Boraschi D (1987). In vivo immunostimulating activity of the 163-171 peptide of human IL-1 beta. J Immunol (in press).
Oppenheim JJ, Kovacs EJ, Matsushima K, Durum SK (1986). There is more than one interleukin 1. Immunol Today 7: 45-54.

Section VII. Assays for and Detection of Cytokines in Cells, Tissues, and Body Fluids

Monokines and Other Non-Lymphocytic Cytokines, pages 373–376
© 1988 Alan R. Liss, Inc.

INTERLEUKIN-1 IN HUMAN BLOOD: CHLOROFORM EXTRACTION AND RADIOIMMUNOASSAY

Joseph G. Cannon, Jos W. M. van der Meer, Stefan Endres, Gerhard Lonnemann and Charles A. Dinarello

Department of Medicine, New England Medical Center, Boston, MA 02111

INTRODUCTION

Practical methods for determining circulating cytokine concentrations are anticipated to aid in the diagnosis of acute infections or other conditions marked by an acute phase response. Present methods for detecting interleukin-1 (IL-1) depend on laborious bioassays which are only semi-quantitative and nonspecific. Radioimmunoassays (RIAs) have been developed recently which reliably measure human IL-1 (alpha and beta) and tumor necrosis factor (TNF) in cell culture supernatants. This report describes the application of these RIAs to human plasma measurements. Specifically, several extraction methods are evaluated for their ability to eliminate plasma factors which interfere with the RIAs.

METHODS

The RIAs for IL-1 beta (Lisi et al., 1987), IL-1 alpha (Lonnemann et al., 1987), and TNF (van der Meer et al, 1987) use polyclonal antibodies developed in rabbits against human recombinant proteins. The cytokines were labeled with ^{125}I by a modification of the chloramine T method. The sensitivities are typically 80, 40 and 10 pg/ml for IL-1 beta, alpha and TNF, respectively. Blood samples were collected in vacuum tubes containing EDTA (1.5 mg/ml) and aprotinin (0.67 TIU/ml). The plasma was centrifuged at high speed to remove platelets and stored at -70°C. Plasma was extracted by mixing with 2 parts chloroform (or other reagents), agitating for 5 minutes on a multisample vortexer, and centrifuging in an microfuge. The aqueous phase was then tested in the RIA.

RESULTS AND DISCUSSION

For a rapid empirical screen of extraction methods, ^{125}I-labeled cytokines were added to whole blood. The blood was briefly mixed, centrifuged and the separated constituents measured in a gamma counter. Virtually all of the radioactivity was detected in the plasma. Next, a variety of reagents including methanol, chloroform, acetone, talc and Florisil were added to the plasma in order to precipitate or adsorb factors which may interfere with the RIAs. These treatments (except chloroform) trapped the radioactivity in an insoluble precipitate. However, mixing plasma first with an equal volume of 50 mg/ml fucose or 1.8 mg/ml 8-anilino-1-napthalene sulfonic acid (ANS) before precipitating with methanol retained most of the radioactivity in the aqueous phase (Table 1). Fucose competes with IL-1 for binding on uromodulin (Hession et al., 1987) and ANS releases T_3 from thyronine binding protein. These results suggest that IL-1 and TNF bind to carriers in the plasma which precipitate with solvent extraction: ANS and fucose dissociated the cytokines from the carriers and the free IL-1 and TNF did not precipite. Chloroform appeared to accomplish the same objective without diluting the plasma.

Table 1. Precipitation of radiolabeled cytokines (%)

	IL-1 ß	IL-1 alpha	TNF
Methanol	8 7	8 9	8 8
+ Fucose	3 5	1 7	2 2
+ ANS	1 8	1 7	1 2
Chloroform	2 1	9	2 2

Table 2. Recovery of unlabeled cytokines by RIA (pg/ml)

	IL-1ß added (125 pg/ml)	TNF added (80 pg/ml)
ANS/Fucose/Chloroform	231 + 33	- -
Chloroform	121 + 45	83 + 5
	(n = 6)	(n = 8)

Figure 1. Comparison of extraction methods

The chloroform extraction method was tested further using plasma samples containing graded concentrations of exogenous IL-1 beta. Both chloroform alone, and chloroform combined with fucose and ANS, yielded IL-1 beta measurements which agreed over a wide range of concentrations with the amount of IL-1 beta added (Figure 1). Further tests involving addition of low concentrations of IL-1 beta or TNF to plasma from several different donors indicated that chloroform alone provided more accurate measurements of exogenous IL-1 beta (Table 2).

Endogenous immunoreactivity was also detected in extracted plasma. The recoveries listed in Table 2 are differences between spiked and unspiked plasma measurements. This immunoreactivity was not due to nonspecific binding of the plasma extract (tested in the RIA in the absence of anti-serum). The influence of EDTA and aprotinin on the standard curve was negligible. Plasma extracts diluted 1:2 and 1:4 exhibited a linear fall in immunoreactivity, rather than a precipitous disappearance, indicating that the immunoreactivity was not due to spurious, low-titer antibody reactions.

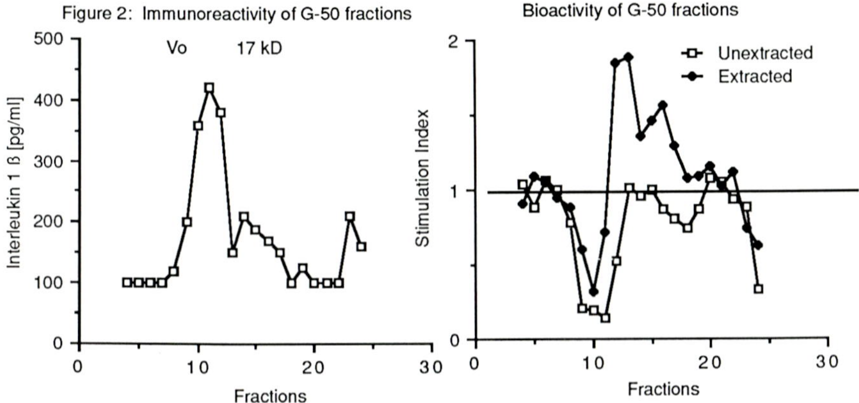

Extracted plasma was chromatographed with Sephadex G-50 (Figure 2) as described previously for detecting IL-1 by bioassay (Cannon and Dinarello, 1985). Immunoreactive material eluted shortly after the void volume, suggesting the presence of 30 kD precursor IL-1 or 17 kD IL-1 bound to carriers. Biological activity measured in portions of the same fractions corresponded to the immunoreactivity. Compared with unextracted plasma, extracted plasma exhibited less inhibitory activity (stimulation index<1) and more IL-1 activity (stimu-lation index>1) in the thymocyte costimulator assay.

Chloroform extraction substantially increased IL-1 beta measurements, had little effect on IL-1 alpha, and a variable, but generally negative effect on TNF measured in plasma from 10 healthy subjects (Figure 3). Heparinized plasma from healthy subjects (n=9) exhibited a similar pattern, however 10

of 16 heparinized plasma samples from patients with infectious
or inflammatory diseases exhibited no IL-1 beta immunoreactivity
until extracted, implying that acute phase plasma may contain
more binding or inhibiting factors than normal plasma.

It remains to be determined how much of the
immunoreactivity shown above represents biologically relevant
forms of cytokines. We anticipate that refinements in labeling
techniques and improved antibody preparations may further
reduce interference from non-cytokine factors in human plasma.

REFERENCES

Cannon JG, CA Dinarello. 1985. Increased plasma interleukin-1
   activity in women after ovulation. **Science** 227:1247-1249.
Lisi PJ, CW Chu, GA Koch, S Endres, G Lonnemann, CA
   Dinarello. 1987. Development and use of a radioimmunoassay
   for human interleukin 1 beta. **Lymphokine Res** 6:229-244.
Lonnemann G, S Endres, JG Cannon, JWM van der Meer, T
   Ikejima, CA Dinarello. 1987. Specific radioimmunoassays
   for inteleukin-1 alpha and beta; the influence of various
   culture conditions on the production of immunoreactive IL-1
   from human mononuclear cells. **J Leukocyte Biol** 42:603.
Hession C et al. 1987. Uromodulin (Tamm-Horsfall glycoprotein):
   A renal ligand for lymphokines. **Science** 237:1479-1484.
van der Meer JWM, S Endres, G Lonnemann, JG Cannon, T
   Ikejima, S Okusawa, JA Gelfand, CA Dinarello. 1987.
   Concentrations of immunoreactive human tumor
   necrosis factor alpha produced by human mononuclear
   cells in vitro. **J Leukocyte Biol**, in press.

Monokines and Other Non-Lymphocytic Cytokines, pages 377–381

A RIA FOR TUMOR NECROSIS FACTOR (TNFα) AND INTERLEUKIN 1β (IL-1β) AND THEIR DIRECT DETERMINATION IN SERUM

Aimée Reuter, Jacques Bernier, Philippe Gysen, Yvonne Gevaert, Renée Gathy, Miguel Lopez, Ginette Dupont, Pierre Damas and Paul Franchimont

Radioimmunoassay Laboratory University of Liege and IRE-MEDGENIX, Fleurus, Belgium

INTRODUCTION

The recent availability of pure recombinant lymphokines and monokines now makes it possible to study their regulation in various immunological processes and host defense mechanisms.

Usually, TNF α and IL-1β are assayed by biological methods. However, these techniques are complex, not specific for a well defined cytokine and time consuming.

- Immunoassay represents an alternative approach for assessing cytokine concentrations in biological fluids. Two enzymo-assays have been carried out for TNFα with detection limits of 5 ng/ml (Yamasaki et al.1986) and 40 pg/ml (Scuderi et al.1986) respectively. For IL-1β one RIA and one ELISA have been developed. Their sensitivities are 100 (Gaffney et al. 1987) and 250 pg/ml (Endres et al.1987) respectively. We have carried out a radioimmunoassay for TNFα and IL-1β and applied it to several pathological conditions.

METHODOLOGY

TNFα radioimmunoassay used polyclonal antibodies raised in rabbits according to a sequential saturation. This antiserum did cross react neither with α, β and γ Interferons, nor Interleukins 1 and 2, nor TNFβ. The assay allowed to detect 2 pg/tube with a precision ranging from 3 to 10% for 10-150 pg/tube concentrations. Within and between- assay coefficients of variation remained below 6 and 11%, respectively.

As regards the IL-1β radioimmunoassay, the polyclonal antibodies did not cross-react with all the cytokines listed above. The assay was able to detect down to 10 pg/tube and its precision ranged from 4 to 11% between 20 and 1000 -g IL-1β/tube. Within and between assay coefficients of variation did not exceed 7 and 13%, respectively.

The recovery of exogenous TNFα and IL-1β added respectively to TNFα-and IL-1β - free serum was complete. Standard curve and dilutions of mononuclear cell culture medium were parallel in both assays.

RESULTS

Patients with heavy burns or multiple injuries had significantly higher TNFα circulating levels than controls and cancerous patients (Table 1). Moreover, this increase in the blood was directly correlated to the severity of the pathology: in

TABLE 1.

SERUM LEVELS OF TNF_α (PG/ML)

SUBJECTS	N	M ± SD
NORMAL SUBJECTS (BOTH SEXES BETWEEN 25 - 65 YEARS)	100	44 ± 8 [D]
PATIENTS		
CANCEROUS PATIENTS	14	39 ± 15 [D]
HEAVY BURNS UBS < 50	12	88 ± 15 [C]
HEAVY BURNS UBS > 50	10	127 ± 22 [A]
MULTIPLE INJURED PATIENTS :	72	
- WITHOUT SHOCK	13	102 ± 19 [B,C]
- WITH SHOCK	59	130 ± 32 [A]
- WITHOUT SEPSIS	24	114 ± 28 [B]
- WITH SEPSIS	48	134 ± 33 [A]
- WITHOUT ARDS	26	117 ± 25 [B]
- WITH ARDS	46	134 + 33 [A]
- WITH ONE OF THESE COMPLICATIONS	18	109 ± 24 [B]
- WITH TWO OF THESE COMPLICATIONS	21	132 ± 31 [A]
- WITH THREE OF THESE COMPLICATIONS	31	141 ± 33 [A]

N = NUMBER OF CASES

M ± SD : MEAN ± STANDARD DEVIATION

VARIOUS LETTERS INDICATE SIGNIFICANTLY DIFFERENCES BETWEEN GROUPS, $P < 0.05$

heavy burns, TNFα was significantly augmented for
U.B.S.> 50 (scaled according to the Unit Burn Standard System). In widespread injuries, there was a
significant correlation between the development of
complications such as shock, sepsis or adult respiratory distress syndrom (A.R.D.S.), considered
separately or combined between themselves, and the
blood TNFα concentrations.
Fig. 1 shows that increase of TNFα is accompanied
with fatal issue of patients developing septic
shock. In the same group of patients, the IL-1β
concentrations remained comparable to those of
controls.

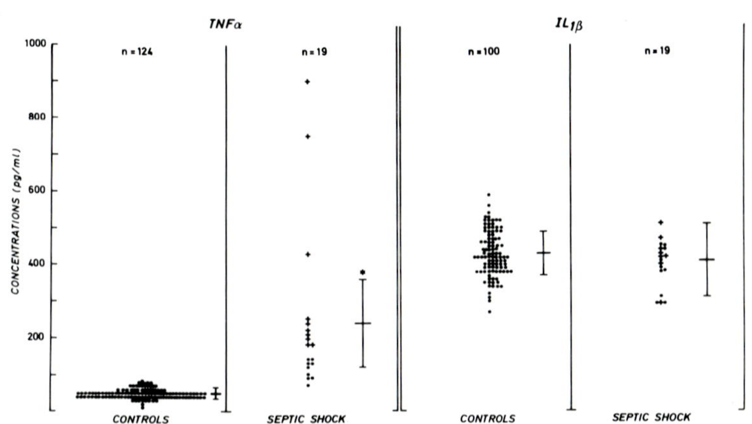

Fig. 1: Concentrations of TNFα and IL-1β in controls
and septic shock + SD. TNFα levels are significantly
increased (P<0.001) whereas IL-1β levels are not
significantly different. + death patients; 0 surviving patients.

    This dissociation between TNFα and IL-1β"syste-
mic" responses is also elicitable in sequential
studies for individual patients (Fig.2). Here again
sera of patients who ultimately died exhibited a
progressive increase of TNFα levels but normal
IL-1β concentrations. In contrast, patients who
recovered, had permanently lower TNFα and normal
IL-1β concentrations.

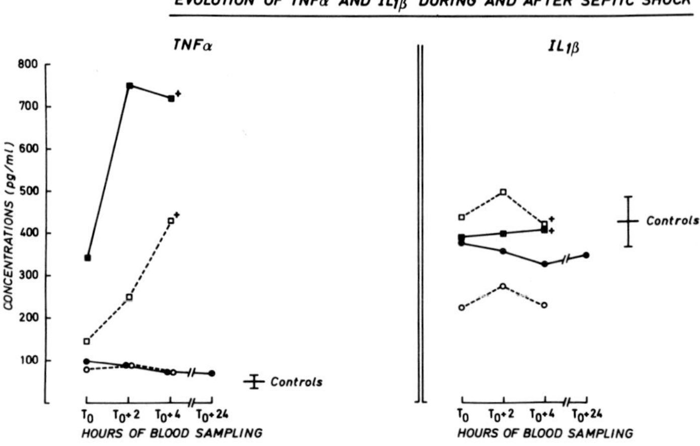

FIG. 2

These findings support the argument that, in patients with either heavy burns or widespread tissue injury:

(1) The TNFα augmentation is bound to be one of the major factors initiating or perpetuating some of complications present in endotoxemic states, such as hypotension, metabolic acidosis, hemoconcentration, renal and pulmonary hemorrhage, since all these effects of TNFα have been already demonstrated in vitro (Tracey, 1986).

(2) In the cases developing septic shock, IL-1β is not likely to be the main agent responsible for the acute inflammatory responses.

(3) Secretion of TNFα and IL-1β by monocytes-macrophages seems to be regulated by different mechanisms.

(4) TNFα could be a reliable marker of the severity of the pathologies reviewed in this article, excepted for cancer patients.

REFERENCES

Endres S, Lonneman G, Van der Meer J et al.(1987). Use of a highly sensitive RIA for measuring intra-individual variations of human monocyte-interleukin 1-β production. Immunobiology 75:48

Gaffney E, Koch G, Tsai S et al.(1987). Quantification of human IL-1β with polyclonal antibody. J Immunol Meth 101:271-277

Scuderi P, LAM K, Ryan K et al.(1986). Raised serum levels of tumor necrosis factor in parasitic infections. The Lancet Dec. 13:1364-1365

Tracey K, Beutler B, Lowry S et al.(1986). Shock and tissue injury induced by recombinant human cachectin. Science 234:470-474

Yamasaki S, Onishi E, Enami K et al. (1986). Proposal of standardized methods and reference for assaying recombinant human tumor necrosis factor. Japan J. Med Sci Biol 39:105-118

Monokines and Other Non-Lymphocytic Cytokines, pages 383–385

GENERATION OF NEUTRALIZING MONOCLONAL ANTIBODIES SPECIFIC FOR HUMAN INTERLEUKIN-1 BETA

David A. Wunderlich, Thomas J. Lobl, Jefferson W. Paslay and Ann E. Berger

Departments of Cell Biology, (D.A.W., A.E.B.) Hypersensitivity Diseases (J.W.P) and Biopolymer Chemistry (T.J.L.), The Upjohn Company, Kalamazoo, Michigan 49001

INTRODUCTION

Interleukin-1 (IL-1) is a leukocyte derived cytokine which mediates diverse immunobiological functions such as stimulation of thymocyte and fibroblast proliferation, induction of IL-2 production by T cells, and stimulation of B cell maturation (Kraukauer, 1986 and Kluger, 1985). Both forms of IL-1, alpha and beta, have recently been purified and molecularly cloned by numerous investigators (March, 1985). Using recombinant human IL-1β, we have generated mouse monoclonal antibodies (MAbs) which neutralize IL-1β biological activities and block binding of IL-1β to its receptor on target cells.

RESULTS AND DISCUSSION

Immune spleen cells from CAF_1 mice immunized with recombinant human IL-1β were fused with SP-2/0 mouse myeloma cells to generate eight monoclonal antibodies reactive wtih human IL-1β. These 8 MAbs, designated B1, B2, B3, B4, B5, B6, B7, and B8 were all reactive with recombinant human IL-1β and nonreactive with recombinant human IL-1α as measured using enzyme linked immunoadsorbant assays (ELISA). In addition, MAbs B1, B2, B3, B4, B6, and B8 detected the characteristic 17,000 M.W. IL-1β molecule in Western blotting experiments.

Competitive binding sutdies were carried out to define the relationship between sites on IL-1β recognized by the MAbs. IgGs purified from ascitic fluids of MAbs

B1, B2, B3, B4, B6, and B8 were labeled with biotin and reacted with IL-1β in ELISA after preincubation of the IL-1 with saturating amounts of IgGs of B1, B2, B3, B4, B6, and B8. Bound biotinylated MAb was detected with peroxidase conjugated streptavidin and enzyme substrate. None of the MAbs competed with biotinylated B1 for binding to IL-1β and B1 IgG did not inhibit the binding of biotinylated B2, B3, B4, B6, or B8 to IL-1β. MAbs B2, B3, B4, B6 and B8 did however inhibit the reaction of each of their biotinylated forms with IL-1β. These results suggest that at least two distinct non-overlapping epitopes (A B1 epitope and a B2, B3, B4, B6, and B8 epitope) on IL-1β are being recognized by the MAbs.

In view of the fact that the anti-IL-1β MAbs are reactive with at least two antigenic determinants on the IL-1 molecule, we have developed a two site sandwich ELISA which can detect and quantitate IL-1β. MAb B1 IgG was adsorbed to ELISA wells followed by IL-1β (or unknown). Bound IL-1β was detected using biotinylated MAb B2, perioxidase labeled streptavidin and enzyme substrate. Detection of IL-1β (as reflected by OD.405 measurement) is linear from 0.5 ng to 10 ng IL-1β per mL. The detection limit of the assay is approximately 600 pg IL-1β/mL. The use of any other combination of the antibodies resulted in an assay with less sensitivity.

The anti-IL-1β MAbs were also tested for their ability to inhibit the IL-1β induced production of IL-2 by the murine IA5 cell line. IgGs of MAbs B1, B2, B3, B4, B6, and B8 all inhibited the IL-1β induced production of IL-2 by IA5 cells. MOPC-21, a control IgG, had no effect. MAb B1 was the most potent inhibitor, with 24 ng IgG/mL yielding half-maximal inhibition (approximately a 40 fold excess of IgG to IL-1β on a molar basis). MAbs B3, B6 and B8 gave 50% inhibiton at 56, 140, and 76 ng IgG/mL, respectively. MAbs B4 and B2 were much less active, 30% inhibition was seen only when B4 and B2 were used at 1 μg IgG/mL.

MAbs B1, B3, and B4 were also tested for the ability to specifically block binding of ^{125}I labeled IL-1β to intact YT.NCI target cells. IgGs derived from these MAbs displayed substantial inhibitory activity. The inhibition appeared to be specific since control IgG

(MOPC-21) was inactive and the MAbs inhibit binding of ^{125}I-IL-1β but not ^{125}I-IL-1α to YT.NC.1 cells. There was no apparent correlation between activity in biological or binding assays and estimated antibody affinity constants.

MAb B1 was also tested for its ability to react with synthetic IL-1β analogues. Peptides corresponding to C-terminal fragments of the 17 kD IL-1β native sequence were synthesized on an Applied Biosystems Automated peptide synthesizer using customized programs (Lobl, 1987). Individual peptides corresponding to amino acids 85-153, 75-153, 64-153, 56-153, 46-153, 35-153, 30-153, 24-153, 18-153, 12-153, and 6-153 were tested for their ability to inhibit the binding of MAb B1 to IL-1β in ELISA. Only the nearly full length (a.a. 6-153) synthetic analogue reacted with MAb B1. This reactivity correlated with biological activity of the synthetic analogues. The findings that full length IL-1β appears to be necessary for both bioactivity and MAb binding, and MAbs directed at distinct sites on the IL-1β molecule inhibit biological activity would suggest that the MAbs may be detecting conformationally determined epitopes on the IL-1β molecule.

REFERENCES

Kraukauer T (1986). Human Interleukin 1. In "CRC Critical Reviews in Immunology," Vol. 6, Boca Raton: CRC Press, pp 213-244.

Kluger MJ (1985). "The Physiologic, Metabolic, and Immunologic Actions of Interleukin 1." New York: Alan R. Liss.

March CJ, Mosley B, Larsen A, Ceretti DP, Braed G, Price V, Gillis S, Henney CS, Kronham SK, Grabstein K, Conlon PJ, Hopp TP, Cosman D (1985). Cloning, sequence and expression of two distinct human Interleukin 1 Complementary DNAs. Nature 315:641.

Lobl TJ, Diebel MR, Yem AW (1987). On resin biotinylation of chemically synthesized proteins for convenient one step purificaiton. Anal. Biochem. Manuscript submitted.

Monokines and Other Non-Lymphocytic Cytokines, pages 387–392

IMMUNOASSAY, BIOASSAY AND IN SITU HYBRIDIZATION OF MONOKINES IN HUMAN ARTHRITIS

GW Duff[1], E Dickens, N Wood, J Manson, J Symons
S Poole[1], F di Giovine.
Univ. Edinburgh, Dept. Medicine, R.D.U., Northern
General Hospital, Ferry Road, Edinburgh EH5 2DQ,
UK and [1]N.I.B.S.C., UK.

INTRODUCTION

Rheumatoid arthritis (RA) is a common disease of
unknown cause. Synovial lining of the joint proliferates
and eventually destroys cartilage and bone. Extra-articular
pathology also occurs at many sites, particularly when
circulating anti-immunoglobulins (rheumatoid factors) are
present. Usually, RA is a chronic inflammatory process
lasting many years with intermittent flares of increased
joint inflammation and systemic acute phase responses.

The idea that soluble factors from inflamed joints
could enter the circulation to stimulate systemic responses
was established when Bodel and Hollingsworth (1967) found
"endogenous pyrogen" in RA synovial exudate fluid (SF) and
the potential for joint damage of "mononuclear cell factor"
(Dayer et al, 1979) and "catabolin" (Saklatvala and Dingle,
1980) became clear in the following decade.

The recognition that IL1 was probably responsible for
all these factor activities (Oppenheim and Gery, 1982) soon
led to its detection in fractionated SF (Fontana et al,
1982; Wood et al, 1983). Using bioassays, however, it has
been impossible to measure IL1 reliably in whole SF because
of interference by SF constituents with biological responses
to IL1. The need for extensive separation made larger-scale
clinical studies impractical. Now, with the availability of
antibody-based assays, we have confirmed the presence of
both IL1 beta and IL1 alpha in most SF from patients with RA
and other arthritic diseases. Immunodetectable IL1 beta in

the range 0.25 to 12ng/ml was present in 86 of 92 SF, and
IL1 alpha at .025-1.5ng/ml in 21 of 31 SF. Table 1 shows
comparative levels of IL1 alpha and beta in representative
SF samples.

Table 1

IL1 alpha and beta levels by RIA (ng/ml) in RA SF

IL1 beta	5.8	3.8	3.4	3.3	2.1	1.5	1.5	1.3	1.2
IL1 alpha	1.5	.05	0	.04	0.3	.06	.03	0.1	0

We have also measured TNF alpha in SF using the L929
cytotoxicity bioassay (Flick and Gifford, 1984). In contrast
to IL1, only about 30% of 120 samples contained L929
cytotoxicity neutralized with mab to TNF alpha. These
bioassay results have been confirmed with an
immunoradiometric assay for TNF alpha (di Giovine et al,
1987). Unlike IL1, TNF appears to be biologically active in
synovial exudate but this may just reflect the use of
different cell types (T cells vs connective tissue cells) in
bioassays for these cytokines. Table 2 shows the range of
TNF bioactivity in SF from different arthritic diseases.

Table 2

TNF alpha bioactivity in SF from arthritic diseases

TNF(u/ml)(a)	RA(c)	OA	RT	AS
<4	40(b)	6	2	1
4-16	16	3	4	1
16-28	2	1	1	1
>28	1	1		

(a) L929 units neutralized with mab to hr TNF alpha
(b) Number of patients in this TNF range
(c) Type of arthritis: RA-rheumatoid; OA osteo; RT-
     reactive; AS-ankylosing spondylitis

The extent that our results reflect a pathological
rise in cytokine concentration is difficult to determine
since normal SF is generally unavailable. However, in a
case of septic arthritis, there were large reductions in
levels of IL1 alpha, IL1 beta and TNF alpha after

treatment, when the joint was returning to normal, compared to initial levels during active disease (Table 3).

Table 3

Immunoreactive cytokine levels (ng/ml) in SF from bacterial arthritis

	ILl alpha	ILl beta	TNF alpha
Day 1	0.11	8.088	1.225
Day 14	<0.025	4.024	0.437

To determine if ILl and TNF genes were activated in synovial cells during the disease, we performed in situ hybridizations. Synovial tissue from RA patients was obtained during joint surgery and immediately frozen in nitrogen. Thin sections were fixed and probed for cytokine mRNA's using 32 P-labelled cDNA for ILl alpha, ILl beta and TNF alpha. Non-specific binding was controlled with plasmid DNA and the presence of cytokine mRNA in tissue was checked by Northern or slot analysis. Many tissues showed preferential binding of individual probes, again providing evidence for specificity. Synovial cells most frequently showed hybridization with ILl beta probe (Figure 1). Positive cells were usually large and occurred in stromal areas remote from lymphocyte-rich follicles and were often seen as pairs or in small groups (Figure 2).

FIGURE 1
A.   B.

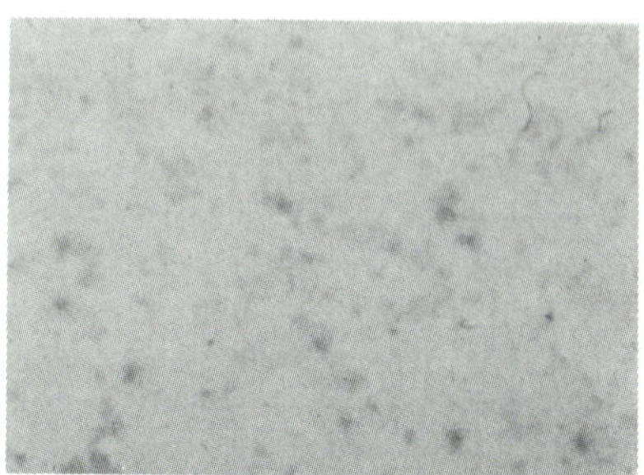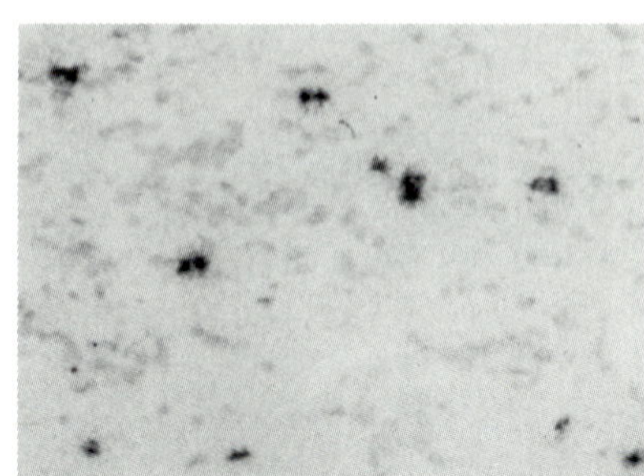

RA synovial tissue sections probed with: (A) plasmid DNA; (B) human ILl beta cDNA. Probes were random-prime labelled with 32P.

FIGURE 2

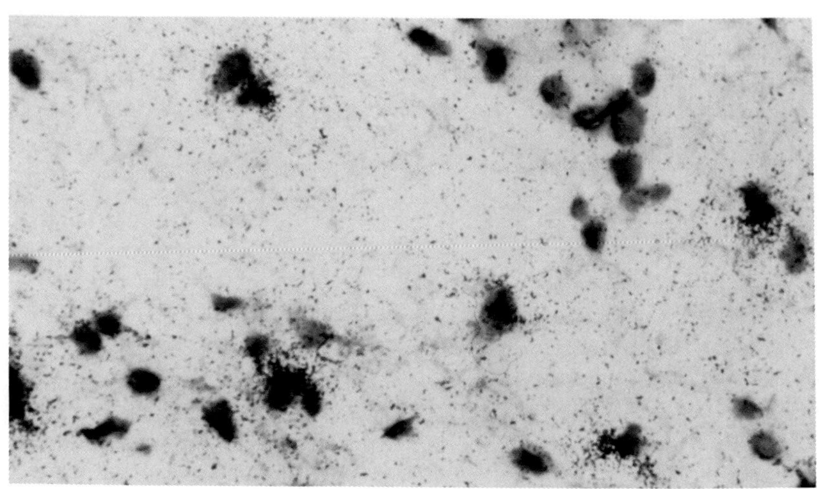

RA synovial tissue section probed for IL1 beta. Control probe (plasmid DNA) and human TNF alpha cDNA did not bind to this sample.

Immuno-phenotyping of consecutive sections identified cells in these areas that stained with Leu M3 mab which reacts with 90% of synovial macrophages. Cells positive for IL1 alpha and TNF alpha mRNA occurred less often (not shown). IL1 alpha localization was similar to IL1 beta but TNF alpha cells often appeared near to blood vessels.

DISCUSSION

IL1 (alpha and beta) and TNF alpha have been measured upto nanomolar concentrations in SF from RA and other arthritic diseases. TNF was biodetectable in synovial exudate and levels correlated well with IRMA measurements. IL1 in whole SF could only be measured by immunoassay.

Aside from the issue of biological inhibition, immunoreactivity and bioactivity of a peptide ligand, measured ex vivo, will be different at any time (immune recognition is not restricted to receptor binding regions). Inert molecules, both larger and smaller than mature peptide, could react with antibody raised to the mature form. Immunoreactive levels reflect cytokine production over time (rather than what happens to be bioactive at any one moment) and may well be a better indicator of chronic disease activity. For example, SF IL1 beta levels by RIA correlate very significantly with other markers of immune activation such as soluble tac protein (Symons et al, 1987).

Finally, we have shown that cells in the synovium of RA patients are activated for IL1 (alpha and beta) and TNF alpha gene expression. Cells containing mRNA for these cytokines were detected by in situ hybridization in snap-frozen pathological specimens, indicating that IL1 and TNF were produced within the rheumatoid lesion during the course of the disease. IL1 beta was more abundant by quantity and by frequency of detection. Both IL1 and TNF are known to promote cartilage and bone resorption in vitro (Gowen et al, 1983; Saklatvala 1986; Bertolini et al, 1986). Their role in the pathogenesis of arthritic diseases and the opportunities that they present for therapeutic interventions should soon become more clear.

ACKNOWLEDGEMENTS

We are grateful to: Dr Don Carter, Upjohn; Dr Ueli Gubler, Hoffmann-La Roche; Prof W Fiers, Univ Gent; Dr G Adolf, Boehringer Institute; and Dr Alan Shaw, Biogen for generous donation of reagents used in these experiments.

REFERENCES

Bertolini DR, Nedwin GE, Bringman TS, Smith DD, Mundy GR (1986). Stimulation of bone resorption and inhibition of bone formation in vitro by human tumour necrosis factor. Nature, 319, 516.
Bodel PT, Hollingsworth JW. (1967). Pyrogen release from human synovial exudate cells. Br. J. Exp. Path., 49(1), 11.

Dayer JM, Breard J, Chess L, Krane SM (1979). Participation of monocyte/macrophages and lymphocyte in the production of a factor that stimulates collagenase and prostaglandin release by rheumatoid synovial cells.
J. Clin. Invest., 64, 1386.

di Giovine FS, Meager A, Poole S, Duff GW. Immunoreactive cytokines in synovial fluids from patients with rheumatic diseases. (Manuscript in preparation).

Flick DA, Gifford GE (1984). Comparison of in vitro cell cytotoxic assays for tumor necrosis factor.
J. Immunol. Methods, 68, 167.

Fontana A, Hengartner H, Weber E, Fehr K, Grob PJ, Cohen G. (1982). Interleukin 1 activity in the synovial fluid of patients with rheumatoid arthritis.
Rheumatol. Int., 2, 49.

Gowen M, Wood DD, Ihrie EJ, McGuire MKB, Russell RGG. (1983). An interleukin 1-like factor stimulates bone resorption in vitro.
Nature, 306, 378.

Oppenheim JJ, Gery I. (1982). Interleukin 1 is more than an interleukin.
Immunol. Today, 3, 113.

Saklatvala J, Dingle JT. (1980). Identification of catabolin, a protein from synovium which induces degradation of cartilage in organ culture.
Biochem. Biophys. Res. Commun. 96, 1225.

Saklatvala J. (1986). Tumour necrosis factor alpha stimulates resorption and inhibits synthesis of proteoglycan in cartilage.
Nature, 322, 547.

Symons JA, Wood NC, di Giovine FS, Duff GW. (1987). Soluble IL-2 receptor in serum and synovial fluid samples from patients with rheumatic diseases.
Brit. J. Rheumatol., 26(supp. 2): 64A.

Wood DD, Ihrie EJ, Dinarello CA, Cohen PL. (1983). Isolation of an interleukin 1-like factor from human joint effusions.
Arthr. Rheum, 26, 975.

Monokines and Other Non-Lymphocytic Cytokines, pages 393–396
© 1988 Alan R. Liss, Inc.

AN ENZYME IMMUNOASSAY FOR PLATELET-DERIVED GROWTH FACTOR
(PDGF): APPLICATION TO THE MEASUREMENT OF MACROPHAGE-DERIVED
PDGF.

R.K. Kumar, R.A. Bennett and A.R. Brody.

Laboratory of Pulmonary Pathobiology, National
Institute of Environmental Health Sciences,
Research Triangle Park, NC 27709.

We have developed an enzyme immunoassay (EIA) for
platelet-derived growth factor to be able to measure
PDGF-like growth factors secreted by macrophages (Shimokado
et al., 1985). This assay is a nonequilibrium competitive
inhibition EIA which detects residual unreacted antibody
following incubation of a limiting amount of high-avidity
anti-human PDGF (Collaborative Research) with the test
sample. The various steps in this assay are explained in
Fig. 1. Quantitation is by comparison with a standard curve
generated using highly purified human PDGF (R&D Systems).
The EIA exhibited high intra- and inter-assay reproducibility: the coefficient of variation of both replicate samples
and repeated assays seldom exceeded 5%. A typical standard
curve is shown in Fig. 2.

We compared the EIA with a radioreceptor assay similar
to that described by Bowen-Pope and Ross (1985). This assay
was based upon the ability of PDGF-containing samples to
inhibit the subsequent binding of [125] I-labelled PDGF (R&D
Systems) to receptor sites on rat lung fibroblasts in primary culture. The EIA exhibited similar sensitivity and
specificity to the radioreceptor assay and was not subject
to interference by nonspecific cytotoxic components in the
sera and conditioned media being tested. In addition, the
EIA was convenient for processing large numbers of samples
for assay.

We employed the EIA to quantify PDGF in human, rabbit,
rat and fetal bovine sera:

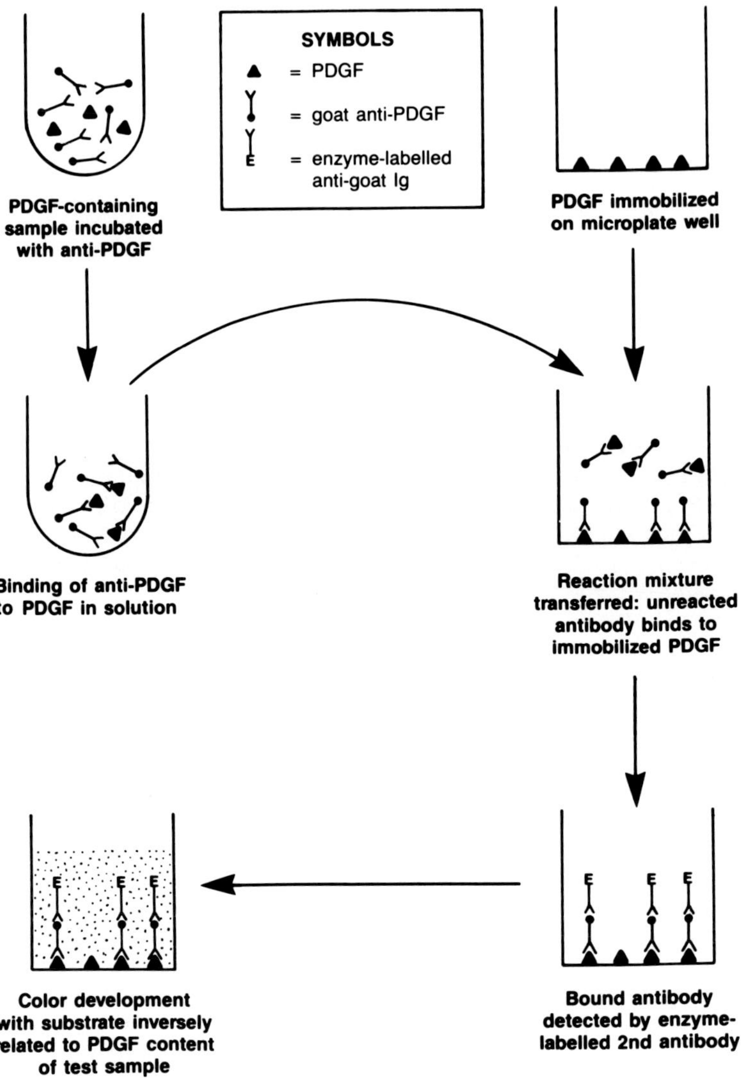

Figure 1.   Diagrammatic representation of the steps involved in the enzyme immunoassay for PDGF.

Serum	PDGF content (ng/ml)	Number of samples
Human	15.4 ± 1.46	10
Rabbit	15.3 ± 1.80	4
Rat	5.5 ± 0.48	6
Fetal Bovine	1.3 ± 0.12	3

PDGF could also be detected in mouse and pig serum (not shown). No PDGF was detected in carefully prepared platelet-poor plasma from rabbits. The entire content of immunoreactive PDGF in sera could be precipitated by 50% saturated ammonium sulfate and subsequently quantitated by the EIA.

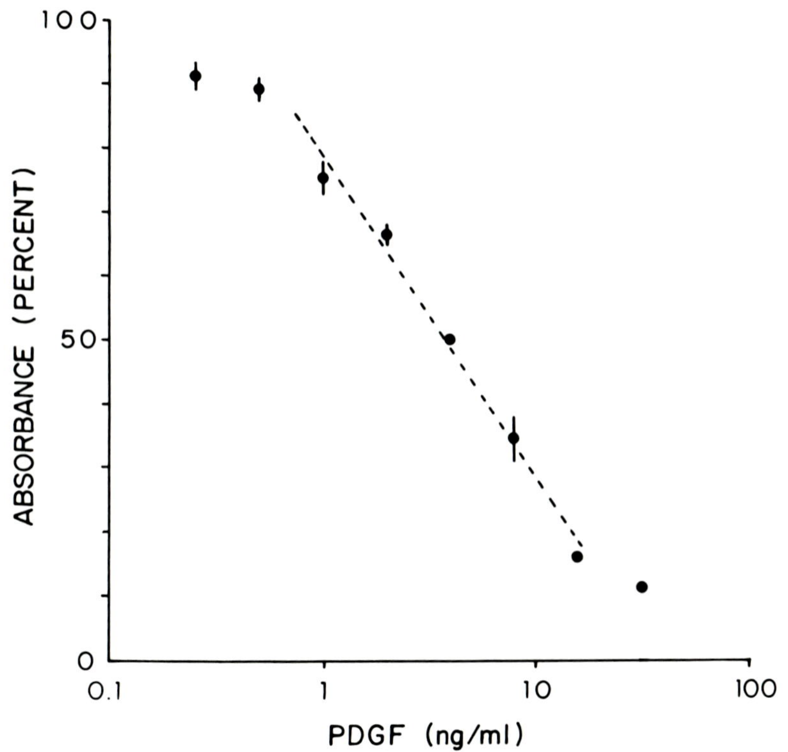

Figure 2. A typical standard curve showing the usable linear range (0.5-16 ng/ml). Error bars represent range of duplicate samples.

We quantitated PDGF-like growth factor in rat alveolar macrophage conditioned media (AMCM) (Bauman et al., 1987) after separation from putative binding proteins by high performance liquid chromatography in 1 M acetic acid. AMCM contained immunoreactive PDGF-like molecules which had a similar elution time to purified human PDGF. The PDGF homologue detected in AMCM bound to receptor sites on rat lung fibroblasts and this binding could be specifically inhibited by preincubation with anti-PDGF (Kumar et al., 1987).

Normal rat alveolar macrophages cultured in serum-free media released immunoreactive PDGF homologue upon stimulation with particulates such as carbonyl iron spheres or asbestos fibers. Quantitation of the release of PDGF-like macrophage-derived growth factor by EIA of fractions obtained by chromatography of AMCM in 1 M acetic acid yielded the following:

Treatment	Immunoreactive PDGF detected
Untreated (n=9)	122 ± 21 pg/10^6 cells/24h
Carbonyl iron spheres	368 pg/10^6 cells/24h
Asbestos fibers	572 pg/10^6 cells/24h

Ongoing studies in our laboratory focus on the production of a PDGF-like growth factor by lung macrophages in vivo following inhalational exposure to toxic environmental agents such as asbestos.

[Dr. Kumar is on leave from the School of Pathology, Univ. of New South Wales, Sydney, Australia, supported by Fogarty International Research Fellowship (PHS 1-F05TW03842-1)].

Bauman MD, Jetten AM, Brody AR (1987). Biologic and biochemical characterization of macrophage-derived growth factor for rat lung fibroblasts. Chest 91:15S.
Bowen-Pope DF, Ross R (1985). Methods for detecting the platelet-derived growth factor receptor. Methods Enzymol 109:69.
Kumar RK, Bennett RA, Brody AR (1987). Rat alveolar macrophages produce a homologue of platelet-derived growth factor. FASEB J (in press).
Shimokado K, Raines EW, Madtes DK, Barrett TB, Benditt EP, Ross RA (1985). A significant part of macrophage-derived growth factor consists of at least two forms of PDGF. Cell 43:277.

Monokines and Other Non-Lymphocytic Cytokines, pages 397–400
© 1988 Alan R. Liss, Inc.

A FLUOROMETRIC ENZYME-LINKED IMMUNOSORBENT ASSAY (F ELISA)
FOR TGF-BETA

Benjamin S. Leung and Li Zhou

Department Ob/Gyn University of Minnesota
Medical School, Minneapolis, Minnesota 55455

INTRODUCTION

Preparation of polyclonal and monoclonal antibodies to
the TGF-β molecule has been frustrated by the low immunogenicity of this polypeptide, possibly due in part to its
highly conserved primary structure among different species,
its ubiquity in tissues and body fluids, and its potent immunosuppressive activity. Recently, Flanders et al (1987)
successfully raised polyclonal antibodies to TGF-β by using
synthetic peptides corresponding to the different regions of
the TGF-β molecule. These antisera are invaluable for studies
relating to the various biological roles of TGF-β. However,
it is highly desirable to have a panel of monoclonal antibodies against the different epitopes of the TGF-β molecule.
They will facilitate the elucidation of the mechanisms of
TGF-β interaction with and dissociation from the carrier protein or the membrane bound receptors, the understanding of
its synthesis and degradation, and the determination of TGF-β
levels from body fluids. This report describes a simple and
sensetive f ELISA we established for the detection of anti-
TGF-β antibodies from producing hybridomas. This preliminary
result shows that this assay warrants further development for
measuring TGF-β levels in biological fluids when monoclonal
antibodies are available.

MATERIALS AND METHODS

Synthetic peptides correspond to position 50-75 and
78-109 of TGF-β, TGF-β1 purified from human platelets,rabbit
anti-P50-75 and anti-P78-109 antisera were kindly supplied

by K. Flanders, Lab of Chemoprevention, NCI, methylumbelli-
feryl phosphatase from Sigma Chemical Co., (St Louis, Mo),
and 96-well microfluor "W" plates and Microfluor fluorometer
were from Dynatech Lab., (Alexander, Va). Latent TGF-β1 and
carrier protein of TGF-β1 from human platelets were a gift
from C. H. Heldin, Ludwig Institute for Cancer Research,
Uppsala, Sweden.

Antigen was dissolved in 0.1 M sodium carbonate-bicarbon-
ate buffer, pH 9.6, with 0.02% sodium azide, and 100 µl
aliquot of an antigen was immobilized on microfluor titer
plates at 4°C overnight. The plate was washed three times in
phosphate-buffered saline (PBS) containing 0.05% Tween 20.
Non-specific binding was minimized by treating the plate with
0.2% PBS-gelatin solution for 1 hour at room temperature.
Reaction of antigen with capturing antibodies (100 µl) at
various dilutions in PBS-Tween was conducted at room temperature for 1 hour. Following three washings with PBS-Tween,
100 µl of alkaline phosphatase conjugated anti-rabbit IgG
(diluted 1:2000 as specified by the manufacturer) was added
and incubated for 1 hour at room temperature. After thorough
washing (3x) with PBS-Tween, 150 µl of the substrate (4-methyl
umbelliferyl phosphate 1.11 mg/50 ml of 0.1 M sodium carbon-
ate-bicarbonate buffer) was added. Fluorometric reading was
made on a Microfluor fluorometer 10-20 minutes after the
reaction.

RESULTS

Antisera to synthetic peptides P50-75 and P78-109 have
been characterized by both radioimmunoassay and colorimetric
ELISA by Flanders et al (1987). By employing different dilutions of these antisera, we demonstrated that the f ELISA
was sensitive to less than 1 ng of coated antigens, and the
dose-response curves were fairly linear at the levels of
antigens added (Fig 1A & B). Sera dilutions of 16,000-fold
remained reactive in this f ELISA. These antisera were
specific only to the corresponding immunogen; virtually no
cross-reactivity of anti-P78-109 was observed on the other
proteins such as mEGF (Collaborative Res. Corp., Bedford, MA),
synthetic peptides corresponding to positions P22-43 or P34-50
of TGF-alpha (from G. Schultz, Louisville, Ky); latent TGF-β
complex, or purified TGF-β carrier protein (Table 1). It
required more than 1000-fold of these peptides to achieve a
ED$_{50}$ binding activity. Anti-P50-75 crossreacted with the
TGF-β native molecule, and the reactivity parallelled that

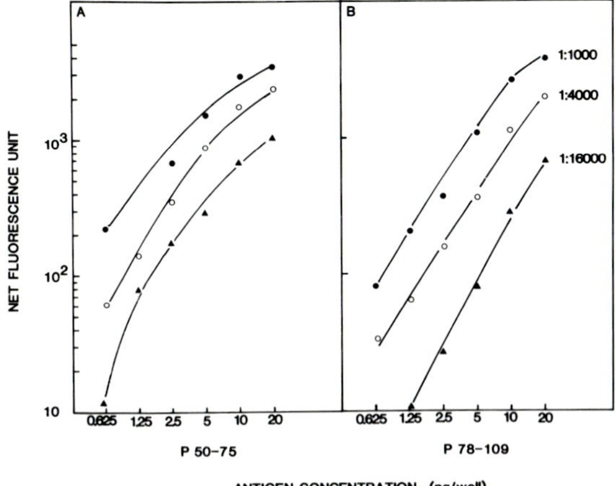

Fig. 1.   Reactivity of Anti-P50-75 (A) and Anti-P78-109 (B) to the corresponding peptide immobilized on microtiter plates at concentrations shown.

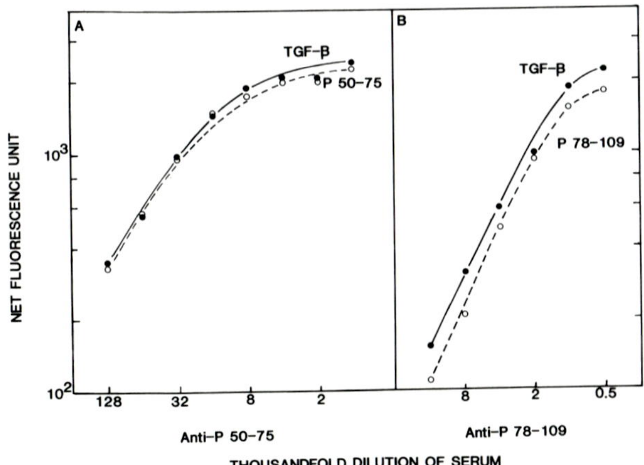

Fig. 2.   Reactivity at various dilutions of anti-P50-75 and Anti-P78-109 (B) to the TGF-β native peptide and the corresponding synthetic peptides. In Fig 2A, P50-75 at 5, ng/well and TGF-β at 2.5 ng/well were used. In Fig 2B, twice the concentration of antigens was used. Background bindings (37-170 FU) were subtracted from curves.

observed for P50-75 (Fig 2A). Similar result was obtained
for anti-P78-109 antisera (Fig 2B).

TABLE 1. Cross reactivity of anti-P-78-109 antiserum

<u>Antigens</u>		ED_{50} (ng)
TGF-β	P78-109	5
	P50-75	>1000
TGFα	P22-34	>1000
	P34-50	>1000
mEGF		>1000
L-TGF-β*		>1000
x-TGF-β**		>1000

* latent form of TGF-β1 purified to homogeneity from human
   platelet.

** carrier protein of TGF-β1 purified to homogeneity from
   human platelet.

REFERENCE

Flanders KC, Roberts AB, Ling N, Fleurdelys BE, Sporn MB
(1987). Antibodies to peptide determinants in transforming
growth factor-beta and their applications. Biochemistry
(submitted).

ACKNOWLEDGEMENT

This research was supported in part by grants from the
Minnesota Medical Foundation, Grant No. MMF-SMF-536-36 and
the Milheim Foundation, Grant No. 10-09551-00.

Monokines and Other Non-Lymphocytic Cytokines, pages 401–403
© 1988 Alan R. Liss, Inc.

EPILOGUE

At the close of the symposium on The
Physiologic, Metabolic, and Immunologic Actions of
Interleukin-1 (4-6 June, 1985, Ann Arbor, MI), I
indicated the paradoxical roles for interleukin-1
(IL-1) were it to mediate effective responses by
the body to two disparate crises, injury and
infection. For IL-1 to be of use to the host
following injury, it would have to prevent the
immune system from responding to occult tissue
antigens exposed by the injury and to support the
repair of injured, usually peripheral, tissues. In
contrast, during infection an enhanced immune
system has survival value and wasting of
peripheral tissues appears to provide essential
nitrogen for antibody, white blood cell and acute-
phase protein synthesis. One answer to the dilemma
is to suggest that the systemic consequences of
IL-1 action might be modified, in some fashion, by
the nature of the local events that triggered IL-1
synthesis and release, so that the disparate needs
of both healing wounds and proliferating
lymphocytes could be met by the same metabolic and
physiologic alterations.

The above solution to the problem involves
two assumptions. The first is that virtually every
systemic metabolic , physiologic and immunologic
event, and many local events, which occur during
infection and following injury are directly or
indirectly mediated by IL-1. The second is a
corollary of the first, that the systemic
metabolic and physiologic responses to either
injury or infection are quantitatively identical,
varying in intensity only to the extent of the
injury or to the perceived level of microbial
challenge. In fact much of the data from injured
and infected patients and many of the studies of
IL-1 action in vivo and in vitro support these
assumptions. Yet there are differences that need
to be accounted for. One is the anergy which
accompanies severe injury and which if it persists
may lead to infection. Another is the altered
acute-phase protein patterns, e.g., severely

burned and severely burned-infected patients
appear to have significant differences in their
plasma protein patterns such to allow one to
distinguish between these two patient groups. The
third is the so-called "primacy of the wound" by
which is meant that wound healing, at least for a
time,appears to take precedence over other
processes. For example, growth in the severely
injured adolescent may be retarded until wound
repair is well underway.

Transforming growth factor beta (TGF beta)
which can be derived from platelets, exhibits
immunosuppressive and angiogenic effects, while
promoting fibroblast collagen and fibronectin
synthesis. TGF beta thus is a candidate for the
role of primary mediator of anergy and of local
repair responses in the severely injured patient.
Interferon beta 2, also known as hepatocyte-
stimulating factor and now as interleukin-6 (IL-
6), is primarily derived from fibroblasts,
epithelial cells and keratinocytes. IL-6 appears
to be able to induce the hepatic synthesis of
many, perhaps of all the known acute-phase
proteins, a number of which are thought to
participate in wound healing. IL-1 also stimulates
the synthesis of some plasma proteins. The
interaction of IL-1 and IL-6 in vitro depends upon
the protein studied, enhancement in the case of
alpha1-acid glycoprotein and haptoglobin,
inhibition of synthesis in the case of fibrinogen.
IL-6 has been found in the plasma of burn
patients. The interactions of IL-1 and IL-6 may
explain the differences in plasma protein in
burned vs burned-infected patients. Together, TGF
beta and IL-6 may account for the "primacy of the
wound".

The foregoing is an example wherein the
confusion of cytokines of which we complained at
the start of the workshop, could give rise to a
cornucopia of treatment possibilities. If only one
molecule, e.g., IL-1, directly or indirectly
controlled all of the body's metabolic,
physiologic and immunologic responses to all
stresses and stimuli, it would be difficult, if
not impossible, to reduce or ablate inappropriate
responses or enhance beneficial activities without

untoward or adverse effects. Instead, the presence
of an array of molecules derived from different
cells and tissues and apparently elicited by
different stimuli, some molecules with
overlapping, but not identical, activities, others
with antagonistic, additive or synergistic
activities as a function of circumstance,
admittedly makes elucidation of host defense
mechanisms in sickness and injury
difficult.However, this diverse array of molecules
also allows the possibility of finely tuning our
treatment of illnesses and injuries through the
use of drugs and biologics in physiologic rather
than pharmacologic amounts.

Michael C. Powanda

The opinions or assertions contained herein
are the private views of the author and are not to
be construed as official or as relecting views of
the Department of the Army or the Department of
Defense (AR 360-5)

Index

α1-Acid glycoprotein, 15, 35, 37, 38, 402
ACTH, 125
Actin filaments, stress fibers, 288
Actinomycin D, 114
Acute phase reactants, 15, 17–18, 26,
    401–402
    hepatocyte/hepatoma, induction in, 35–38
Adenovirus E1A oncogene sensitization of
    NIH 3T3 cells, TNF-α, 243–248
Adult respiratory distress syndrome, 379
Advanced glycosylation end products (AGE),
    macrophages, TNF and, 145–149
A549 cells, 252
Albumin, 35–37
    excretion, IL-1 and TNF amplification of
        glomerulonephritis, 345, 346
Alkaline phosphatase, 264
Amadori product,146
Aminopyrine, 341
Amyloid A, 15, 340
Amyloidosis, ω-3 fatty acids and, 154
Amyloid P protein, serum, 15
Ankylosing spondylitis, 388
ANS, 374
Antibody-mediated glomerulonephritis, IL-1
    and TNF amplification, 343–347
Antichymotrypsin, 15
Anti-CSF-G and CSF-M antisera, 304
Anti-IL-1 monoclonal antibodies, 2, 45
Anti-p65 antibody, 232
α₁-Antitrypsin, 33
Antiviral activity with IFNs, TNF-α,
    251–253
A172 glioblastoma, 256
Apoptosis, TNF-mediated cytolysis, 285–290
Aprotinin, 375
Arachidonic acid, 224–226
    metabolism, cyclooxygenase pathway,
        128
Arachidonic acid metabolites
    omega-3 fatty acids and decreased IL-1
        production, 153, 156
    IL-1
        enhancement by IFNγ and cyclohexi-
            mide, monocytes, 114
        gene expression regulation, 61–66
    TNF-α, gene expression regulation,
        61–66
    see also specific metabolites
Arginine residue, IL-1β receptor, 194, 195

Arthritis, osteo-, 388; *see also* Rheumatoid
    arthritis
Atherosclerosis, ω-3 fatty acids and, 154
A375 melanoma cells, 74, 76, 215
A23187 calcium ionophore, 223, 224

Bacillus subtilis, 320, 322, 326
Basement membrane, glomerular, IL-1 and
    TNF amplification of glomerulone-
    phritis, 343, 344
B-cell stimulating factor-2 (BSF-2), 3, 6, 15,
    21, 24, 29, 35, 37, 38; *see also* Inter-
    feron-β₂
BHT, 254
Blood vessels
    glomerular capillary thrombosis, 346
    IL-1 mRNA localization, 92
Bone
    IL-1 mRNA localization, 92
    turnover, 261–266
Bone marrow
    blast progenitor cells in vitro, IL-1,
        297–300
    IL-1 mRNA localization, 91
    transplantation, 305
Brain, IL-1 mRNA localization, 92
Breast carcinoma, T47, 24, 25
Burkitt's lymphoma, 183
Burns, 402
    TNF-α, 378–380

Cachectin. *See* Tumor necrosis factor *entries*
Calcium, 217, 219–221, 238
Calcium ionophore A23187, 223, 224
Calmodulin kinase, 232
    inhibitor, W7, 57–59
Cancer marker, TNF-α as, 380
Capillary thrombosis, glomerular, IL-1 and
    TNF amplification of glomerulone-
    phritis, 346
Cardiac myxoma, 8, 9
Cartilage, IL-1 mRNA localization, 92
Catabolin, 387
Catalase, TNF-α cytotoxic activity, 253, 254
cDNA cloning, IL-1, 73–77
    amino acid sequences, 75–77
    cf. other species, 76, 77
Cerebral malacia, 347
Ceruloplasmin, 15
CESS cells, 6, 8, 23, 24

CE-2 fibrosarcoma, IL-1β effect, 365–370
CFU-blasts, 297–300
CFU-GEMM, 308, 310
CHAPS, 188, 189
Chemotactic agent, TGF-β as, 314
Chloramphenicol acetyltransferase (CAT), 33
    pro-IL-1β gene expression, *cis* and *trans*
        acting elements, 47–49, 51, 52
Chloroform extraction, IL-1β, 373–376
CHO DHFR cells, 22, 24, 26
Chromatography, HPLC, IL-1 phosphoryla-
    tion, PBMCs, 231
Chromosome 2, mouse, 42, 43
Chromosome 7, 21, 31
Circular dichroism, 192, 194
cis acting elements, pro-IL-1β gene expres-
    sion, 47–53
Collagenase, 131, 217, 323
Collagens I and II, gene expression induc-
    tion, TGF-β, 313–316
Colony-stimulating factors. *See* CSF *entries*
COLO-16 cell line, 18, 49, 51, 52
Complement
    component factor B, 15
    C3, 15, 26
Con A, 125, 127–129
COS1 cells, 74, 77
Covalent disulfide binding to α₂-macroglobu-
    lin, IL-1, 209–212
C reactive protein, 15, 33
Crosslinking, IL-1 receptor, 168–171, 176
CSF, monocyte-specific, stimulation of
    monocyte lineage cells, 301–305
CSF-1, 240, 304, 305, 307–309
CSF-G, 303, 307–310
    radioprotection, synergism with IL-1,
        360, 362, 363
CSF-GM, 83, 119, 121, 145, 307–310
    radioprotection, synergism with IL-1,
        360, 362
    recombinant, myeloid cells, signal induc-
        tion in, 235–241
    O₂– production, 237, 240
CSF synergism in radioprotection, IL-1,
    359–360, 362–363
C3HA cells, 285–288
Cyclic AMP, 221, 232
    induction, PEPCK, 267, 269, 270, 271
    TNF-α, gene expression regulation,
        67–72
Cyclic GMP, 221
Cycloheximide, 245
    enhancement, monocytes, IL-1, 113–118
        IL-1β mRNA, 116–118
        translation, 117–118
Cyclooxygenase
    inhibitors, 64

pathway, arachidonic acid metabolism,
    128
Cyclophosphamide, 341
Cysteine, 188
Cysteine proteinase, 15, 35, 37
Cytochrome P-450-dependent liver drug me-
    tabolism depression, IL-1 and TNF
    synergism, 337–341
Cytolysis mediated by apoptosis without nu-
    clear disintegration, TNF, 285–290
Cytolytic T lymphocytes, 167
Cytotoxic activities, TNF-α, 253–254

Decay-accelerating factor, 102
2-Deoxyglucose, 105
Dexamethasone, 17, 19, 32, 62
    IL-1 and TNF depression of liver drug
        metabolism, 337, 339, 341
    IL-1 gene transcription and translation,
        83–87
    quantitation, FITC, 87
Diabetes mellitus
    insulin-dependent, IL-1 and TNF syner-
        gism and, 291, 294
    omega-3 fatty acids and, 154
Diabetic myelin, 147
Diazepam, 341
Dichroism, circular, 192, 194
Digestive tract, IL-1 mRNA localization, 92
Disulfide binding, covalent, IL-1 to α₂-mac-
    roglobulin, 209–212
Disulfide bond essential for binding, IL-1 re-
    ceptors, 185–190
Dithiothreitol, 185–189
Docosahexaenoic acid, 153
Dot blot assay, IL-1 mRNA quantitative anal-
    ysis, 79, 81
Drug metabolism, liver, IL-1 and TNF
    depression, 337–341

Eicosapentaenoic acid, 153–157
Electrophoresis
    band shift assays, pro-IL-1β gene
        expression, *cis* and *trans* acting
        elements, 49–53
    IL-1 covalent disulfide binding to α₁-
        macroglobulin
        PAGE, 210
        SDS-PAGE, 210–211
    IL-1 phosphorylation, PBMCs, SDS-
        PAGE, 231
    IL-1 receptor, 169–171, 177, 182
EL 4 (thymoma) cells, 175–177
    assay, 84
    IL-1 receptors, 185–188, 204–206
    IL-1β-stimulated, linoleic acid release,
        223–228

EL4 cf. RAJI cells, IL-1 receptor differ-
ences, 179–183
Scatchard analysis, 180, 181
specificity, 180
EL4-CTLL conversion assay, 110, 111
ELISA, 383, 384
fluorometric, TGF-β, 397–400
IL-1β, 377
TNF, 146
Endocytosis, IL-1 receptor, 180
Endoplasmic reticulum, rough, IL-1 plasma
membrane anchoring mechanism, 102
β-Endorphin inhibition, PMNCs, IL-1β,
125–129
and IFNγ inhibition, 125–128
Endothelium, IL-1 mRNA localization, 92
Enzyme immunoassay, platelet-derived
growth factor, 393–396
Epidermal growth factor (EGF)
cross-reactivity with TGF-β, 400
IFN-β_2 gene expression, 31
IFN-γ regulation, 159–162
receptor, 159–160
on hemopoietic cells, 161
inducible, on lymphocytes, 159–162
Epstein-Barr virus, 183
Erythropoietin, 307, 308, 310
Escherichia coli, 191, 192, 198, 205
Eskimos, dietary ω-3 fatty acids, 154
ETAF, 52
Ethanol, 239
Ethylene vinyl acetate (EVA), 329–333
N-Ethylmaleimide, 186–189

FACS, 275
Factor B complement component, 15
Fatty acids, omega-3, dietary, and decreased
IL-1 production, 153–157
Fc receptors, monocyte, IL-1 effects,
281–284
FFI, 146
Fibrinogen, 15, 18, 35–38, 340, 402
Fibroblast growth factor, 159
Fibroblasts
L929, mouse, 121, 215, 247
proliferation, substance P enhancement,
131–135
LPS, 133, 134
Fibronectin gene expression, induction,
TGF-β, 313–316
Fibrosarcoma CE-2, IL-1β effect, 365–370
FITC, 219, 275
IL-1 gene transcription, 87
IL-1 secretion kinetics, LPS-activated
monocytes, 100
FMLP, 236, 237, 239
c-*fos*, 58
F17 cells, 286–288

G-CSF. *See* CSF-G
GIF, 74, 76, 77
Glioblastoma, A172, 256
Glomerular basement membrane, IL-1 and
TNF amplification of glomerulonephritis, 343, 344
Glomerular capillary thrombosis, IL-1 and
TNF amplification of glomerulone-
phritis, 346
Glomerulonephritis
antibody-mediated, amplification, IL-1
and TNF synergism, 343–347
omega-3 fatty acids and, 154
Glucocorticoid(s), 17, 19, 32, 62, 233, 255,
256, 288
IL-1 and TNF depression of liver drug
metabolism, 337, 339, 341
IL-1 gene transcription and translation,
83–87
quantitation, FITC, 87
induction PEPCK in hepatoma cells, IL-1
and TNF synergism, 267–271
Glucocorticoid-antagonizing factor, 267
Glycoprotein, α-1 acid, 15, 35, 37, 38, 402
Glycosaminoglycans, 314–316
Glycosylation
advanced end products (AGE), macrophage receptor, TNF and, 145–149
IL-1, 148–149
IL-1
plasma membrane anchoring mecha-
nism, 104–106
receptor, 175
GM-CSF. *See* CSF-GM
Gold in rheumatoid arthritis, 209
Granulomatous inflammation induction, IL-1,
329–333
IFNγ, 331–332
Growth inhibition kinetics and receptor bind-
ing, IL-1, 213–216
IL-1β, 214–216

Haptoglobin, 15, 402
Heart, IL-1 mRNA localization, 92
HeLa cells, 33, 49, 51
Helper factors, skin graft-induced, 167, 171,
172
Hemopexin, 15, 17
Hemopoietic cells, EGF receptor, 161
Hemopoietic progenitors
interferon-β2, 21, 25–26
selective growth inhibition, TGF-β, 307
Hepatocyte/hepatoma, induction in, acute
phase reaction, 35–38
Hepatocyte-stimulating factor (HSF), 15–19,
21–23, 29, 35, 38, 340; *see also* In-
terferon-β_2

Hepatoma cells
    acute phase reaction induction, 35–38
    H4IIE rat, 268
    PEPCK in, IL-1and TNF synergism,
        267–271
H4IIE rat hepatoma cell line, 268
Histamine, 257–259, 319–321
Histidine decarboxylase locus, IL-1 genes,
    mouse chromosome 2, 44
HIV (HTLV), 6, 8, 253
HLA-DR (Ia), 120; *see also* MHC class II
HL-60 cells, 237–241
HSB-2 subclones, leukemia-derived, IL-1
    and IL-2 receptor induction, 217–222
H7, protein kinase C inhibitor, 56–58
HTLV (HIV), 6, 8, 253
Human chorionic somatomammotropin,
    365–366
Hybridization in vitro, IL-2 RNA, 114; *see*
    also In situ hybridization
Hybridoma growth factor, 3, 5, 15, 21, 22,
    23, 25; *see also* Interferon-β_2
Hybridoma/plasmacytoma growth factor, 3;
    see also Interferon-β_2
Hybrids, somatic cell, IL-1 genes, mouse
    chromosome 2, 42
Hydrogen peroxide, TNF-α, 253, 254
4-Hydroxyperoxycyclophosphamide (4-HC),
    297

Immunoglobulin G, 281–283, 383, 384
Immunoprecipitation, IL-1 receptor, 167–173
Indomethacin, 126, 127, 257
Infection, interferon-β2, 21–26
Inflammation
    chronic granulomatous, IL-1 induction,
        329–333
    chronic vs. "recycling" acute, 333
    increased vascular permeability, IL-1
        role, 319–323, 325–328
    interferon-β_2, 21–26
Inositol phosphates, CSF-GM, recombinant,
    signal induction in myeloid cells,
    236–241
In situ hybridization
    IL-1 gene expression, mRNA tissue local-
        ization, 89–92
    tissues listed, 91–92
    rheumatoid arthritis synovial fluid, IL-1
        and TNF in, 389–391
Insulin
    IL-1 and TNF synergism and, 292–294
    receptor, 177
Insulin-dependent diabetes mellitus, IL-1 and
    TNF synergism and, 291, 294
Interferon(s)
    antiviral activity, with, TNF-α, 251–253

IL-1β synthetic nonapeptide effect on
    cellular immunoreactivity and CE-
    2 fibrosarcoma growth, 366, 368,
    370
and monocyte-specific CSF, stimulation
    of monocyte lineage cells, 302,
    303
Interferonα, 251, 252, 255, 277
    antiviral activity with, TNF-α, 251–256,
    257, 259
Interferonβ, 217, 251, 252, 277
Interferonβ_2, 3–5, 15–19, 35, 36, 340
    genetics, 21, 31
        gene expression regulation, 31–33
    hemopoietic progenitors, 21, 25–26
    infection, 21–26
    inflammation, 21–26
    multiple forms, 29–31
    see also Interleukin-6
Interferonγ, 9, 83, 137, 139, 146, 147, 217,
    218, 221, 277, 292
    enhancement, monocytes, IL-1, 113–118
        IL-1β-mRNA, 116–118
        translation, 117–118
    epidermal growth factor regulation,
        159–162
    IL-1 effects on monocyte Fc receptor
        expression, 281–284
    inhibition, and β-endorphin, 125–128
    in vivo immune system effect, cf. TNF-
        α, 349–353
    and LPS effects on monokine transcrip-
        tion and translocation, 119–122
    TNF-α, gene expression regulation,
        67–72
Interleukin-1 (α and β), 5, 9, 15, 17, 18, 19,
    21, 26, 35, 37, 38, 401
    amino acid sequences, 75–77, 181,
        191–193, 203
    bone marrow blast progenitor cells in vi-
        tro, 297–300
    cDNA cloning, rat, 73–77
        cf. other species, 76, 77
    covalent disulfide binding to α_2-macro-
        globulin, 209–212
    CSF synergism in radioprotection,
        359–360, 362–363
    cycloheximide enhancement, monocytes,
        113–118
        IL-1β-mRNA, 116–118
        translation, 117–118
    and omega-3 fatty acids, dietary, 153–157
    gene expression detection by mRNA tis-
        sue localization, C57BL/6 mice,
        89–92
        tissues listed, 91–92
    gene expression regulation, arachidonate
        metabolites, 61–66

genes, 109
gene transcription and translation, glucocorticoid effect, 83–87
  quantitation, FITC, 87
granulomatous inflammation induction,
  329–333
  IFNγ, 331–332
growth inhibition kinetics and receptor
  binding, 213–216
IFN-β_2 gene expression, 30–33
IFN-γ enhancement, monocytes, 113–118
  translation, 117–118
and IL-2 production, 217–222
IL-2 receptor induction by leukemia-derived HSB-2 subclones, 217–222
inflammation, increased vascular permeability role, 319–323, 325–328
LAF bioassay, 74, 76, 77
and macrophage AGE receptor, 148–149
macrophage cell line, generation in,
  131–135
monoclonal antibodies against, 45
monocyte Fc receptor expression,
  281–284
monocyte-specific CSF, stimulation of
  monocyte lineage cells, 302, 303
mRNA
  expression, second messenger inhibitor effects, mouse macrophages, 55–59
  quantitative analysis, monocytes/mac-
   rophages, 79–82
muramyl dipeptide induction, 141–144
phosphorylation, human PBMC response,
  229–234
plasma membrane anchoring mechanism,
  101–107
  amino acid sequence, 101
pro-. *See* Pro-IL-1 *entries*
production
  autoregulation, human mononuclear
   cells, 109–112
  TNF-α and IFN-γ effects on immune
   system, 351–352
rheumatoid arthritis, 131, 132, 135, 209
  in situ hybridization, 389–391
  synovial fluid, 387–388, 391
secretion in response to IL-2, PBMC,
  137–139
secretion kinetics, α cf. β, LPS-activated
  monocytes, 97–100
substance P enhancement of fibroblast
  proliferative activity, 131–135
and TNF induction in YT cells, IL-2 receptors, 273–278
Interleukin-1α, 8, 17, 35, 37, 38, 191, 197,
  203, 216, 261, 268, 292, 294, 320,
  322, 323, 333, 338, 373, 375, 383

and β genes, RFLPs and linkage, mouse
  chromosome 2, 41–46
and IL-1 receptor, 168, 170, 175, 176,
  185–188
listeriosis, murine, effects on pathogenesis, 355–357
see also Interleukin-1 (α and β)
Interleukin-1β, 8, 17, 18, 35, 37, 38,
  219–221, 230, 251, 257–258, 274,
  276, 282, 292, 294, 320, 322, 323,
  330, 331, 333, 338
ELISA, 377
β-endorphin inhibition, PMNCs, 125–129
  and IFNγ inhibition, 125–128
growth inhibition kinetics and receptor
  binding, 214–216
and IL-1 receptor, 175, 176
LPS and γ-IFN effects on transcription
  and translocation, 120, 121
monoclonal antibodies against, generation, 383–385
mRNA and IFNγ, 116–118
nonapeptide, synthetic, effect on cellular
  immunoreactivity and fibrosarcoma CE-2 growth in BALB/c
  mice, 365–370
production of mRNA by mast cells,
  258–259
RIA
  and chloroform extraction from
   blood, 373–376
  determination in serum, 377–380
receptor binding site map, human,
  191–195, 200–201
-stimulated EL4 thymoma cells, linoleic
  acid release, 223–228
structure–function relationship, humans,
  monoclonal antibodies, 197–201
see also Interleukin 1 (α and β); Pro-IL-
  1β gene expression, *cis* and *trans*
  acting elements
Interleukin-1 and TNF synergism, 258–259
actions on osteoblast-like cells, 261–266
cytochrome P-450-dependent liver drug
  metabolism depression, 337–341
glomerulonephritis, antibody-mediated,
  amplification, 343–347
induction of IL-2 receptor expression on
  YT cells, 273–278
inhibition of glucocorticoid induction of
  PEPCK in hepatoma cells,
  267–271
macrophage AGE-receptor, 148–149
pancreatic beta-cell toxicity, 291–294
radioprotection, mice, 359–361, 363
Interleukin-1 receptor
  crosslinking, 168–171, 176

disulfide bond essential for binding, 185–190
EL-4 thymoma cell line, 185–188, 204–206
endocytosis, 180
glycosylation, 175
IL-1α, 168, 170, 175, 176, 185–188
IL-2β, 175, 176
immunoprecipitation, 167–173
phosphorylation, 175, 176
protein kinases in signal transduction, 175
RAJI cf. EL4 cells, 179–183
  Scatchard analysis, 180, 181
  specificity, 180
SDS-PAGE, 169–171, 177, 182
structure and properties, 175–177
trans-retinoic acid effects, 203–206
xenogeneic antiserum, 168, 172–173
Interleukin-2, 5, 83, 159, 167, 169, 177, 274, 277, 332, 333, 383
IL-1-dependent, 217–222
IL-1β synthetic nonapeptide, CE-2 fibrosarcoma, 367, 368
production, IL-1β-stimulated EL4 cells, 223–228
RNA blot analysis, 218
stimulation of IL-1 secretion, PBMCs, 137–139
toxicity, 138
trans-retinoic acid effect, 205
Interleukin-2 receptor
IL-1 and TNF induction in YT cells, 273–278
induction by leukemia-derived HSB-2 subclones, IL-1, 217–222
Northern blots, IL-2R mRNA, 276
RNA blot analysis, 218
YT cells, induction, 273–278
Interleukin-3, 83, 240, 304, 307–313
Interleukin-4, 9, 309
Interleukin-6, 3–10, 15, 17, 22, 23, 29, 35–38, 402
biological properties, 8
mouse, 6
physicochemical properties, 7
see also Interferon-β_2
In vitro hybridization, RNA, IL-1 enhancement by IFNγ and cycloheximide, monocytes, 114
IPTG, 24

26kDa protein, 3–5; see also Interferon-β_2
K562 cell line, 175, 176, 215
Kidney, IL-1 mRNA localization, 92
Klebsiella pneumoniae, 355

LAF activity, 294
LAF bioassay, IL-1, 74, 76, 77

Lectin-like receptor mannose-dissociable, IL-1 plasma membrane anchoring mechanism, 103, 104–107
Leukemia-derived HSB-2 subclones, IL-1 and IL-2 receptor induction, 217–222
Leukotriene B4, 337, 340
Limulus amebocyte lysate (LAL) assay, 119, 330, 360
Linoleic acid release, EL4 thymoma cells, IL-1β-stimulated, 223–228
Lipocortin, 255, 256
Lipopolysaccharide (LPS), 47, 50, 51, 55–59, 63, 64, 360, 363
-activated monocytes, IL-1 secretion kinetics, 97–100
IFNβ_2 gene expression, 31, 32
and IFN-γ effects on monokine transcription and translocation, 119–122
IL-1
  effects on monocyte Fc receptor expression, 281–284
  enhancement by IFNγ and cycloheximide, monocytes, 113–118
  gene transcription, 84–87
  mRNA quantitative analysis, 81
  and TNF amplification of glomerulonephritis, 344–347
  and TNF depression of liver drug metabolism, 337–340
Salmonella minnesota, 125, 127–129
-stimulated macrophages, IL-1 plasma membrane anchoring mechanism, 101–107
  amino acid sequence, 101
TNF-α
  gene expression regulation, 67–72
  and IFN-γ effects on immune system, 351
Liposomal MDP, induction of IL-1, 141–144
Listeria monocytogenes, 355–357
Listeriosis, murine, effects on pathogenesis, IL-1α, 355–357
Liver
  drug metabolism, IL-1 and TNF depression, 337–341
  IL-1 mRNA localization, 92
L929 mouse fibroblasts, 215, 247
  cytotoxicity assay, 121
Lung, IL-1 mRNA localization, 92
Lupus erythematosus, systemic, 353
Lupus nephritis
  omega-3 fatty acids and, 154
  mouse NZB $\times$ NZW F$_1$ model, 349–353
Lymph nodes, IL-1 mRNA localization, 91
Lymphocytes, EGF receptor, inducible, 159–162; see also T cells

Lymphoma
    Burkitt's, 183
    EL 4. *See* EL 4 *entries*
    YAC-1, 366
Lymphotoxin, 211, 285, 288
Lysosomes, IL-1 plasma membrane-anchoring mechanism, 103

α_2-Macroglobulin, 15, 18, 35–38
    IL-1 covalent disulfide binding to, 209–212
    IL-1 genes, mouse chromosome 2, 44
Macrophage(s)
    AGE receptor, TNF and, 145–149
        IL-1, 148–149
    IL-1
        mRNA quantitative analysis, 79–82
        and TNF depression of liver drug metabolism, 338
    LPS-stimulated, IL-1 plasma membrane-anchoring mechanism, 101–107
        amino acid sequence, 101
    second messenger inhibitor effects, IL-1 and TNFα mRNA expression, 55–59
    see also Monocytes
Macrophage-activating factor, 211
Macrophage cell line, IL-1 generation in, 131–135
Macrophage-derived vasopermeability factor, 322
    from U937 cells, 325–328
Malacia, cerebral, 347
Mammary cell line, MDA-MB-415, 213, 215, 216
Mannose-dissociable lectin-like receptor, IL-1 plasma membrane anchoring mechanism, 103, 104–107
Mast cells, mRNA production and TNF-α and IL-1, 258–259
MCF-7 cells, 285
MDA-MB-415 mammary cell line, 213, 215, 216
Melanoma cell line A375, 74, 76, 215
2-Mercaptoethanol, 185–187
Metallothionein-II, 255
Methylamine, 209–211
MHC class I, 23
    TNF-α, 255, 256
MHC class II
    HLA-DR (Ia), 120
    induction, TNF-α and IFN-γ effects on immune system, 349–350, 352
    TNF-α, 255, 256
β_2-Microglobulin, 116, 255, 256
M1 cell line, 215
Monoclonal antibodies, anti-IL-1 generation, 383–385

genes, mouse, 45
and structure–function relationship, 197–201
Monocytes
    CSF stimulation, 301–305
    Fc receptor expression, IL-1, 281–284
    IL-1 enhancement by IFNγ and cycloheximide, 113–118
        IL-1β-mRNA, 116–118
        translation, 117–118
    IL-1 mRNA quantitative analysis, 79–82
    LPS-activated, IL-1 secretion kinetics, 97–100
    see also Macrophage *entries*
Monocyte-specific CSF, 301–305
Mononuclear cells, IL-1 autoregulation, 109–112; *see also* PBMCs
Muscarinic M$_2$ receptor, 241
Muscle, IL-1 mRNA localization, 92
Mutagenesis, site-specific, IL-1β receptor, 194
myc, 244
c-*myc*, 58
Myelin, diabetic, 147
Myeloid cells, signal induction in, cSF-GM, recombinant, 235–241
    O_2- production, 237, 240
Myxoma, cardiac, 8, 9

Naloxone, 125–127, 129
NEM, 186–189
Nephritis, lupus
    ω-3 fatty acids and, 154
    mouse NZB × NZW F$_1$ model, 349–353
Nephrotoxic nephritis, rats, 343–347
Neurokinin-A and -B, 132, 134
NIH 3T3 cells, sensitization by adenovirus E1A oncogene, 243–248
NK cells, 217, 274, 294
    IL-1β synthetic nonapeptide effect, CE-2 fibrosarcoma, 365, 367
Northern blot analysis
    IL-1 gene
        expression regulation, 65
        transcription, 86
    IL-2R mRNA, 276
    TNF-α gene expression regulation, 65
NSF-60 cell line, 309

OCTA-binding factor, pro-IL-1β gene expression, 48, 51
2′,5′-Oligoadenylate synthetase, 23, 255
Omega-3 fatty acids, dietary, and decreased IL-1 production, 153–157
Oncogenes and susceptibility to cytolysis, listed, TNFα, 244; *see also specific oncogenes*
Ornithine decarboxylase, 69

Osteoarthritis, 388
Osteoblast-like cells, IL-1 and TNF synergism, 261–266
Osteocalcin, 264
Ovary, IL-1 mRNA localization, 92
Oxygen production, CSF-GM, recombinant, signal induction in myeloid cells, 237, 240

Pancreas
    beta-cell toxicity, IL-1 and TNF synergism, 291–294
    IL-1 mRNA localization, 92
Parotid secretory protein locus, IL-1 genes, mouse chromosome 2, 44
PBMCs
    IL-1 phosphorylation, 229–234
    IL-2 stimulation of IL-1 secretion, 137–139
d-Penicillamine, rheumatoid arthritis, 209, 211, 212
PEPCK in hepatoma cells, glucocorticoid induction, IL-1 and TNF effects, 267–271
Peptides, synthetic, TGF β, 398, 399
Peyer's patches, IL-1 mRNA localization, 91
Phalloidin, 288, 289
Phosphatidyl inositols, 217
Phosphatidylserine, 238
Phosphoenolpyruvate carboxykinase (PEPCK), 267–271
    cyclic AMP induction, 267, 269, 270, 271
Phospholipase A_2, 223, 224, 225, 227, 255
Phosphorylation
    human PBMC response, IL-1, 229–234
    IL-1 receptor, 175, 176
Phytohemagglutinin, 219–222
Plasma membrane-anchoring mechanism, IL-1, 101–107
    amino acid sequence, 101
Plasminogen activator, 131
Platelet-derived growth factor, 21, 145, 159, 211, 261
    enzyme immunoassay, 393–396
    IFNβ_2 gene expression, 31, 32
PMA, 219–221, 223, 224, 226, 227, 232, 256–258
Polymorphonuclear cells (PMNCs), IL-1β inhibition by β-endorphin, 125–129
    and IFNγ inhibition, 125–128
P protein, amyloid, 15
Prednisolone, 231
Pro-IL-1, 101–105
    α, 102, 103, 106
Pro-IL-1β gene expression, *cis* and *trans* acting elements, 47–53
    CAT gene, 47–49, 51, 52

electrophoresis, band shift assays, 49–53
    OCTA-binding factor, 48, 51
    repressor factor, 48
Proliferation assays, IL-1β receptor, 192, 193
Promethazine, 321
Pro-opiomelanocortin (POMC), 125, 129
Prostaglandin(s), 89, 217
    IL-1 and TNF synergism, 261–265
Prostaglandin E_2, 126–129, 131, 199, 257–259, 262
    IL-1 gene expression regulation, 62–66
    IL-1 protein production autoregulation, mononuclear cells, 112
    LPS and γ-IFN effects on transcription and translocation, 121
    TNF-α gene expression regulation, 62–66, 68
Proteinase inhibitor $\alpha 1$, 15
Protein, 26 kDa, 3–5; *see also* Interferon-β_2
Protein kinase(s)
    p65 phosphorylation, 232–233
    in signal transduction, IL-1 receptor, 175
Protein kinase C, 217, 219, 220, 222, 232
    CSF-GM, recombinant, signal induction in myeloid cells, 236–238, 240
    H7 inhibitor, 56–58, 219, 232
    translocation, IL-1β-stimulated EL4 cells, 223–228
Pseudomonas aeruginosa, 355
p65 (IL-1 protein), 230–233
    amino acid sequence, 231
    antibody to, 232
    protein kinases phosphorylating, 232–233
    Western blots, 232
Pulse-chase analysis
    IL-1 gene transcription, 84
    IL-1 secretion kinetics, LPS-activated monocytes, 99

Radiation effect, IL-1β synthetic nonapeptide effect on cellular immunoreactivity and CE-2 fibrosarcoma growth, 370
Radioimmunoassay (RIA)
    and chloroform extraction from blood, IL-1β, 373–376
    determination in serum of IL-1β and TNF-α, 377–380
    omega-3 fatty acids and decreased IL-1 production, 155, 156
    IL-1
        protein production autoregulation, mononuclear cells, 110, 111
        in synovial fluid, rheumatoid arthritis, 387–388, 391
    TNF-α, 373, 374

Radioprotection, IL-1 synergism with
    CSF, 359–360, 362–363
    TNF, 359–361, 363
RAJI cf. EL4 cells, IL-1 receptor, 179–183
    Scatchard analysis, 180, 181
    specificity, 180
ras, 244, 255
RAW 264 cells, 68–70
Repressor factor, pro-IL-1β gene expression,
    48
RFLPs
    IL-1 genes, mouse, 41–46
    TNF-α cf. -β, 350, 351
Rheumatoid arthritis
    omega-3 fatty acids and decreased IL-1
        production, 153, 154
    gold in, 209
    IL-1, 131, 132, 135, 209, 387–391
        in situ hybridization, 389–391
    d-penicillamine, 209, 211, 212
    substance P, 131, 132, 135
    synovial fluid, 387–391
    TNF, 387–391
RNA blot analysis, IL-2, 218
RNA in vitro hybridization, IL-1 enhance-
    ment by IFNγ and cycloheximide,
    monocytes, 114
RNA, messenger
    IL-1β, IL-1 enhancement by IFNγ and
        cycloheximide, monocytes,
        116–118
    IL-1, second messenger inhibitor effects,
        mouse macrophages, 55–59
    IL-2R, 276
    localization, IL-1 gene expression, 89–92
        tissues listed, 91–92
    production, mast cells, IL-1β, 258–259
    quantitative analysis, monocytes/macro-
        phages, IL-1, 79–82
    TNF-α, mast cell production, 258–259
Rough endoplasmic reticulum, IL-1 plasma
    membrane-anchoring mechanism, 102

Salmonella minnesota lipopolysaccharide,
    125, 127–129
Schwartzman reaction, 325
Second messenger inhibitor effects, IL-1 and
    TNFα mRNA expression, macro-
    phages, mouse, 55–59
Shock, septic, 379, 380
Site-specific mutagenesis, IL-1β receptor,
    194
Skin, IL-1 mRNA localization, 91, 92
Skin graft-induced helper factors, 167, 171,
    172
Somatic cell hybrids, IL-1 genes, mouse
    chromosome 2, 42

Somatomammotropin, human chorionic,
    365–366
Southern blots, IL-1 genes, mouse chromo-
    some 2, 42, 43
Spleen, IL-1 mRNA localization, 91
Spondylitis, ankylosing, 388
SP6 in vitro transcription system, 80
src, 244
Staphylococcus aureus, 6, 168
Stress fibers, actin filaments, 288
Substance P, 259
    enhancement of fibroblast proliferative
        activity, IL-1, 131–135
        LPS, 133, 134
    rheumatoid arthritis, 131, 132, 135
"Suicide" program induction, TNF, 285
Suprarenal gland, IL-1 mRNA localization,
    92
SV40 enhancer, 50–52
Synovial fluid, rheumatoid arthritis, mono-
    kines in, 387–391
Systemic lupus erythematosus, 353

Tac antigen, 219, 221, 222
T cells, 217, 227–228
    cytolytic, 167
    helper, 167
Testis, IL-1 mRNA localization, 92
T47 breast carcinoma, 24, 25
TGF-α, 159–162
    cross-reactivity with TGF β, 400
TGF-β, 255–259, 261, 402
    1 cf. 2, 307, 308, 310, 311
    chemotactic agent, 314
    collagens I and II gene expression induc-
        tion, 313–316
    ELISA, fluorometric, 397–400
    fibronectin gene expression, induction,
        313–316
    hematopoietic progenitor cells, selective
        growth inhibition, 307
    IFNβ_2 gene expression, 31
    peptides, synthetic, 398, 399
THP-1 cell line, 47, 49–53
Thy-1, 102
Thymoma. *See* EL 4 *entries*
Thymus, IL-1 mRNA localization, 91
Thyroid, IL-1 mRNA localization, 92
TPA, 236–238
trans acting elements, pro-IL-1β gene
    expression, 47–53
Transcriptional rate, IL-1 enhancement by
    IFNγ and cycloheximide, monocytes,
    114, 116–118
Transcription system, SP6 in vitro, 80
Translation, IL-1 enhancement by IFNγ and
    cycloheximide, monocytes, 117–118
Translocation, protein kinase C, IL-1β-stim-
    ulated EL4 cells, 223–228

Trans-retinoic acid
    IL-1 receptors, 203–206
    IL-2, 205
Trypsinization, IL-1 plasma membrane-anchoring mechanism, 105, 106
Tumor necrosis factor (TNF), 5, 8, 15, 17, 21
    cytolysis mediated by, apoptosis without nuclear disintegration, 285–290
    ELISA, 146
    IFN β_2 gene expression, 29–33
    LPS and γ-IFN effects on transcription and translocation, 120, 121
    macrophages, AGE receptor, 145–149
    "suicide" program induction, 285
    see also Interleukin-1 and TNF synergism
Tumor necrosis factor α, 35, 37, 38, 83, 87, 292–294
    adenovirus E1A oncogene sensitization of NIH 3T3 cells, 243–248
    antiviral activity with IFNs, 251–253
    cf. β, 138, 292, 350, 351
    burns, 378–380
    cancer marker, 380
    cellular gene regulation by, 254–256
    cytotoxic activities, 253–254
    IL-1 role in inflammation, 322, 323
    interferon-γ, alternate effects on in vivo immune system, 349–353
    oncogenes and susceptibility to cytolysis, listed, 244
    radioimmunoassay, 373, 374
        determination in serum, 377–380
    receptor, 245–247

rheumatoid arthritis, synovial fluid, 388–390
    in situ hybridization, 389–391
    synthesis regulation, 256–258
Tumor necrosis factor α, gene expression regulation
    arachidonate metabolites, 61–66
    cyclic AMP, 67–72
    interferon-γ, 67–72
    lipopolysaccharide, 67–72
    mast cell production of mRNA, 258–259
    mRNA expression, second messenger inhibitor effect, mouse macrophages, 55–59
Tumor necrosis factor β, 138, 292, 350, 351

U937 cell line, 49, 51, 52, 325–328
Uterus, IL-1 mRNA localization, 92

Vaccinia growth factor, 159–162
Varicella zoster virus, 127, 129
Vascular permeability, IL-1 role, 319–323, 325–328
Vasopermeability factor, macrophage-derived, 322
    U937 cells, 325–328
Vitamin D, 337

Western blots, p65, 232
W7, calmodulin kinase inhibitor, 57–59

Xenogeneic antiserum, IL-1 receptor, 168, 172–173

YAC-1 lymphoma, 366
YT cells, IL-2 receptor, 273–278